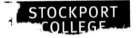
Complementary Therapies for Pharmacists

Complementary Therapies for Pharmacists

Steven B Kayne

BSc, PhD, MBA, LLM, DAgVetPharm, FRPharmS, FCPP, MPS(NZ), FNZCP FFHom (Hon)

Honorary Consultant Pharmacist, Glasgow Homeopathic Hospital

Visiting Lecturer in Complementary Medicine, University of Strathclyde, Glasgow

Pharmacy Dean, Faculty of Homeopathy, London

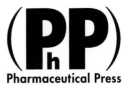

Pharmaceutical Press

Published by the Pharmaceutical Press
1 Lambeth High Street, London SE1 7JN, UK

© Pharmaceutical Press 2002

First published 2002

Text design by Barker/Hilsdon, Lyme Regis, Dorset
Typeset by Type Study, Scarborough, North Yorkshire
Printed in Great Britain by TJ International, Padstow, Cornwall

ISBN 0 85369 430 3

A catalogue record for this book is available from the British Library

For Calum, Eilidh and Tara

Contents

Foreword

The use of complementary medicines by the public has grown enormously over the last few years and pharmacists have greatly expanded their sales of medicinal products in this area. A recent survey of community pharmacists on the use of complementary medicines showed that 99% of respondents reported that one or more types of complementary remedies were sold in the pharmacy in which they practised.[1] This has meant that pharmacists have had to learn, or relearn, about the modern usage of complementary medicines, particularly herbal remedies, homeopathic remedies, aromatherapy products and flower remedies.

The House of Lords has also recognised the growth in use and importance of complementary medicine in the public's eyes. Its Select Committee on Science and Technology provided a Report on Complementary and Alternative Medicine and drew attention to the importance of herbal medicine and homeopathy as two of the 'big five' therapies (the others were osteopathy, chiropractic and acupuncture).[2] They went on to say that there was a real need for evidence in this area and that further research would require much work and resources. However, they said that if a therapy did gain a critical mass of evidence to support its efficacy, then the National Health Service and the medical profession should ensure that the public has access to it and its potential benefits. The growth of the use of complementary medicine is therefore likely to continue.

By their very nature, complementary medicines are often taken with orthodox medicines and the public may well believe that there are no interactions. This is often far from the truth, e.g. as with St John's wort, and publications such as the *British National Formulary* warn prescribers that complementary therapy may affect conventional therapy.

There is no doubt that the public trusts pharmacists to offer informed advice on the use of such complementary medicines and the profession expects pharmacists to ensure that they are competent in any area in which such advice is given. Therefore, pharmacists are now required by the Royal Pharmaceutical Society of Great Britain to offer advice on homeopathic or herbal medicines or other complementary therapies or medicines only if they have undertaken suitable training or have specialised knowledge. There is also a requirement not to recommend any remedy where pharmacists have any reason to doubt its safety or quality. They must therefore have a very good knowledge in complementary medicine if they are to provide good advice on what to buy and how to use these medicines and so protect the public from dangerous products.

This book is therefore timely and is written for pharmacists by a pharmacist who is an acknowledged expert in the subject. Dr Kayne has taken the largest areas of interest (homeopathy, herbal remedies and aromatherapy) and given a down-to-earth, practical explanation of the important issues to pharmacists. He gives a balanced view, very much aimed at giving the evidence for the use of these therapies. It will come as no surprise to the reader that Dr Kayne is not only a very experienced practitioner, but also an accomplished teacher and writer.

As you read through the book, you will find that it is not so much a textbook as a well-referenced source book of up-to-date information. It is written in an easy-to-read style and is basically what is called a 'good read'. I am sure that it will remain on pharmacists' shelves for many years, so that it can be referred to regularly as well as used as a refresher course when necessary.

Enjoy reading it.

Prof Tony Moffat FRPharmS
Chief Scientist, Royal Pharmaceutical Society of Great Britain
July 2001

References

1. Barnes J. *Uncovering Potential Problems Associated with Complementary Remedies: A Survey of Community Pharmacists*. London: Royal Pharmaceutical Society of Great Britain, 1999.
2. House of Lords Select Committee on Science and Technology. *Complementary and Alternative Medicine*, 6th report 1999–2000 [HL123]. London: Stationery Office, 2000.

Preface

This book has been a long time in the writing. My friends at the Pharmaceutical Press have been extremely supportive, waiting patiently as I found myself shooting off at tangents to pursue fascinating aspects of the subject material. There was another perhaps more acceptable reason why it took so long; the rapidly changing environment in which complementary and alternative medicine (CAM) is now offered both in the UK and in the rest of Europe has meant constant updating of the text. For example, the Report of the House of Lords Scientific Committee[1] is having an important effect on CAM in the UK.

There is no doubt that we have come a long way since I started out in homeopathy in the late 1960s. I have never adopted a crusading approach to any of the disciplines that collectively make up what we describe as CAM, preferring to use them alongside orthodox pharmacy. In the early days I was labelled as a bit of an eccentric at best and an outright nutter at worst for even flirting with what was often described as 'quackery'. Now I think it is fair to say that the majority of colleagues accept that CAM does have a part to play in modern pharmacy practice (although exactly what part may be open to discussion), despite one or two sceptics who still make their extreme views known in correspondence to the pharmaceutical journals.

Many of the concepts applicable to CAM are consistent with those advocated by pharmaceutical care programmes and fit in well with our day-to-day activities. CAM is about much more than using minute quantities of medicines or sticking pins along imaginary meridians; it about an emphasis on whole-body health rather than just treating localised illness, so long the main aim of orthodox medicine. The latter position is changing, making the integration of CAM and orthodox medicine more possible.

There is still one major barrier against total integration. All CAM disciplines suffer from a lack of good-quality research-based evidence supporting their use. Given the paucity of resources and the patient-oriented approach to practice, this is to be expected. I have provided snapshots of available evidence throughout the book but there is no doubt that much needs to be done before many reasonable doubts from the scientific community can be satisfied. Mind you, there is a substantial body of opinion that says if observational studies indicate safe and effective outcomes, and patients are happy with their progress, why bother with science? Notwithstanding this argument, sooner rather than later, the demands for the wider availability of CAM under the UK National Health Service will lead to the involvement of the two clinical evaluation agencies in Britain, and the CAM community will be obliged to respond.

This book is divided into four parts, dealing with:

- general aspects of CAM, highlighting the various concepts and issues of delivery common to all its wide-ranging disciplines
- the four disciplines most appropriate to pharmacy practice (homeopathy, herbalism, aromatherapy and flower therapy) in detail, giving some guidance as to how pharmacists may integrate their use into their practice
- traditional Chinese and Indian medicine
- other CAM therapies about which pharmacists may be asked.

CAM is often perceived as being totally safe by the public; this is a false assumption. To assist pharmacists in assessing cases of potential adverse reactions that may present in the pharmacy or hospital environments sections dealing with this aspect are included. There are some difficulties associated with the practice of traditional therapies of which colleagues (particularly those practising in areas with large immigrant populations) should be aware.

Although written primarily for pharmacists in the UK I hope that health professionals and colleagues in other parts of the world will also find the book of interest. Comments on the text are welcome. Please feel free to contact me by e-mail on Skayne9665@cs.com.

Steven Kayne
Glasgow, July 2001

Reference

1. House of Lords Select Committee on Science and Technology. *Complementary and Alternative Medicine*, 6th report 1999–2000 [HL123]. London: Stationery Office, 2000.

About the author

Steven Kayne has recently retired from community pharmacy practice after almost 30 years and now acts as honorary consultant pharmacist at Glasgow Homeopathic Hospital. He is a visiting lecturer in complementary medicine at the University of Strathclyde, Glasgow and Pharmacy Dean of the UK Faculty of Homeopathy, London. He teaches and writes on a wide variety of pharmacy-related topics both in the UK and overseas, and serves on a number of government and professional advisory bodies and examination boards. Steven is an elected member of the Scottish Executive of the Royal Pharmaceutical Society of Great Britain and a Governor of the College of Pharmacy Practice. He is also a Freeman of both the City of Glasgow and the City of London.

Acknowledgements

I should like to express my thanks to Mrs Mary Gooch and her staff at the library of the Glasgow Homeopathic Hospital for their kind attention to my numerous requests for literature searches and to my elder son, Lee Kayne PhD MRPharmS LFHom (Pharm), for his advice and computing skills. Finally, I should like to thank the staff at my publishers for their assistance over the 3 years it took to produce this book.

Abbreviations

ADHD	attention deficit hyperactivity disorder
ADRs	adverse drug reactions
AIDS	acquired immunodeficiency syndrome
AK	applied kinesiology
BAHM	British Association of Homeopathic Manufacturers
BHomP	*British Homeopathic Pharmacopoeia*
BMA	British Medical Association
BPC	British Pharmaceutical Conference
BSA	body surface area
CAM	complementary and alternative medicine: this term is used in this book to cover all non-orthodox disciplines, whether a product or medicine is involved or whether the intervention involves a procedure or therapy without accompanying medicine
CEAs	cost-effectiveness analyses
CHM	Chinese herbal medicine
DMSA	meso-2,3-dimercaptosuccinic acid
EBC	Economic Botany Collections
EEC	European Economic Community
EFA	essential fatty acid
ESCOP	European Scientific Cooperative on Phytotherapy
EU	European Union
FDA	Food and Drug Administration
GGHOS	Glasgow Homeopathic Hospital Outcome Scale
GHP	*German Homeopathic Pharmacopoeia*
GP	general practitioner
GSL	general sales list
HAs	health authorities
HIV	human immunodeficiency virus
MCA	Medicines Control Agency
MtrPs	myofascial trigger-points
NAHAT	National Association of Health Authorities and Trusts
NHP	Nottingham Health Profile

NHS	National Health Service
NIH	National Institutes of Health
NMQP	non-medically qualified practitioner
NSAIDs	non-steroidal anti-inflammatory drugs
OM	orthodox medicine: this term covers all conventional interventions
OTC	over-the-counter
PCGs	Primary-care Groups
PLRs	product licences of right
QALYs	quality-adjusted life years
QOL	quality of life
RCT	randomised controlled trial
RCVS	Royal College of Veterinary Surgeons
RPSGB	Royal Pharmaceutical Society of Great Britain
SMT	spinal manipulation therapy
SSRI	selective serotonin reuptake inhibitors
TCM	traditional Chinese medicine
WHO	World Health Organization
WWF	Worldwide Fund for Nature

Note

There is a trend in the UK to use the word 'homeopathy' rather than the traditional 'homoeopathy'. The former spelling is used throughout this book except in the titles of the Royal London Homoeopathic Hospital, the Bristol Homoeopathic Hospital and the Society of Homoeopaths which still prefer to use the traditional spelling.

Part One

Introduction to CAM

1

The concepts of CAM

Introduction

The art and science of medicine

Throughout history there have been two separate traditions of the practice of medicine. One is the so-called 'art of healing'. It usually involves its own specialised brand of training and relies mainly on a prescriber's intuition and patient perceptions of successful outcomes. The second tradition, the 'science of healing', is based on technological and scientific ideas and leaves much less opportunity for practitioners to express an innovative and intuitive approach to medicine, but generally it has a more predictable result.

In the past, the phrase 'art of medicine' was often applied to the practice of complementary and alternative medicine (CAM). Practitioners have used the phrase to cover up a good deal of muddled thinking and uncritically accepted prejudices. The term is perhaps most misleading when applied to aspects of medical practice that are amenable to empirical study but about which sufficient data have not been accumulated. Practitioners have commonly used the word 'philosophy' in a similar context, for example, they might say: 'My philosophy on using antihistamines for allergies is to use . . .'. Implicit in such usage is the erroneous assumption that what has been labelled a matter of philosophy or personal opinion is thereby exempt from rigorous evaluation. This view has hampered the progress of CAM. However, the situation is changing with the growing importance of evidence-based medicine to purchasers, providers and patients alike.

In an address to the Third Royal London Homoeopathic Hospital International Conference in February 2001, Dr Robert van Haselen told the audience that there has not always been a clear and strict division between art and science.[1] He stated that the purpose of anatomical images from the Renaissance until the nineteenth century had as much to do with aesthetics and disclosing the 'divine architecture' as with the intention of medical illustration. Medical science was more closely linked with a 'naturalistic observation' than with 'intervention' and this was the dominant view until well into the nineteenth century. Since then, scientific and non-scientific medicine have interacted. In some cases this interaction has had positive results, with one supplying features that the other has lacked; thus homeopathic remedies may be used alongside orthodox medicines to treat different aspects of the same disease. Complementary therapies usually stress the idea of restoring a patient's overall wellness rather than merely seeking a reduction in any particular clinical symptom.

Unfortunately, for most of the twentieth century there was considerable suspicion, and even scepticism, voiced by members of the scientific community when referring to CAM. Orthodox medicine insists that the evidence supporting CAM is flimsy or absent.[2] Some treatments are not supported by any randomised clinical trials at all. In other cases there are trials that are methodologically flawed and without robust conclusions. Sceptics claim that the inability to explain the mechanisms of action of most complementary disciplines equates with a simple placebo response at best, and quackery at worst. Ironically, it has been suggested that quackery – medicine practised in the market-place by commercial operators – could also be considered an alternative medicine.[3] After all, it was viewed by the public as offering a different method of treating common ailments. Not surprisingly, this view is not promoted widely! CAM proponents point out that many orthodox interventions are not proven to be effective beyond reasonable doubt, yet they are in routine use.

Modern scientific thinking believes that knowledge should be pursued using the following criteria:[4]

- objectivism – the observer is separate from the observed
- reductionism – complex phenomena can be explained in terms of simpler component phenomena
- positivism – all information can be derived from physically measurable data
- determinism – phenomena can be predicted from scientific laws and environmental conditions.

Complementary medicine just does not fit into this mould. Most complementary disciplines have developed from patient-oriented studies – observational and anecdotal information assembled over hundreds, and in some cases thousands, of years. This does not answer the very real criticisms about the lack of detailed evidence of effectiveness or concerns over possible dangers.

Stimulating the body's own ability to heal – a possible mechanism for CAM

What does healing mean? There can be no doubt in the minds of CAM practitioners that healing means restoring an unwell patient to his or her own particular state of wellness – definitely not seeking to treat a condition in isolation. Does healing mean actively treating, that is a meaningful intervention provided by a practitioner? One aspect of healing that is common to all the therapies that collectively make up CAM is the belief that they work by stimulating the body to heal itself. This response can be initiated by administering carefully chosen interventions – medicines or a physical procedure – or by the practitioner alone during a well-structured consultation. The power of consultation with a skilled practitioner can be an important element in initiating a healing response in humans and perhaps in animals too. It is an interesting argument that, if this is indeed the case, i.e. if the interaction is so important, then self-treating with CAM, including the purchase of over-the-counter (OTC) medicines without advice, might exclude a major source of the healing process.

One could also consider whether a definition of healing should include a reference to individuals' intrinsic genetic or acquired ability to withstand disease themselves, without external intervention. There are many examples of the body's ability to heal itself if given the chance.

Hippocrates was born on the Greek island of Kos. During his lifetime it is said that people came to him in their thousands to seek his advice for their ills. They found a temple of healing dedicated to the god Asclepius. Inside the stone walls of the temple and beside bubbling mineral springs the medical pilgrims experienced a ritual relaxation programme called incubation or temple sleep. Hippocrates made little use of drugs, relying on fomentations, bathing and diet. Diet was very simple and included vinegar and honey. Above all, Hippocrates did not attempt to interfere with nature: no attempts to modify or block biochemical pathways here. He knew that many diseases were self-limiting. He is said to have believed that 'our natures are physicians of our diseases'.

Further examples of the power to self-heal come from modern times. Proportionately more soldiers died of their wounds in Vietnam than in the Falkland Islands conflict between the UK and Argentina. In Vietnam helicopter evacuation was quick and casualties were given blood transfusions and kept warm. In the Falklands evacuation was often impossible due to the appalling weather. Doctors could not reach soldiers on exposed moorland to administer transfusions. However, many casualties survived despite injuries that could have been expected to kill them. Without transfusion, natural clotting mechanisms were not disturbed and haemorrhage was less severe. The cold weather complemented the normal effects of shock, slowing body mechanisms.

A second example comes from an African prostitute. Despite the fact that over the past 20 years one or two of the eight men she serviced each day had HIV, the girl has never become infected. While many people are dead and dying of AIDS in Africa, there are about 200 sex workers, all of whom should be dead by now but who appear to be disease-free. Are these girls genetically protected? When these girls give up their repeated exposure to the deadly virus they seem to lose their immunity. The spiritually minded might say that divine providence is at work, offering protection during the working life of these girls.

A final example of what might be called intrinsic self-treatment is provided by asthma. In the UK one in 10 adults and one in seven children suffer from asthma and it is now the most common chronic childhood disease in many developed countries. By contrast, it is almost unheard of in parts of Africa where there is more exposure to germs in childhood, and families are bigger. It has been suggested that young children in a family are less likely to have asthma problems than older siblings. Fewer babies would develop asthma, hayfever and other allergic diseases in the first place if they were exposed to dirt. Parents who are overly concerned with hygiene may be weakening their children's resistance. This comes as good news to grubby little boys and girls everywhere!

The foregoing is by way of providing evidence that there does seem to be an intrinsic ability – genetic or acquired – to self-heal one's body. Stimulating or encouraging this ability in some way might therefore be a reasonable approach to healing. This is the aim of most CAM disciplines.

Classification of CAM

CAM is a term applied to over 700 different treatments and a large variety of diagnostic methods. A distinction is sometimes made between CAM, which involves the use of medicines or other products, and complementary and alternative therapy, which includes those interventions that rely on procedures alone. This book uses the term CAM to describe all types of non-orthodox medicine.

The British Medical Association (BMA) report on alternative therapies, published in 1986, identified 116 complementary medical treatments that were used 'reasonably often' in the UK; this number has probably increased considerably by now.[5] These treatments include an uncertain number of traditional ethnic therapies. Many are well known, others are exotic or mysterious, and some may even be dangerous.

The different approaches in CAM have been classified as follows:[6]

- complete systems of healing, including acupuncture, chiropractic, herbalism, homeopathy, naturopathy and osteopathy
- specific therapeutic methods, including aromatherapy, massage and reflexology
- psychological approaches and self-help exercises, including relaxation, meditation and exercise
- diagnostic methods, including iridology and kinesiology.

In their report published in 2000[7] the House of Lords Select Committee on Science and Technology divided CAM therapies into three groups (Table 1.1):

- Group 1 embraces disciplines that have an individual diagnostic approach and well-developed self-regulation of practitioners. Research into their effectiveness has been established and they are increasingly being provided on the National Health Service (NHS). The report says that statutory regulation of practitioners

Table 1.1 House of Lord's classification of complementary and alternative medicine (CAM) disciplines[7]

Group 1	Group 3A
Acupuncture	Anthroposophical medicine
Chiropractic	Ayurvedic medicine
Herbal medicine	Chinese herbal medicine
Homeopathy	Eastern medicine
Osteopathy	Naturopathy
	Traditional Chinese medicine
Group 2	
Alexander technique	**Group 3B**
Aromatherapy	Crystal therapy
Flower remedies	Dowsing
Hypnotherapy	Iridology
Massage	Kinesiology
Meditation	Radionics
Nutritional medicine	
Reflexology	
Shiatsu	
Spiritual healing	
Yoga	

of acupuncture and herbal medicine should be introduced quickly and that such regulation may soon become appropriate for home-opathy.
- Group 2 covers therapies that do not purport to embrace diag-nostic skills and are not well regulated.
- Group 3 covers other disciplines that are either long-established but indifferent to conventional scientific principles (3A) or lack any credible evidence base (3B).

There have been criticisms of this classification. The inclusion of Chinese herbal medicine in Group 3A, for example, has drawn criticism,[8] with claims that this ignores the existence of research that has shown this therapy's usefulness in many disorders and supports its provision in state hospitals throughout China, alongside conventional medicine. It is sug-gested that, although the research is of variable quality, it should not be ignored. Furthermore, promising trials have been carried out in the west, including two successful double-blind placebo-controlled trials of a Chinese formula for atopic eczema that concluded 'there is substantial clinical benefit to patients who had been unresponsive to conventional treatment.'[9,10]

The main recommendations of the House of Lords report, which deal with training, professional regulation and research, are discussed in Chapters 2 and 3.

The approach to healing

The perception of CAM and orthodox medicine

The following terms have been applied to describe the two approaches to healing:[11]

orthodox	unorthodox, unconventional
conventional	alternative
established	fringe
scientific	natural
proven	unproven

All of these words communicate a particular viewpoint. Some betray the preconceptions of people who apply them to the practice of medicine.

In the first column, the words 'orthodox' and 'conventional' clearly imply a certain correctness in the approach to healing. 'Established' simi-larly suggests a degree of authority has been applied, perhaps by learned bodies or even society as a whole. 'Scientific' and 'proven' imply an expected – almost guaranteed – successful outcome.

In contrast, in the second column we find 'unorthodox', which can be defined as being 'alternative', 'fringe', 'natural' or 'unproven'. From a sociological viewpoint unconventional therapy refers to medical practices that are not in conformity with the accepted standards of the medical community and are therefore not taught at medical schools. 'Alternative' is a neutral word meaning 'presenting a choice'. 'Fringe' and 'unproven' are words associated with a wish to marginalise the subject. Used in this context, 'natural' could mean unstandardised.

Over recent years orthodox medicine has become better at curing and helping with diseases but worse at relieving illness and sickness, and providing comfort. One of the key roles of CAM is in the management of illness and sickness, and the provision of human comfort.[12]

Complementary and alternative approaches

The words complementary and alternative are often used interchangeably. In the UK, health professionals prefer to use the former only because it implies an ability to complement or complete other treatments. There is evidence to show that this is what happens in practice. Users of CAM are not necessarily seeking alternatives as a result of direct dissatisfaction, but are likely to use complementary therapies in parallel,[13] except in the case of purchasing OTC homeopathic medicines in a pharmacy.[14] Alternative, on the other hand, implies a choice between two courses of action, for example treating a patient with orthodox (or allopathic) medicine or with homeopathy. In fact, there are many instances where patients can benefit from using the best of both worlds. It is not unusual for homeopathic physicians in the UK to prescribe an antibiotic and a homeopathic remedy (e.g. Belladonna) on the same prescription form. In some cases CAM practitioners may use more than one complementary discipline concurrently. For example, asthma may be treated by a whole range of therapies, including relaxation, breathing exercises and yoga, as well as with neutraceuticals, homeopathy and acupuncture.[15]

It is significant that the 1986 BMA report was entitled *Alternative Therapy*,[5] while six years later the next report had the title *Complementary Medicine*.[16] A similar trend in the literature can be observed over the same period of time. In the early 1990s a British pharmacy multiple launched an involvement in what it initially called alternative medicine, changing its promotional material to use the term complementary medicine within a few months.

Support for the complementary notion of healthcare is far from universal. The term 'CAM' has been rejected in one publication because it 'includes therapies like homeopathy which in their purest form are based on philosophies that fundamentally conflict with medical orthodoxy'.[17] The term 'alternative medicine' is used in this book and defined thus:

> Alternative medicine can be taken to encompass all the healthcare practices that at any specific point in time generally do not receive support from the medical establishment in the British context, whether this be through such mechanisms as orthodox medical research funding, sympathetic coverage in the mainstream medical journals or routine inclusion in the mainstream medical curriculum.[17]

The term 'alternative' is also preferred in the USA because not all alternative therapies complement allopathic medicine.[18] The opposite approach has been expressed by a paper in which the authors' aim was to determine the association between the use of non-conventional and conventional therapies in a representative population survey.[19] A total of 16 068 people of 18 years of age or older were involved in the study. Participants were asked about their visits to non-conventional and conventional practitioners during the previous year (1996). From the resulting data it was estimated that:

- 6.5% of the US population had visited both types of practitioner during the year studied
- 1.8% visited only non-conventional practitioners
- 59.5% visited only conventional practitioners
- 32.2% visited neither type of practitioner.

It appeared therefore that non-conventional therapies were being used to complement orthodox treatments rather than to replace them.

CAM is often used alongside orthodox medicine to treat different aspects of the disease. Rarely are the two therapies used to treat exactly the same symptoms. In fact evidence suggests that many Americans use CAM in addition to, rather than as an alternative to, orthodox medicine.[20]

The following definition of CAM has been suggested by colleagues working at Harvard Medical School:[21]

> Alternative medicine refers to those practices explicitly used for the purpose of medical intervention, health promotion or disease prevention which are not routinely taught at US medical schools nor routinely underwritten by third-party payers within the existing US health care system.

It may be misleading to make a firm distinction between the terms 'complementary' and 'alternative', as it is the precise context within which a therapy is being used that will determine just how it should be defined at any one time.[22]

Not all proponents of complementary medicine agree with the terms 'complementary' and 'alternative'. They believe that the use of such terminology serves to emphasise the gap between the orthodox and CAM approaches. They would prefer to see the various CAM therapies referred to as specialities within an integrated medical system of practice and not grouped together under a separate label.

Definitions

Trying to construct a definition that covers such a heterogeneous group of therapies is difficult. Many of the therapies are well known while others may be exotic, mysterious or even dangerous. Some relaxation techniques, massage therapies, special diets and self-help groups could be considered to be lifestyle choices rather than true therapeutic interventions, although it could be argued that an enhanced feeling of wellbeing is sufficient to warrant the inclusion of a procedure in the latter.

Often CAM is described by what it is not, rather than what it is. Thus, it may be described as 'not taught formally to health professionals' or 'not scientifically tested'.

Complementary medicine has been defined in several different ways. One definition is:

> Complementary medicine is a diagnosis, treatment and/or prevention which complements mainstream medicine by contributing to a common whole, by satisfying a demand not met by orthodoxy or by diversifying the conceptual framework of medicine.[23]

This definition poses at least two questions: what is meant by 'mainstream' and whom does complementary medicine seek to satisfy?

Another rather more comprehensive definition has been provided by the Cochrane Collaboration.[24] The Cochrane Collaboration is an international organisation that aims to help people make well-informed decisions about healthcare by preparing, maintaining and promoting the accessibility of systematic reviews of the effects of healthcare interventions. The main output of the Collaboration is through the Cochrane Library, an electronic database that is updated quarterly and distributed on CD-Rom and via the internet.

The Cochrane definition of CAM is:

> CAM is a broad domain of healing resources that encompasses all health systems, modalities and practices and their accompanying theories and beliefs,

other than those intrinsic to the politically dominant health systems of a particular society or culture in a given historical period.

CAM includes all such practices and ideas self-defined by their users as preventing or treating illnesses or promoting health and well-being. Boundaries within CAM and between the CAM domain and that of the dominant system are not always sharp or fixed.

A definition that implies a degree of flexibility, which is to be preferred, particularly in the pharmacy environment, is:

CAM is a group of non-orthodox and traditional therapies that may be used alone, or to complement orthodox or other non-orthodox therapies, in the treatment and prevention of disease in human and veterinary patients.

It is appropriate to offer definitions of three further terms at this stage.

Patients   By convention anyone who is unwell is usually called a patient, a term derived from the Latin *patior*, 'to suffer'. Throughout this book this is used as a generic term to identify people who are unwell, whether they are to be treated by orthodox or complementary medicine. This is not meant to imply that other words such as 'client' or 'customer' are inappropriate in certain circumstances, merely that one word is used to prevent confusion.

Disease   Disease is used in this book in its orthodox sense to mean the following related items, collectively recognised as having a separate coexistence and origin:

- a group of subjective problems reported by the patient (symptoms)
- objective alterations in body functions, usually identified by a trained observer (signs)
- the results of various investigations or procedures (investigations).

It has been pointed out that disease and health are commonly thought of as distinct opposites.[25] In fact, both may be considered to be facets of healthy functioning, each necessary for the other and each giving rise to the other. Thus, disease may be thought of as a manifestation of health. It is the healthy response of an individual striving to maintain equilibrium within the body. Disease can be viewed as a meaningful state that can inform health professionals how to help patients heal themselves. People's problems then become 'diseases of meaning'.

Health The World Health Organization (WHO) defines health as follows:

> Health is a state of complete physical, mental and social well-being, and not merely the absence of disease or infirmity.[26]

It is difficult to see how this could possibly be achieved without a holistic approach to health delivery.

The holistic approach to healing

Virtually all CAM practices claim to be holistic, that is to treat the whole person rather than a condition in isolation. This is one of the most – if not the most – important features of CAM.

Definition

The origin of the word 'holism' is attributed to Jan Christian Smuts (1870–1950), a South African botanist and philosopher with the distinction of having the international airport at Johannesburg named in his memory. Smuts, who was Prime Minister of his country after the First World War, wrote a book entitled *Holism and Evolution*[27] in which he described holism as 'the principle which makes for the origin and progress of wholes in the universe'. He further explained his idea thus:

- Holistic tendency is fundamental in nature.
- Holism has a well-marked ascertainable character.
- Evolution is nothing but the gradual development and stratification of a progressive series of wholes, stretching from the inorganic beginnings to the highest levels of spiritual creation.

The concept of holism is much older, dating back to Cicero (106–43 BC), to whom the following has been attributed:

> A careful prescriber before he attempts to administer a remedy or treatment to a patient must investigate not only the malady of the person he wishes to cure, but also his habits when in health, and his physical condition.

The precise definition of what is now understood by a holistic approach seems to vary between practitioners.[28] Some practitioners consider holism to be the ability to integrate different treatments for different needs, such as using herbal medicine for a specific ailment, acupuncture for chronic pain or hypnosis to stop smoking. A small minority stress that holism implies links between individual and environment, and suggest treatments that would not only balance the internal parts of an individual but also the relationship between the individual and the environment. More generally, however, practitioners and patients define holism as treatment of the whole person – an approach that considers body, mind and spirit as a single unit.

Holistic medicine has been described in the following terms:[29]

- a response to the person as a whole entity (body, mind and spirit) within that person's own environment (family, culture and ecological status)
- a willingness to use a wide continuum of treatments, ranging from surgery and drugs to nutrition and meditation
- an emphasis on a participatory relationship between practitioner and patient
- an awareness of the impact of the health of the practitioner on the patient.

The holistic approach and CAM

A holistic approach to healthcare leads to a highly individual approach that results in patients with apparently similar symptoms being treated in very different ways. Conversely, it also means that particular treatments may be used to treat widely different conditions.

When a patient visits a complementary practitioner for the first time, the consultation may well last for over an hour, although about 40 min is more usual.

Fortunately, methods exist to allow counter prescribing of complementary medicines in the pharmacy environment, without the need for a protracted consultation. However, this does restrict the range of conditions that can be treated realistically to acute self-limiting problems, except where pharmacists have special advanced skills and the appropriate facilities to allow indepth consultations; treatment always remains within personal limits of competency.

Gathering information

The CAM practitioner needs to obtain information on how the patient functions in a normal state of well-being, in addition to hearing about the symptoms that prompted the visit, so that the patient may be returned to his or her own state of good health. Environmental and social factors also have to be considered. To obtain this information, patients are often asked a list of seemingly unrelated questions on their first visit, including the following examples:

- What type of food do you like – sweet, salty, spicy or bland?
- What type of weather conditions do you prefer – hot, cold, wet, dry, etc.?
- Do you like to be with other people or do you like to be alone?
- Are you a gregarious extrovert type of person or are you quiet and introverted?
- Do you dream and if so, can you remember the main subjects involved?

Patients' style of handwriting and colour preferences can be useful in establishing various personality traits, and therefore in choosing an appropriate therapy.[30] Personality and demeanour are important as they can determine how a patient is treated. This procedure is known in orthodox medicine, but is usually practised covertly. For example, in a US study, medical staff were found to have given placebos to unpopular patients who were suspected of exaggerating their pain or who had failed to respond to traditional medication.[31] The holistic practitioner acknowledges that people have different personalities and takes this fact into consideration overtly when treating them.

Practitioners may be interested in any modalities, i.e. what makes the condition feel better or worse, or whether the condition is better or worse at certain times of the day. The exact site of the problem will be identified. In response to the patient's statement 'I have a sore throat' the practitioner may ask 'Is it worse on the right or left side?' Individualised treatment appropriate to patients can then be chosen, the aim being to return them to their own particular state of good health.

The consultation

It is probably not possible to describe a typical consultation even within one discipline, let alone generalise across all CAM consultations. Consultations are so varied that any differences are only stereotypical, misleading or meaningless. Table 1.2 speculates on how a consultation with a CAM practitioner might differ from one with a conventional healthcare professional.

Essentially the difference lies in the focus of the approach to healthcare. This is depicted in Figure 1.1. CAM seeks to focus on overall health, while the focus of orthodox medicine is essentially disease-oriented.

Table 1.2 Speculative differences between complementary and alternative medicine (CAM) and orthodox medicine consultations

Component	CAM	Orthodox medicine
Time	More	Less
Touch	More	Less
History-taking	Holistic, expansive	Specific, behavioural
Patient's role	Conscious, participatory	Passive
Decision-making	Shared with patient	Practitioner tends to make decisions (paternalistic)
Bedside manner	Empathic, warm	'Professional', cool
Language used	Subjective, simple words	Objective, uses jargon

Social considerations

In the early days of the current wave of interest in CAM, some researchers were of the opinion that the holistic approach was inappropriate because it provided an individualistic solution to problems of health, rather than seeking to alter the social structure that promoted an unhealthy environment.[32] The sociological literature often highlights the fact that in concentrating on an individual the needs of the wider

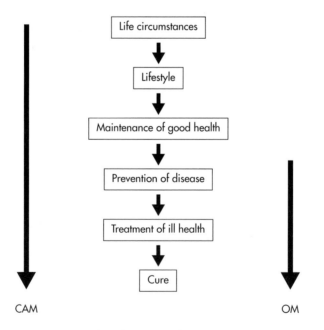

Figure 1.1 Representation of the factors involved in complementary and alternative medicine (CAM) and orthodox medicine (OM) healthcare systems.

community may be overlooked.[33] When responsibility is shifted to a single person, the social structures that constrain individual behaviour and lifestyle choices may be obscured. This emphasis on such weaknesses in the holistic view may be one reason for its lack of acceptance by orthodox practitioners in the past.

Notwithstanding this opinion, the idea of individualising treatments is gaining acceptance and it is likely that modern biotechnology will provide the opportunity for future orthodox medicines to be tailored to patients' specific requirements.[34]

Change of emphasis

With this change in emphasis a situation is developing in which orthodox medicine and CAM are apparently swapping positions. As orthodox medicine moves towards more individualised interventions, CAM (or at least those disciplines practised in the pharmacy environment) appears to be moving from its traditional holistic base to a more disease-centred approach. OTC remedies with multiple constituents, giving specific indications for use on the label, are being produced in many countries for mass distribution. At present European regulations prevent such claims from being made as far as homeopathy is concerned, but that position is set to change in the future. The trend is therefore likely to accelerate, providing a source of concern to many practitioners who feel the special status of CAM is being eroded.

References

1. Van Haselen R. Reuniting art with science: impossibility or necessity? In: *Proceedings of the 3rd International Conference*. London: RLHH & Parkside Health, 2001: 7.
2. Ernst E. Quadruple standards? *Focus Altern Complement Ther* 2000; 5: 1–2.
3. Porter R. *Health for Sale – Quackery in England 1660–1850*. Manchester: MUP, 1989: 128.
4. Micozzi M. *Fundamentals of Complementary and Alternative Medicine*. New York: Churchill Livingstone, 1996: 3.
5. *Alternative Therapy: Report of the Board of Science and Education*. London: British Medical Association, 1986.
6. Petroni P C. Alternative medicine. *Practitioner* 1986; 230: 1053–1054.
7. House of Lords Select Committee on Science and Technology. *Complementary and Alternative Medicine*, 6th report 1999–2000 [HL123]. London: Stationery Office, 2000.
8. Dharmananda S. *Controlled Clinical Trials of Chinese Herbal Medicine: A Review*. Oregon: Institute for Traditional Medicine, 1997.

9. Sheehan M P, Rustin M H A, Atherton D J *et al.* Efficacy of traditional Chinese herbal therapy in adult atopic dermatitis. *Lancet* 1992; 340: 13–17.

10. Bensoussan A, Menzies R. Treatment of irritable bowel syndrome with Chinese herbal medicine. *JAMA* 1998; 280: 1585–1589.

11. Buckman R, Sabbagh K. *Magic or Medicine?* London: Macmillan, 1993.

12. Dieppe P. The role of complementary medicine in our society and the implications that this has in research. *Focus Altern Complement Ther* 2000; 5: 109–110.

13. Sharma U. *Complementary Medicine Today: Practitioners and Patients.* London: Routledge, 1992.

14. Kayne S B, Beattie N, Reeves A. Buyer characteristics in the homoeopathic OTC market. *Pharm J* 1999; 263: 210–212.

15. Huntley A, White A, Ernst E. Complementary medicine for asthma. *Focus Altern Complement Ther* 2000; 5: 111–116.

16. Anon. *BMA Report on Complementary Medicine.* London: BMA Books, 1992.

17. Saks M (ed.) *Alternative Medicine in Britain.* Oxford: Clarendon Press, 1992: 4.

18. Lin J H. Evaluating the alternatives. *JAMA* 1998; 279: 706.

19. Druss B G, Rosenbeck R A. Association between use of unconventional therapies and conventional medical services. *JAMA* 1999; 282: 651–656.

20. Eisenberg D M, Kessler R C, Foster C *et al.* Unconventional medicine in the United States. *N Engl J Med* 1993; 328: 246–252.

21. Micozzi M. *Fundamentals of Complementary and Alternative Medicine.* New York: Churchill Livingstone, 1996: 5.

22. Lannoye M P. Amendments to the explanatory statement (part B–A3-0291/94-26.4.94) for the report on the status of complementary medical disciplines to the European Parliament's Committee on the Environment, Public Health and Consumer Protection. In: Richardson J (ed.) *Complementary Therapy in the NHS: A Service Evaluation of the First Year of an Outpatient Service in a Local District General Hospital.* London: Health Services Research and Evaluation Unit, the Lewisham Hospital NHS Trust, 1994.

23. Ernst E, Resch K L, Miller S *et al.* Complementary medicine – a definition. *Br J Gen Pract* 1985; 34: 506.

24. Anon. *Complementary Medicine Information Pack for Primary Care Groups.* London: Department of Health/MHS Alliance, 2000.

25. Jobst K A, Shostak D, Whitehouse P J. Diseases of meaning: manifestations of health and metaphor. *J Altern Complement Med* 2000; 5: 495–502.

26. World Health Organization. Preamble to the Constitution of the World Health Organization as adopted by the International Health Conference, New York, 19–22 June 1946; signed on 22 July 1946 by the representatives of 61 states (Official Records of the World Health Organization, no. 2, p. 100) and entered into force on 7 April 1948. http://www.who.int/m/topicgroups/who_organization/en/index.html.

27. Smuts J C. *Holism and Evolution.* New York: Macmillan, 1926.

28. Coward R. *The Whole Truth. The Myth of Alternative Health.* London: Faber & Faber, 1989.

29. Pietroni P C. Holistic medicine: new lessons to be learned. *Practitioner* 1987; 231: 1386–1390.

30. Mueller J. Handwriting as a symptom. *Allgem Homoöpath Z* 1993; 238: 60–63.
31. Goodwin J S, Goodwin J M, Vogel A V. Knowledge and use of placebos by house officers and nurses. *Ann Intern Med* 1979; 91: 112–118.
32. McKee J. Holistic health and the critique of western medicine. *Soc Sci Med* 1988; 26: 775–784.
33. Labonte R, Penfold P S. *Health Promotion Philosophy. From Victim Blaming to Social Responsibility*. Vancouver: Western RO Health & Welfare, 1997: 7.
34. Davies M. From genomics to the clinic: the challenge for molecular science. *Pharm J* 2000; 265: 411–415.

2

Practice and delivery of CAM

The demand for complementary medicine

Patients' requirements for healthcare

It has been stated that patients have four main requirements for health-care, whatever system of medicine they choose:[1] effective treatment and care, good relationship with practitioner, provision of information and remaining in control of treatment.

Personal experience suggests that concerns about safety and side-effects are also important patient requirements.

Effective treatment and care

There are two terms commonly used to describe the outcome of any given treatment: efficacy and effectiveness.

Efficacy Efficacy is measured under standard scientific conditions (usually a randomised clinical trial). It is the normal requirement before the Medicines Control Agency will consider granting a licence for the release of a medicine to the market. Several methodological problems are encountered in setting up clinical trials in complementary and alternative medicine (CAM) and these are discussed in Chapter 3.

Effectiveness This is more patient-oriented and refers to a clinical outcome measured (or perceived) under field conditions. Thus, if a homeopathic medicine is given to a patient who is then seen to improve, one would say the remedy was effective rather than efficacious. Theoretical justification is not usually an issue. There is no doubt that what is perceived as being effective differs widely between patients, and in many cases between patient and prescriber too. Part of this divergence may be due to the fact that it is possible to identify two treatment outcomes. The first, an improvement in the clinical characteristics of the condition being treated, can be assessed in terms of any or all the following:

- resolution of symptoms
- less discomfort
- a need to take less medication.

The second outcome concerns the patient's overall feeling of wellness. This is largely subjective and may vary from day to day. Patients differ in their ability to deal with disease and this may be reflected in the success or otherwise of treatment (see section dealing with placebo response in Chapter 3).

Some CAM disciplines are more difficult to assess than others; determining a mechanism of action may be impossible. This topic will be expanded when each therapy is discussed in later chapters.

Good relationship with practitioner

This includes such features as a feeling of comfort, getting support and sympathy, being told the truth, getting valid explanations, being treated as a person, etc. (unpublished results).

Provision of information

Information should be given about the condition and treatment of the condition for which advice is being sought. A review of a number of studies found that better outcomes were achieved when patients had received more information.[1]

Remaining in control of treatment

Health professionals have found themselves in the position of having to respond reactively to requests for advice and treatment. Governments have begun to acknowledge that patients have the right to be treated as they wish.

Does CAM fulfil these requirements? – the motivation for using CAM

The reasons that motivate consumers to seek out CAM are multifactorial. There is no doubt that orthodox medicine (OM) is unequalled for the care of many physical ailments, particularly those related to trauma, emergency medicine and terminal disease. However, OM is less effective in preventing the development of disease, in altering the course of chronic physical disease and in addressing the mental, emotional and spiritual needs of an individual. Efforts at prevention in OM have generally focused on screening programmes designed to detect early disease such as cervical smear programmes, mammography clinics, and cholesterol and blood pressure checks, rather than on primary prevention. The non-specific symptoms and signs that are the frequent forerunner to many major diseases are given less attention.[2]

A study of patients receiving homeopathy at three London clinics sought to identify reasons why they chose this particular complementary therapy.[3] A total of 268 patients took part in the study, of whom 201 (74.9%) were female. Eighty-nine patients were attending the British School of Osteopathy, 92 were attending a large acupuncture centre in London and the remaining 87 attended the Royal London Homoeo-pathic Hospital.

The following were identified as being the most common reasons across the three groups:

- 'The emphasis is on treating the whole person.'
- 'I believe complementary medicine will be more effective for my problem than OM.'
- 'I believe that CAM will enable me to take a more active part in maintaining my health.'
- 'OM was not effective for my particular problem.'

In fact, a total of 20 reasons were identified and the authors classified them into five groups: value of CAM, OM is ineffective, adverse effects of OM, communication between patient and practitioner, cost and avail-ability. Overall, it would seem that the swing towards CAM is due to patients' requirements for healthcare to be satisfied to a large extent.

The reasons why people choose to use homeopathic medicines have also been suggested as a basis for understanding the source of future demand.[4] From a marketing perspective, reasons can be divided into 'push' and 'pull' factors. Push factors are essentially clinical in nature. They relate to the perceived dangers of using conventional medicines, such as drug toxicity, which may encourage patients to seek safer alternatives. Pull factors are those that encourage people to use comple-mentary treatments (usually for particular complaints). These may be social (advice from family and friends), financial (considered to be good value for money) or due to patients' beliefs that CAM is a good form of treatment.

The risk–benefit ratio

At a time when conventional medicine continues to achieve spectacular successes in understanding and treating a plethora of new diseases with ever more ingenuity, there is an undertone of public dissatisfaction with OM. With a growing emphasis on the quality of healthcare, iatrogenic illnesses and adverse events, significant professional and public attention has been focused on the issue of drug safety and the risk–benefit ratio. A recent meta-analysis estimated that in the USA 6.7% of hospitalised patients experience serious adverse drug reactions and that more than 100 000 Americans die annually from drug-induced conditions. One leading hospital spends more than $5m each year as a result of adverse drug events. These and other similar studies are described in a book that details many aspects of medical harm.[5]

It has been suggested that some patients may think of unconventional therapies as a type of risk-free supplementary insurance that buys a higher state of wellness and a symptom-free, stress-free existence.[6]

In 1985 the public was assured that:

> Drugs are remarkably safe. Few patients would refuse an elective surgical operation with a risk of less than 1:10 000. Yet for medicines much greater safety is demanded and achieved.[7]

In fact the seeds of discontent with OM predated this statement by some 30 years. The most significant event affecting complementary medicine was the terrible tragedy of thalidomide. Although the first child afflicted by thalidomide damage to the ears was born on Christmas day 1956 it took about 4½ years before an Australian gynaecologist, Dr W G McBride of Huntsville, New South Wales, suspected that the drug was the cause of various abnormalities in three children he had seen at a local hospital and brought the matter to the notice of his colleagues in a short letter to the *Lancet*.[8] Until then patients picked up prescriptions from their doctors, visited their local pharmacy to obtain the medicine and went home fully expecting to get better. Adverse drug reactions, called 'side-effects', were relatively unknown, at least to patients. However, following thalidomide, regulatory authorities the world over became aware of the dangers of approving drugs without adequate testing procedures. From this time on, consumers began asking questions about the risks as well as the benefits of a particular drug.

Perceptions of unacceptable drug risks have been known to affect people's choice of treatment for some time.[9] There is considerable evidence that the public consider complementary medicines to offer a more satisfactory health–benefit ratio.

The attitudes and perceptions of a sample of Swedish adults with respect to a number of common risks have been studied.[10] Respondents characterised themselves as persons who disliked taking risks and who resisted taking medicines unless forced to do so. Prescription drugs (except for insomnia and antidepressant treatments) were perceived to be generally high-benefit and low-risk. The results for herbal medicine and acupuncture showed an extremely low perceived risk (only slightly higher than vitamins) and a perceived benefit approximately equal to vitamins, oral contraceptives and aspirin.

In a survey of patients from the UK, Germany and Austria it was found that the two most frequent reasons for using CAM were a desire to use all options in healthcare and the hope of being cured without any side-effects.[11]

Disenchantment with OM: the new approach to healthcare

In the period after World War II health for most people was something that only became an important issue when they fell ill.[12] Health and illness were considered to be beyond one's control. The roles had always seemed clear. Patients walked into the surgery looking worried and awkwardly described their symptoms. Doctors looked wise and explained what was wrong,[13] dispensing health together with the local chemist. Illness was either the result of an unfortunate chance meeting with some passing bacterium or virus, or due to a genetic predisposition. The mood was almost fatalistic. There was, of course, a general view that people should protect their health by maintaining appropriate standards of hygiene, but the overall responsibility for promoting well-being was seen as resting with the state.

In the last few decades there has been a move from paternalism to consumerism in health policy.[14] Patients are now being treated more as consumers who make demands and have individual needs that must be satisfied. The internet is revolutionising the way patients talk to health professionals. Because of the amount of health information on the worldwide web, many patients are likely to describe what they think the problem is and ask the doctor or pharmacist whether he or she agrees or not. More than 40% of the 10.6 million internet users have sought health-related information, making it second only to pornography in popularity. Most of the tens of thousands of health sites originate in the USA; 17 million American adults have surfed for health information online in the past year.

Some doctors complain that they are being plagued by a new type of hypochondriac, dubbed the cyberchondriac, a condition in which patients arrive at the surgery armed with piles of information to try to prove that they have a certain illness. A quick internet search for information on back pain illustrates the problem. Search for the word 'backache' using the Excite search engine, for example, and you are presented with a list of 2643 sites.

UK health reforms in recent years have served to define consumerism in terms of:

- the maximisation of patient choice
- the provision of adequate information about proposed treatment plans
- taking patients' preferences into account
- carrying out surveys on patient satisfaction.

Patients are given information and encouraged to complain if services do not meet their expectations. The Patients' Charter, published by the Ministry of Health in 1991, implied that people should be treated as healthcare customers.[15] Important considerations are issues such as communication, staff attitudes and consultation environments. With widespread discussion of these matters in the media, it is not surprising that OM should become a target for discontent in some people's minds and that they should demand other types of treatments. As early as 1978 patients are thought have turned to homeopathy as a result of a dissatisfaction with allopathic medicine.[16] The medical establishment is well aware of the growing demand for CAM. In 1995 an article in the *British Medical Journal* observed: 'If general practice is going to ask people their views it will need to value the replies and be prepared to look for ways of responding to them'.[17]

Some of the possible reasons for the development of widespread discontent with OM amongst users of CAM are:[18]

- OM has culturally distanced itself from the consumers of its services.
- OM has failed to match its promises with real breakthroughs in combating disease created by modern lifestyles.
- OM has alienated patients through unsympathetic or ineffectual practitioner/patient interaction.

With the advent of healthcare consumerism, and as a result of a finite health budget, the public are now encouraged to be largely responsible for their own health. This does not only apply to self-treating trivial ailments. It means having a 'responsible' lifestyle too. If you smoke 60 cigarettes a day, you are likely to go to the back of the queue for heart bypass surgery, if indeed you are considered at all. This is indicative of the responsibilities now expected of the population. If the public accept this argument, should healthcare professionals not respond accordingly? Healthcare should be a two-way dialogue in many people's minds. This notion has always been part of the CAM doctrine.

Dissatisfaction with the OM consultation

The holistic approach to treatment offers a high quality of personal attention and care. A whole range of aspects of an individual's life are considered – aspects that a general practitioner (GP) conducting a busy surgery with limited resources would normally ignore. Furthermore, it gives an individual a feeling of participating in health decisions and thus allows some measure of control over one's care. This point is now also being accepted by OM, if rather slowly. Legal opinion is moving towards the position that doctors should discuss healthcare decisions with patients, inviting them to indicate preferences where options are available.

One study asked three groups of CAM patients and an OM group to compare the consultation styles of GPs and CAM practitioners.[19] CAM practitioners were generally perceived as having more time to listen. Another study tested the hypothesis that patients judge the manner of non-medically trained complementary practitioners more favourably than that of their GPs.[20] A questionnaire was sent out to 3384 individuals suffering from symptoms described as arthritis, who had responded to a feature in a popular women's magazine. A little under 30% of the questionnaires were returned and of these, 333 respondents (25%) said they had consulted both a complementary practitioner and a GP. In answer to the question 'Were you satisfied or dissatisfied with your treatment?' the complementary practitioners scored more highly. As far as friendliness was concerned, however, the GPs appeared to be ahead of the complementary practitioners.[21] It was acknowledged in the paper that the group was self-selected and therefore could be considered to be biased in favour of CAM.[20]

Consultations with CAM practitioners are often patient-led and loosely structured, as opposed to the usually highly structured, time-constrained, physician-led OM consultation. The patient's problem is often explored at length, with a mutually acceptable approach being fully explained before being chosen. This approach has been frequently described as being 'far more sympathetic than OM' by patients. Furthermore, CAM practitioners tend to be more relaxed, less formal in their approach and more casually dressed to try and encourage a sense of rapport with their patients. All this does not necessarily mean that patients will receive a more accurate diagnosis or a more successful outcome. However, in my experience a participatory type of consultation is generally more acceptable to the patient and often leads to improved compliance with the treatment regimens.

A consistent patient concern is the concealment of information about diagnosis and treatment by OM doctors. It has been pointed out[22] that such practices date back to Hippocrates, who instructed physicians 'to perform duties calmly and adroitly, concealing most things from the patient while you are attending to him'. Old habits die hard!

The growing emphasis on a systems approach to medical treatment may reduce the potential conflict between the patient and a practitioner's reputation, as well as the escalating costs to the National Health Service (NHS). Responsibility for a patient's welfare may no longer rest with a single physician but with a team of health professionals, each dealing with a different aspect of medicine. In general, complementary practitioners tend to take total ownership of a problem, giving a heightened sense of security to patients who then have to tell their story to only one person.

Belief in the value of CAM as an appropriate approach to healthcare

It may be that the discontent with OM is due not just to the failings of conventional medicine itself, but to a new consciousness of the value of involving the individual in his or her well-being and a new sense of the value of being 'natural'. Patients are no longer willing to be treated in a paternalistic 'I know best' manner with standardised medication. They want a sensitive recognition of themselves as an unwell person, rather than accepting treatment for a disease in isolation.

Laypersons' views of medicine may vary from the theories generally accepted by practitioners of orthodox medicine.[23] Such beliefs may well influence their choice of healthcare.[24]

The motives of 38 patients attending a centre specialising in CAM have been studied in depth.[25] A high proportion of the patients were suffering from long-term chronic diseases and had been unable to find satisfactory relief using OM. Some were uninterested in the philosophy of CAM and were keen to get better by whatever means available, while others were more interested in the techniques by which their health was to be improved.

In a two-part study an attempt was made to measure the depth of commitment to CAM quantitatively using factor analysis and correlation measures.[26] In the first study a total of 79 undergraduates were asked to consider 35 statements, of which 12 were sympathetic to CAM and 23 were expressing antagonism or scepticism towards it. The statements were arranged beside a Likeart scale, ranging from 1 (strongly agree) to 6 (strongly disagree). In the second study, the number of statements was reduced to 19, and the responses of 24 students recorded. Subsequently a further five statements were removed, leaving a 14-statement scale requiring clinical validation.

It has been said that CAM – in particular, homeopathy – appeals to patients who feel that attention should be paid to the underlying causes of ailments rather than just the symptoms.[27] The different health and illness beliefs of patients choosing traditional and alternative medicine have been studied.[28] Two groups of patients, one visiting a GP and the other a homeopath, were matched in physical and social characteristics. They were invited to complete a questionnaire measuring several items, including perceived susceptibility to disease and illness, their own control over health and how they perceived the efficacy of traditional (by which the authors meant orthodox) versus alternative therapy. The major difference between the two groups was that the homeopathic group were much more critical of and sceptical about the efficacy of OM. They believed their general health could be improved.

Decreased efficacy of orthodox drugs

It is known that some drugs appear to become less efficacious the longer they are used to treat a particular condition. Skin conditions treated with steroids fall into this category; as time proceeds patients often claim that the efficacy of the various topical preparations falls. One study determined that the failure of OM was nearly always the main reason for trying CAM given by a sample of 56 patients attending a CAM centre.[29]

In one of a series of studies that has contrasted the beliefs, behaviours and motives of users of OM and CAM, different attitudes towards health and illness among a German adult working population have been examined.[30] A group of 202 subjects recruited from several OM and CAM therapeutic centres completed a questionnaire that assessed a number of beliefs, including control over one's health and the perceived efficacy of orthodox versus complementary medical treatment. Overall the CAM group compared to the OM group were more critical and sceptical of the effectiveness of OM; they were likely to express less satisfaction with their orthodox physician's treatment, felt that their doctors were less concerned with their well-being and listened to them less and they viewed their GPs as being less effective in their treatment.

In Israel a survey of CAM practitioners revealed that the most frequently cited reason for patients turning to CAM was a disappointment with conventional medicine.[31]

Perceived effectiveness

The perceived effectiveness of acupuncture, herbalism, homeopathy, hypnosis and osteopathy in the treatment of 25 common complaints ranging from cancer to the common cold has been examined.[32] Conventional medicine was clearly seen by the majority of respondents as being more effective in the treatment of most major illnesses. On the other hand, CAM was seen to be most useful in specific conditions, including depression, stress and stopping smoking (where hypnosis was considered to be superior to conventional medicine), and in the treatment of common colds and skin problems. Amongst those people with a strong belief in CAM, herbalism and homeopathy were seen as being valuable in chronic and psychological conditions; homeopathy was favoured in the treatment of allergies. Acupuncture and osteopathy were both perceived as valuable in the treatment of back pain, while hypnosis was seen as useful in the treatment of a variety of psychological problems and considered to be superior to orthodox procedures. Overall, herbalism appeared slightly more popular than homeopathy and acupuncture. It has been suggested that rheumatological patients perceive CAM to have certain advantages over OM. Between 64% and 94% of persons attending North American rheumatology clinics use some form of CAM.[33] The fact that people are able to specify which complementary therapies are likely to be effective in which conditions should make researchers cautious about using CAM as an umbrella term.

Referral guidelines that were created for staff working in the Lewisham Hospital NHS Trust in south London and published in a report on the first year of providing complementary services are shown in Table 2.1.[34] The guidelines reflected ongoing evaluation and other sources of effectiveness data for the four disciplines offered by the Trust, and gave an indication of those interventions likely to be the most successful for a given condition.

Table 2.1 Lewisham Hospital National Health Service Trust complementary referral guidelines[34]

Condition	Treatment
Arthritis	Acupuncture, homeopathy, osteopathy
Back and neck pain	Acupuncture, osteopathy
Digestive disorders	Acupuncture, homeopathy
Gynaecological (dysmenorrhoea)	Acupuncture, homeopathy
Headaches, migraine	Acupuncture, homeopathy
Musculoskeletal (pain and functional problems)	Acupuncture, osteopathy
Upper respiratory tract disease, asthma and hayfever	Acupuncture, homeopathy

Financial reasons

There are two financial issues: the cost of CAM when prescribed under the NHS or at the expense of another third party and the out-of-pocket expense to the final consumer.

Cost of prescribed CAM   CAM often claims to offer therapies that are good value for money. Hard evidence of this is sparse; many of the figures that do exist suffer from considerable limitations. Pharmacoeconomic methodology has only recently evolved and few studies have applied the principles rigorously to CAM.

Economic evaluations such as cost-effectiveness analyses (CEAs) are intended to inform decision-makers about the relative efficiency of different interventions, including CAM.[35] In order to be able to make generalisations, economic evaluations should use the same metric to assess health benefits, e.g. quality-adjusted life years (QALYs). However, the recurrent conditions for which CAM is typically used suggest that the health benefits of CAM will manifest themselves primarily as quality-of-life improvements that appear in CEAs as 'utilities' attached to health states. Appropriate utility measures will therefore be critical to the production of valid CEAs of CAM therapies.

As competition for healthcare expenditure grows, the importance of economic evaluation to healthcare providers and purchasers is becoming more evident. CAM must provide the necessary data to facilitate comparison with orthodox therapies. In measuring the costs of any therapy, both direct and indirect costs should be included; in OM indirect costs are usually significantly greater than direct costs. Indirect costs include days lost at work and the cost of providing caregivers during rehabilitation.

The existing methods of assessing CAM costs have been investigated and some potential outcome measures for CAM considered in a wide-ranging review article.[36] Four methods for the economic evaluation of treatment have been developed for OM care and could be applied to CAM:

- cost minimisation – compares the cost of alternative methods of healthcare
- cost-effectiveness – relates costs to outcome, measured as days lost at work and similar physical units
- cost utility – relates cost to QALYs
- cost benefit – relates cost to outcome in economic benefits.

There are several examples of studies of cost minimisation. One study showed that 22 homeopathic GPs working within the UK NHS issued 12% fewer prescriptions than average and that the mean cost of ingredients was reduced by 20p per item.[37] Unfortunately, there were several serious limitations to the study, not least being that the sample was too small to allow generalisations to be made. No allowance was made for extended consulting time. When it was published the survey gained widespread attention in the media and the results certainly contributed to discussions on widening the availabilty of homeopathy in the NHS. The cost of a consultation (which can last six times longer than an orthodox consultation)[38] is considerably more expensive to the NHS than the standard 4-min OM consultation. In a retrospective study treating a sample group of 89 rheumatoid arthritis patients with CAM, it was concluded that the costs of using CAM appear to be most sensitive to the time spent with the patient by the doctor.[39]

In fact, homeopathic remedies may potentially save the NHS a lot more than 20p for a similar course of treatment (Table 2.2). However, the recent substantial switch towards generic prescribing in the UK

Table 2.2 Comparative costs of medicines for a typical 30-day course of treatment

Therapeutic category	Example of orthodox medicine	Cost (£)	Example of homeopathic medicine 6c (125 tablets)	Cost (£)
Antihistamine	Loratadine 10 mg	7.57	Euphrasia	2.50
Anxiolytic	Oxazepam 15 mg	2.80	Aconite, Argent nit	2.50
	Paroxetine 20 mg	17.76		
Antidiarrhoeal	Loperamide 2 mg	2.85	Arsen alb, Podophyllum	2.50
Antirheumatic	Diclofenac 50 mg	4.86	Rhus tox, Bryonia	2.50
Hypnotic	Zopiclone 7.5 mg	3.65	Coffea, Passiflora	2.50
Diuretic	Spironolactone 50 mg	4.78	Apis	2.50

means that this differential is less striking than it used to be. If the potential cost of treating adverse drug reactions with OM (particularly for long-term therapy) is taken into account, then the savings can still be meaningful.

Savings have also been identified amongst German dental surgeons following the use of homeopathic Arnica 12x prior to dental surgery.[40] Unfortunately, no time period was stated. Savings of about £45 per patient have been reported following the use of acupuncture instead of drugs.[41]

In a US study of work in the cost-effectiveness category[42] a total of 208 practitioners involved in primary care of back pain were recruited. The group comprised physicians, chiropractors, orthopaedic surgeons and nurse practitioners. The practitioners treated 1633 consecutive patients who presented with untreated back pain of less than 10 weeks' duration. Use of medication was significantly lower and patient satisfaction significantly higher among the patients treated by chiropractors than in all other groups. There was no difference between the groups in time to functional recovery.

In order to determine cost utility, effective outcome measures are necessary, but there are certain difficulties in measuring quality of life and calculating its financial value. The Nottingham Health Profile (NHP) provides one method of gathering the required data. It uses a questionnaire comprising 38 questions covering patients' energy, physical mobility, emotional reactions, social isolation, pain and sleep. This tool was used to study the effects of acupuncture in stroke patients in an open controlled study.[43] There was a clear trend in favour of acupuncture improving the quality of life with respect to mobility and emotion.

Cost–benefit measures in purely financial terms what a treatment costs and what it achieves. In the above study[43] it was calculated that hospital costs were on average $26 000 less for patients treated with acupuncture than for controls.

It has been concluded that the systematic economic evaluation of CAM is still in its infancy.[36] It is vital that appropriate standardised outcomes are developed so that an accurate picture of treatment costs can be provided. It is unlikely that CAM will be integrated into the mainstream of therapeutics until such action has been taken.

In the UK there is some advantage to the patient of having prescribed homeopathic remedies as part of an NHS treatment, because in nearly all cases the cost of the remedy will be less than the UK prescription tax (currently approximately £6 per item) and pharmacists will generally invite the 20% of patients who are liable to pay the tax to buy the remedies over-the-counter (OTC) at the lower retail price.

Out-of-pocket purchase As far as OTC medicine purchases are concerned, the average cost of a CAM remedy is generally less than the average sale in a community pharmacy or health store. This can act as an incentive to the purchaser. CAM remedies bought by pet owners for veterinary use similarly are perceived as being good value, especially as the vet's fees are avoided.

There does not appear to be any literature on how the cost of attending CAM practitioners affects the demand, although the classic buyer profile seems to indicate that persons with higher amounts of disposable income are more likely to purchase private treatment.

The 'green' association

It has been argued that a heightened awareness of green issues has resulted in an increasing dissatisfaction with traditional orthodox cures.[18] Many of the CAM disciplines are considered to be natural and the remedies made from non-synthetic sources. This appeals to the sensitivities of the environmentalist lobby.

Encouragement by media and self-study materials

Almost every popular journal and most newspapers have run features on CAM in the last 5 years. Many relate in graphic detail almost magical cures achieved by people who had given up the idea of ever feeling well again.

A rich source of written patient education material comes from publications with more focused readerships than the popular magazines. They are self-help-oriented and may be directed towards issues involving gender or age group, or medical problems. Several doctors and other health professionals have taken a lead in offering consumer guides to healthcare. Disciplines such as aromatherapy, herbalism, homeopathy, exercise and relaxation all readily lend themselves to self-treatment.

Cultural reasons

The mobility across national borders of people whose cultural backgrounds emphasise the use of holistic forms of medicine is another reason for increased demand for CAM. Thus, migrants from the Indian subcontinent and China bring their customs with them when they migrate. Either from an inherent mistrust of western medicine or from a misunderstanding of what it can achieve, such people prefer to continue using traditional methods that have proved successful over many centuries.

The effect of opinion leaders

It is likely that role models have a significant effect in leading people to use CAM. Film stars and royalty are particularly active in promoting their particular discipline either by taking on some capacity within an organisation or in newspaper and magazine articles. The British royal family, especially HM the Queen Mother, who is Patron of the British Homeopathic Association, have used homeopathy widely and the spinoff has been noted.

The use of CAM

A survey of the prevalence of CAM in the UK in 1980–81[44] showed that there were approximately 13 million visits to practitioners annually; it was estimated that there were 7500 such practitioners in the UK, about 30% of the number of GPs. The data from a review of some later surveys carried out on the users of complementary medicine in the UK[45] are reproduced in Table 2.3.

However, relying on market research data is not always appropriate, for there are often shortcomings in the way in which the data are collected.[46] A review, adjudged to be the most rigorous investigation to date,[45] provides an estimate for the lifetime use of acupuncture, chiropractic, herbal medicine, homeopathy and hypnotherapy in England of more than one in four adults.[47] If reflexology and aromatherapy are included, the figure moves up to one in three. In any year it is estimated that 11% of the adult population visited a CAM therapist for one of the named therapies.

If the popularity of four examples of CAM are compared across several countries, some interesting differences emerge.[48] There is likely

Table 2.3 Surveys on use of complementary and alternative medicine (CAM) in the UK[45]

Survey	% sample ever used CAM	% sample used CAM in past year	No. of therapies surveyed
Gallup 1986	14	No data	6
Which? 1986	No data	14%	5
MORI 1989	27% (including OTC medicines)	No data	13
Thomas 1993	16.9 (33 if OTC is included)	10.5	6

OTC, over-the-counter.

to be some disparity in the definitions of what is meant by CAM and the selection of therapies assessed. Table 2.4 shows that consumer surveys carried out in the early 1990s demonstrated positive public attitudes to CAM in many European countries, with France and Germany leading the way. In Spain, the UK and the USA, the most popular treatments appear to be the manipulative disciplines. Herbal medicine is more popular than homeopathy in the UK.

The above-mentioned review by Zollman and Vickers[45] shows a rather different result for the UK. Four of the five studies considered placed the popularity of the disciplines in the order: acupuncture, chiropractic, herbalism, homeopathy and osteopathy. The remaining study by MORI in 1989 did not ask about herbalism and recorded faith healers as third choice but was otherwise identical.

The recognised patterns of users of CAM have been listed as:[45]

- earnest seekers – these users have an intractable health problem for which they try many different forms of treatment
- stable users – people who use one type of therapy for most of their healthcare problems or have one main problem for which they use a regular portfolio of CAM therapies
- eclectic users – people who choose different therapies depending on individual circumstances
- one-off users – people who use CAM for limited experimentation.

Another study examined whether people thought neurotics were more likely to get better when using CAM rather than orthodox medicine.[49] Homeopathy was perceived as being more effective for treating patients

Table 2.4 A comparison of complementary and alternative medicine (CAM) usage (% population)[48]

% population using	All CAM	Acupuncture	Chiropractic /osteopathy	Herbalism	Homeopathy
Belgium	31	19	19	31	56
Denmark	23	12	23	No data	28
France	49	21	7	12	32
Germany	46	No data	No data	No data	No data
Netherlands	20	16	No data	No data	31
Spain	25	12	48	No data	15
UK	26	16	36	24	16
USA	34	3	30	9	3

with unstable psychological characteristics and OM was seen as more effective for treating patients with stable psychological characteristics.

In the USA, the estimated number of visits made during 1990 to providers of unconventional therapy was greater than the number of visits to all primary-care medical doctors nationwide, and the amount spent on CAM was comparable to the amount spent by Americans for all hospitalisation.[50] There were limits to the representativeness of the sample used in this study, which was carried out by telephone. People living in houses without a telephone and non-English speakers were excluded. The sample was largely made up of whites. Extrapolations from a further survey carried out in 1997 suggested a 47.3% increase in total visits to alternative-medicine practitioners from 427 in 1990 to 629 million in 1997, thereby exceeding total visits to all US primary-care physicians.[51] The authors concluded that the substantial increase in use and expenditure between 1990 and 1997 was attributable primarily to an increase in the proportion of the population seeking alternative therapies rather than increased visits per patient.

The profile of a CAM user in the USA has been defined following a 1998 survey that included a total of 1035 individuals randomly selected from a panel who had agreed to participate in mail surveys and who lived throughout the USA and had used CAM in the previous year.[52]

The survey concluded that CAM users tend to:

- be better educated
- be of poorer health status
- have a belief in body, mind and spirit in health
- have had a transformational life experience
- have a commitment to the values of environmentalism, feminism, personal growth psychology and spirituality, love of the foreign and exotic
- be reporting anxiety, back problems, chronic pain or urinary tract problems.

Outstanding questions still exist about:

- the relationship between CAM use and health status
- the role played by the media and the internet in influencing the choice to use CAM
- whether or not CAM users were more likely to be psychologically distressed
- the extent of CAM use among ethnic minority populations.

The study was criticised because it did not test respondents' views on dissatisfaction with OM. Lord Baldwin, a member of the Parliamentary Group for Alternative and Complementary Medicine, suggested that it could be implied from the results that patients' choices have little to do with dissatisfaction with conventional healthcare,[53] but he did not believe this was the case.

The extent to which demographic and health-related variables are related to visits to a CAM practitioner has also been investigated.[54] Overall visits to CAM providers (9%) were lower than reported in other surveys. Gender, education, age, geographic location and race (Hispanics and African Americans proved to be less likely to visit CAM providers than whites) were statistically significant predictors of visits to CAM providers. Individuals in poorer health and those suffering from mental, musculoskeletal and metabolic disorders also tended to be more likely to have visited a CAM provider. Although the choice of alternative versus orthodox treatment appears to be a complex phenomenon, these data suggest that the heaviest users of CAM therapies tend to be individuals with comorbid, non-life-threatening health problems.

An interesting study in Hawaii estimated the prevalence of CAM use and its relation to quality of life among cancer patients from diverse ethnic backgrounds.[55] Given the ethnically diverse population in Hawaii, it provided an excellent model for the study. CAM use was highest among Filipino and Caucasian patients, intermediate for native Hawaiians and Chinese, and significantly lower among Japanese. Some ethnic preferences for CAM followed ethnic folk medicine traditions, e.g. herbal medicines by Chinese, Hawaiian healing by native Hawaiians, and religious healing or prayer by Filipinos. CAM users reported lower emotional functioning scores, higher symptom scores and more financial difficulties than non-users. This study detected ethnic differences in CAM use, in particular a low use among Japanese patients, and supports the importance of cultural factors in determining the frequency and type of CAM therapies chosen.

In 1995 the percentage of the Canadian population who saw an alternative practitioner during the previous year was estimated at 15%.[56] In Australia approximately half the population have used CAM,[57] while in Israel the figure was around 6% in the mid-1990s.[58] With substantial immigration from Eastern Europe in recent years this latter figure is likely to increase.

What sort of conditions are most often treated with CAM?

Over three-quarters of patients presenting to practitioners of the major CAM disciplines have musculoskeletal problems as their main complaint. Neurological, psychological and allergic disorders are also common.[36] Homeopathy and herbalism are used more often by patients with asthma, skin conditions and menstrual problems.

In the USA high levels of CAM use tend to occur among individuals with chronic conditions, particularly where pain is a central component (such as arthritis, low back problems and headaches), mental health problems (particularly anxiety, depression and insomnia), cancer and acquired immunodeficiency syndrome (AIDS). A substantial amount of CAM use also appears to be for health maintenance, wellness and prevention of disease.

The use of CAM along with conventional cancer therapy is well known. However, little is known about the use of alternative treatment in pediatric oncology. A Dutch study to determine which medical and demographic characteristics distinguish users of CAM from non-users was conducted in a pediatric oncology sample of children with different survival perspectives.[59] The parents of 84 children with cancer (43 patients in first continuous remission and 41 patients who had suffered a relapse or second malignancy) participated in the study and were surveyed with respect to the use of alternative treatment. The survival perspective appeared to be the most important variable distinguishing users of alternative treatment from non-users. Twenty-six families (31%) had used or were using alternative treatment, of which 19 were families of children with cancer who had suffered a relapse (46%), and seven were families of children with cancer in remission (16%). The most common types of CAM used were based on homeopathy and anthroposophy.

References

1. McIver S. *Obtaining the Views of Primary and Community Health Care Services*. London: Kings Fund Centre, 1993.
2. Watkins A B. Contemporary context of complementary and alternative medicine. Integrated mind–body medicine. In: Micozzi M S (ed.) *Fundamentals of Complementary and Alternative Medicine*. New York: Churchill Livingstone, 1996: 49–63.
3. Vincent C A, Furnham A. Why do patients turn to complementary medicine? An empirical study. *Br J Clin Psychol* 1996; 35: 37–48.
4. Kayne S B. *Homoeopathic Pharmacy: An Introduction and Handboook*. Edinburgh: Churchill Livingstone, 1997: 10–12.
5. Sharpe V A, Faden A I. *Medical Harm*. New York: CUP, 1998.

6. Campion E W. Why unconventional medicine? *N Engl J Med* 1993; 328: 282–283.
7. Asscher W. Risk–benefit analysis in medical treatment. *BIRA J* 1985; 4: 54–56.
8. McBride W G. Thalidomide and congenital abnormalities. *Lancet* 1961; ii: 1358.
9. Von Wartburg W P. Drugs and perception of risks. *Swiss Pharmaceut* 1984; 6: 21–23.
10. Slovak P, Kraus N, Lapps H, Major M. Risk perception of prescription drugs: report on a survey in Sweden. *Pharm Med* 1989; 4: 43–65.
11. Ernst E, Willoughby M, Weihmayr Th. Nine possible reasons for choosing complementary medicine. *Perfusion* 1995; 11: 356–359.
12. Eisenberg D M, Kessler R C, Foster C *et al*. Unconventional medicine in the United States. *N Engl J Med* 1993; 328: 246–252.
13. Crompton S. Quackery and the internet. *London Times* 1999; December 14.
14. Klein R. *The Politics of the National Health Service*, 2nd edn. Harlow: Longman, 1989.
15. *The Patients' Charter*. London: HMSO, 1991.
16. Avina R L, Schneiderman L J. Why patients choose homoeopathy. *West J Med* 1978; 128: 366–369.
17. Neve H, Taylor P. Working with the community. *BMJ* 1995; 311: 590–591.
18. Bakx K. The 'eclipse' of folk medicine in western society. *Soc Health Illness* 1991; 13: 17–24.
19. Furnham A, Vincent C, Wood R. The health beliefs and behaviours of three groups of complementary medicine and a general practice group of patients. *J Altern Complement Med* 1995; 1: 347–359.
20. Ernst E, Resch K L, Hill S. Do complementary medicine practitioners have a better bedside manner? *J R Soc Med* 1997; 80: 118–119.
21. Resch K L, Hill S, Ernst E. Use of complementary therapies by individuals with 'arthritis'. *Clin Rheumatol* 1997; 16: 391–395.
22. Katz J. *The Silent World of Doctor and Patient*. New York: Free Press, 1984: 4.
23. Helman C. *Culture, Health and Illness*, 2nd edn. Oxford: Butterworth-Heinemann, 1990.
24. Furnham A. The A type behaviour pattern, mental health and health locus of control beliefs. *Soc Sci Med* 1983; 17: 1569–1572.
25. Finnegan M. The Centre for the Study of Complementary Medicine: an attempt to understand its popularity through psychological, demographic and operational criteria. *Complement Med Res* 1991; 5: 83–88.
26. Finnegan M. Complementary medicine: attitudes and expectations, a scale for evaluation. *Complement Med Res* 1991; 5: 79–81.
27. English J M. Homoeopathy. *Practitioner* 1986; 230: 1067–1071.
28. Furnham A, Smith C. Choosing alternative medicine: a comparison of the beliefs of patients visiting a general practitioner and a homoeopath. *Soc Sci Med* 1988; 26: 685–689.
29. Moore J, Phipps K, Mercer D, Lewith G. Why do people seek treatment by alternative medicine? *BMJ* 1985; 290: 28–29.
30. Furnham A, Kirkcaldy B. The health beliefs and behaviours of orthodox and complementary medicine clients. *Br J Clin Psychol* 1996; 35: 49–61.

31. van Haselen R A, Graves N B, Dahiha S. The costs of treating rheumatoid arthritis patients with complementary medicine: exploring the issue. *Complement Ther Med* 1999; 7: 217–221.

32. Vincent C, Furnham A. The perceived efficacy of complementary and orthodox medicine: preliminary findings and development of questionnaire. *Complement Ther Med* 1994; 2: 128–134.

33. Boisset M, Fitzeharles M A. Alternative medicine use by rheumatology patients in a universal health care setting. *J Rheumatol* 1994; 21: 149–152.

34. Richardson J. *Complementary Therapy in the NHS: A Service Evaluation of the First Year of an Outpatient Service in a Local District General Hospital.* London: Health Services Research and Evaluation Unit, the Lewisham Hospital NHS Trust, 1994.

35. Meenan R. Developing appropriate measures of the benefits of complementary and alternative medicine. *J Health Serv Res Policy* 2001; 6: 38–43.

36. White A R, Resch K L, Ernst E. Methods of economic evaluation in complementary medicine. *Forsch Komplemenärmed* 1996; 3: 196–203.

37. Swayne J. The cost and effectiveness of homoeopathy. *Br Homeopath J* 1992; 81: 148–150.

38. Fulder S J, Munro R E. Complementary medicine in the United Kingdom: patients, practitioners and consultations. *Lancet* 1985; 2: 542–545.

39. van Haselen R A, Graves N B, Dahiha S. The costs of treating rheumatoid arthritis patients with complementary medicine: exploring the issue. *Complement Ther Med* 1999; 7: 217–221.

40. Feldhaus H-W. Cost-effectiveness of homoeopathic treatment in a dental practice. *Br Homeopath J* 1993; 82: 25–28.

41. Myers C P. Acupuncture in general practice: effect on drug expenditure. *Acupunct Med* 1991; 9: 71–72.

42. Cary T S, Garrett J, Jackman A *et al.* The outcomes and costs of care for acute low back pain among patients seen by primary care practitioners, chiropractors and orthopedic surgeons. *N Engl J Med* 1995; 333: 913–917.

43. Johansson K, Lindgren I, Widner H *et al.* Can sensory stimulation improve the functional outcome in stroke patients? *Neurology* 1993; 43: 2189–2192.

44. Fulder S J, Munro R E. Complementary medicine in the United Kingdom: patients, practitioners and consultants. *Lancet* 1985; 2: 542–545.

45. Zollman C, Vickers A. Users and practitioners of complementary medicine. *BMJ* 1999; 319: 836–838.

46. Vickers A. Use of complementary therapies. *BMJ* 1994; 309: 1161.

47. Thomas K J, Nicholl J P, Coleman P. Use and expenditure on complementary medicine in England – a population based survey. *Complement Ther Med* 2001; 9: 2–11.

48. Fisher P, Ward A. *Complementary Medicine in Europe. Report from Complementary Research: An International Perspective.* COST and RCCAM Conference. Luxembourg: EU Science Research and Development Directorate, 1994: 29–43.

49. Furnham A, Bond C. The perceived efficacy of homeopathy and orthodox medicine: a vignette-based study. *Complement Ther Med* 2000; 8: 193–201.

50. Eisenberg D M, Kessler R C, Foster C *et al.* Unconventional medicine in the United States. *N Engl J Med* 1993; 328: 246–252.

51. Eisenberg D M, Davis R B, Ettner S L *et al*. Trends in alternative medicine use in the United States 1990–1997. *JAMA* 1998; 280: 1569–1575.

52. Astin J A. Why patients use alternative medicine: results of a national study. *JAMA* 1998; 279: 1548–1553.

53. Baldwin Lord. Why patients use alternative medicine. *JAMA* 1998; 280: 1659.

54. Bausell R B, Lee W L, Berman B M. Demographic and health-related correlates to visits to complementary and alternative medical providers. *Med Care* 2001; 39: 190–196.

55. Maskarinec G, Shumay D M, Kakai H, Gotay C. Ethnic differences in complementary and alternative medicine use among cancer patients. *J Altern Complement Med* 2000; 6: 531–538.

56. Millar W J. Use of alternative health care practitioners by Canadians. *Can J Public Health* 1997; 88: 154–158.

57. MacLennan A H, Wilson D H, Taylor A W. Prevalence and cost of alternative medicine in Australia. *Lancet* 1996; 347: 569–573.

58. Berenstein J H, Shmuel A, Shuval J T. Consultations with practitioners of alternative medicine. *Harefuah* 1996; 130: 83–85.

59. Grootenhuis M A, Last B F, de Graaf-Nijkerk J H, van der Wel M. Use of alternative treatment in pediatric oncology. *Cancer Nurs* 1998; 21: 282–288.

3

Provision of evidence for CAM

The provision of CAM

In the UK the common law right to choose one's own treatment for illness has been barely constrained by law.[1] It is currently legal for anyone in the UK to practise complementary medicine without any training, except in the areas of osteopathy and chiropractic, which are protected by statute, as long as they do not claim to be statutorily registered in protected professions such as dentistry, medicine or pharmacy, or supply medicines limited to prescription.

By contrast, in many other European Union countries, as well as the USA, there are few healthcare activities that are allowed without some type of certification. Acupuncturists, herbalists, naturopaths and osteopaths have been prosecuted for practising without appropriate qualifications, and the technical illegality of much complementary practice has meant that it has been pursued informally and disparately, with less opportunity for professional organisations to develop.[2] One of the recommendations of the House of Lords report (see below) was that standardised training courses and accreditation by professional bodies should be developed in complementary and alternative medicine (CAM).

The various routes for delivery of CAM are summarised in Figure 3.1, which includes the factors influencing the decision to choose CAM discussed in Chapter 2. These are clinical considerations, social and financial reasons, and beliefs in holistic therapies. It also shows the progression from self-treating to medical practitioner and the part played by various intermediaries who may be consulted directly or in a chain of consultations as the condition being treated progresses.

Medically qualified physicians

This category covers those who have undergone training at a medical school and are registered medical practitioners. Doctors may use complementary medicine exclusively or, more likely, as an adjunct to their orthodox practice. They may hold a formal postgraduate qualification, or have a lesser course of training or no training at all. In the UK untrained

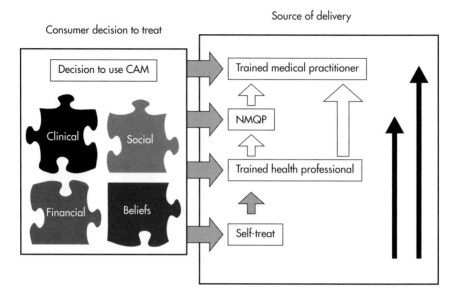

Figure 3.1 Representation of delivery of complementary and alternative medicine (CAM). NMQP, non-medically qualified professional. Black arrows represent consumer decisions. White arrows represent referral to other practitioners.

doctors may issue National Health Service (NHS) prescriptions for homeopathic medicines quite legally without having any real knowledge of the subject. This usually occurs as a reactive response to requests from patients. A *British Medical Journal* editorial noted that CAM is no longer an obscure issue in medicine.[3] Patients are using alternative therapies in addition to conventional care and sometimes do not share this information with their general practitioner (GP). Even if they did, would conventional doctors know how best to advise them about safety issues or about the effectiveness of a particular therapy for their problem? Although many medical schools and training programmes now include teaching on CAM, the approaches are variable and often superficial. This situation is likely to be responsible for resistance amongst some doctors to embrace CAM.

A number of questions have been posed about physicians' attitudes and behaviour towards CAM:[4]

- If the care is provided on a delegated or referred basis, how much does a doctor need to know to make appropriate referrals and supervise delegated treatment?
- If doctors are to treat patients with CAM, what training do they require?

Initiatives to include CAM therapy in medical education at Southampton Medical School and by other bodies in the UK have been described.[4] Teaching in Glasgow has also developed in recent years.[5] The Glasgow module is entitled 'human healing' and is designed to pose more questions than it answers and to challenge our pre-existing ideas. What is human healing? How does it happen, and how can we study it? What is already known? How can we, as doctors, influence healing? Many issues are addressed by studying the therapeutic consultation, with debate and reflection.

Similar changes are occurring in the USA. In 1995 a national conference on complementary and alternative therapy education involving the National Institutes of Health recommended that complementary and alternative therapy should be included in nursing and medical education. Two years later a survey of all 125 US medical schools found that 75 of them offered some form of education on complementary and alternative therapy.[6]

Attitude of GPs to CAM

Resistance to information that directly contradicts conventional wisdom has a long history. Apparently it was not unusual in 1919 for well-known physicians to get up and leave when medical papers were being read that emphasised the germ theory of disease![7] Many physicians still dismiss a patient's questions concerning CAM because they believe it is quackery, without any proof to support this claim.[8] This violates the patient's right to full disclosure of all possible treatment options and encourages patients to use these therapies without their physician's knowledge. As a result, it is estimated that 46% of those using alternative medicine do so without the supervision of their primary-care physicians or alternative medicine practitioners.

Over the years there has been a change in the attitude of the medical profession towards those practising CAM. In 1980 an editorial in the *British Medical Journal* suggested that some aspects of chiropractic ought to be as extinct as 'divination of the future by examination of a bird's entrails' while other CAM practitioners' beliefs were described as being 'irrational'.[9] By 1999 attitudes had changed such that 'a new dawn' was being welcomed and acknowledgement was given that CAM was not 'unproved', there being increasing evidence to show the effectiveness of some treatments in some conditions.[10]

The attitude of UK GPs to CAM may have a significant influence on whether it is made available to patients under the NHS or whether the full cost of treatment has to be borne by the patient. Several studies have been carried out to investigate doctors' attitudes to CAM. In 1988 a random selection of 77 GPs in the Tayside area of Scotland and a cohort of 95 medical students at Dundee University were studied.[11] The disciplines covered in the survey were acupuncture, chiropractic, homeopathy, herbalism, hypnosis and osteopathy. It was found that one in six of the GPs had undertaken training in one or more complementary therapies and a further 47% would like to arrange training in at least one CAM technique. Twenty per cent of GPs currently used CAM in their surgeries. Most thought the techniques included in this survey were useful. The majority of students showed an interest in CAM. Seventy-five per cent would like the subject included in the curriculum. Generally the two groups were enthusiastic about CAM. They appeared to be less concerned with the question 'how does it work?' than with 'does it work?' Another study found 86 of 100 trainee GPs had a positive attitude to non-conventional therapies.[12]

Other research has found that 70% of medical students considered non-conventional therapy useful and 63% were in favour of such therapies being made available on the NHS.[13]

A meta-analysis of 12 surveys addressing the subject of what physicians think of CAM was published in 1995.[14] The results showed a substantial variability between surveys. On average physicians perceived CAM to be moderately effective. Manipulative therapies were believed to be the most useful and/or effective form of CAM, acupuncture was ranked second and homeopathy third. Young physicians judged CAM more optimistically than their older colleagues.

The attitudes of GPs vary with geographic location. Sixty-eight per cent of GPs in the English south-western counties of Devon and Cornwall who responded to a 1997 survey had been involved with CAM in some way during the previous week, and 16% had actually practised it.[15] The doctors were asked to rate the usefulness of various disciplines on a visual analogue scale. The majority of respondents believed that acupuncture, chiropractic and osteopathy were effective and should be funded by the NHS. Surveys in other regions of the UK have shown that the proportion of GPs practising CAM varies from 37% in Avon[16] to 14% in west Dorset, where a total of 11 complementary disciplines was surveyed.[17] Another source states that at least 40% of general practices in the UK provide some complementary medicine services,[18] although the evidence base for their use is limited at best and non-existent at worse. A survey of members and fellows of the Royal College of Physicians has been conducted to determine their use of CAM.[19] Because of a low response rate (23%; n = 2875), the results need to be interpreted with caution, but nevertheless 32% of respondents practised CAM and 41% referred patients to CAM. CAM practice and referral appeared to be similar in private practice and in the NHS, and was most common in palliative care and pain. Female respondents had more positive attitudes to CAM than did male respondents. Overall, respondents thought that more evaluation of CAM was required, that it was not just a fad, that it should not be available on the NHS and that it was not necessarily important that physicians knew about their patients using CAM treatments. There was a distinct level of practice of CAM among hospital physicians, and this required an undergraduate and postgraduate educational strategy.

The reasons for GPs referring or not referring patients for homeopathy have been investigated. It has been concluded that better communication was necessary between the homeopathic community and GPs, and that this could lead to a provision of better healthcare for patients in the future.[20] Some doctors have appointed CAM practitioners to work alongside their surgery staff. In a project closely linked to the idea of integrative medicine, Francis Treuhertz, the English homeopath, was employed in a general medical practice in the 1990s for one day a week.[21] Using the Glasgow Homeopathic Hospital Outcome Scale he found that most of the 500 patients picked in order of arrival at the surgery were returning scores in the 0–4+ range, a continuum stretching from no change to cured, i.e. no patients considered themselves to be worse for treatment.

In a study of 275 physicians practising at two sites in the USA and one in southern Israel, primary-care physicians were found to be more likely than other medical specialists to be knowledgeable about, personally subscribe to and refer patients for alternative therapies.[22] Referral rates were similar across the three sites and were based on patient requests, failure of conventional treatment and a belief that the patient had a psychological illness. Physicians who used alternative therapies for themselves and in their practices had higher rates of referrals.

International rates for the practice of CAM by primary-care physicians vary from 8% in Israel, through 16% in Canada,[23] 30% in New Zealand[24] to an impressive 95% in Germany.[25]

It has been suggested that the following provocative issues should be considered by practitioners:[4]

- How do you feel about your patients using CAM? What do you think their expectations or assumptions regarding your knowledge of CAM might be?

- Are you mostly interested in fundamental questions about whether or not CAM works and its mechanism of action or more curious about its safety, cost-effectiveness and how optimally to combine it with conventional treatments?
- Can you recall the last time a patient mentioned he or she was using CAM? What was your attitude to this? Do you think your attitude has changed in the past 5–10 years? If so, why?
- Reflecting on your undergraduate training, were there opportunities to challenge the basic assumptions and values of medicine to prepare you for a changing working environment?
- Why do you think some doctors choose to do a 3-year part-time training in CAM? If you were to undertake such a course, would you think it would be a challenging experience and would you be well supported by your peers?
- If you had undertaken training in CAM, how might it change your current working practice? Would your current professional organisations be adequate for your ongoing training, regulation and representation needs?
- With an increased proportion of undergraduate teaching in CAM occurring in optional modules, how will those who choose not to do them compensate for these lost opportunities in education? Will it be as part of their specialist or general practice training or through continuing professional development?

Recognising the increasing demand for CAM in modern healthcare, more than 80% of medical students may like further training in these areas.[26]

In the USA a medical school panel has been established at Harvard to develop a Division of Complementary and Alternative Medicine.[27] Its aim will be to pursue research in and evaluation of alternative medicine and to enable Harvard physicians to be well informed about any 'offbeat' therapies they may encounter. Medical schools across the USA are likely to follow this lead. More than 70 US universities now offer some sort of CAM programme.

Pharmacists

Attitude to CAM

Pharmacy has had a long association with herbal medicine. Indeed, it was as a result of concerns about herbal adulteration that regulation came to the profession in the mid-1800s. However, the profession's contact with other CAM therapies has been less harmonious. Homeopathy was the target of much opposition for many years, with reports of acrimonious debates at the Royal Pharmaceutical Society of Great Britain (RPSGB) Council in the 1960s. Following the publishing of an article in the *Pharmaceutical Journal* in 1991,[28] correspondence on the topic continued for many months. The situation has now changed considerably. Appropriate CAM therapies are accepted by the RPSGB as a potential adjunct to the pharmacists' armamentarium and training in the particular disciplines being offered by its members is considered to be mandatory.

The first in a series of fact sheets on complementary and alternative therapies, produced by the Society's Science Committee's working group on complementary medicine, was launched at the British Pharmaceutical Conference (BPC) in Birmingham in September 2000 by Professor William Dawson (chairman of the Science Committee and of the complementary medicine working group).[29] All participants at the conference received a copy of the fact sheet, which was also distributed to pharmacists with the *Pharmaceutical Journal*. The fact sheet provided key information for pharmacists on various aspects of essential oils and aromatherapy preparations containing these oils. Sections on the use and administration of essential oils, and how essential oils should be packaged and stored, were included, together with a summary of clinical research involving essential oils, and aspects of quality and safety relating to their use. Other fact sheets on complementary medicine cover herbal medicine and homeopathy. Plenary sessions on CAM were held at the 1999 BPC (Cardiff)[30] and the 2000 BPC (Birmingham).[31] At the 2001 BPC (Glasgow) two 2-h sessions devoted to the care of cancer patients with CAM were scheduled on the final day. Despite this progress the Council's formal position with regard to homeopathy has remained unchanged since 1988. It is that 'homeopathic remedies have no scientific evidence for their efficacy, only anecdotal and subjective reports' and 'there is no scientific evidence for the efficacy beyond that to be expected from a placebo response'.[32] This would seem to be at odds with the *de facto* position in the profession and in need of revision.

Support for CAM has been carefully screened. In 1997 the Statutory Committee of the RPSGB ruled that any pharmacist who was practising Spagynk therapy was liable to a charge of misconduct and could be struck off the register.[33] In Spagynk therapy patients provide a sample of blood or urine, which undergoes a steam distillation process. The residue is heated and it is claimed that subsequent microscopic examination allows the recognition of certain patterns that can be 'read' by a trained practitioner.

Community pharmacy involvement in CAM

A 1998–99 survey of community pharmacists commissioned by the RPSGB on the use of CAM showed that 99% of respondents reported that one or more types of complementary remedies, including vitamin and mineral supplements, were sold in the pharmacy in which they practised.[34] Of this percentage, 76% sold homeopathic medicines, 86% sold homeopathic remedies, 73% sold essential oils, 43% sold flower remedies and 33% sold anthroposophical medicines. There does not seem to have been any assessment of the number of trained pharmacists who actually offer CAM in their premises proactively. In the past any treatment received in a pharmacy was likely to be a reactive response, given at the request of the patient, rather than a proactive one given at the instigation of the practitioner. With improved availability of training at both postgraduate and undergraduate levels this situation is changing slowly, and many health professionals are beginning to use complementary therapies alongside orthodox medicine (OM). In pharmacy this has generally been confined to herbalism, homeopathy and aromatherapy, although Chinese and Indian medicine is being offered on a limited scale by practitioners of Asian origin.

There seems to be a trend in the UK (as with some GP surgeries) towards refitting pharmacies to include facilities for practitioners trained in the main CAM disciplines (homeopathy, herbalism, aromatherapy, reflexology and chiropractic). One large pharmacy multiple is currently refitting a number of its stores to include a whole floor devoted to the provision of CAM.

There has been some penetration of CAM into hospital pharmacy, with pharmacists encouraging the inclusion of various herbal, homeopathic and aromatherapy products into pharmacy inventories.

Pharmaceutical care and CAM

Many elements of pharmaceutical care are compatible with the practice of CAM and similar techniques are available across both orthodox and non-orthodox disciplines. It would be appropriate for details of CAM involvement by patients to be recorded during a pharmaceutical care interview and consideration given to integrating CAM into the care plan if the patient so wishes.

Training for pharmacists

In England, the Centre for Pharmacy Postgraduate Education, funded by the Department of Health and based at the Department of Pharmacy, Manchester University, has a distance learning workbook and tape package on CAM. Similar bodies serving Scotland, Northern Ireland and Wales also provide training on CAM, some by video link to remote communities. Articles on various aspects of CAM appear in the pharmacy press on a regular basis. In a survey funded by the RPSGB of 1337 community pharmacists in 1997–98, which had a 67% response rate, 40% of pharmacists reported that they had received or undertaken some type of training in complementary medicine at either postgraduate or undergraduate level.[26] Almost all 16 Schools of Pharmacy in the UK offer exposure to CAM.[35] Although most pharmacists involved in CAM use their skills as an adjunct to orthodox pharmacy practice, a few have pursued their studies through bodies providing non-medically qualified practitioner (NMQP) qualifications and conduct consultations on their premises.

Other health professionals

This group comprises persons statutorily registered in the various professions allied to medicine including dentistry, midwifery, nursing, physiotherapy, podiatry, etc., who offer complementary disciplines in addition to their orthodox skills. There is also a growing acceptance of CAM in veterinary medicine, until now the most resistant profession to accepting CAM.

Complementary practitioners

> Sharing responsibility for the care of patients by integrating properly trained and registered complementary therapists alongside what are considered to be more conventional practitioners could, I believe, provide exciting long-term benefits.
>
> HRH the Prince of Wales speaking in 1994

In common with most European countries and the USA, a group of people, often called NMQPs, whose living is derived from the practice of their chosen discipline, are the main providers of CAM in the UK.[36] In 1981 there were only about 13 500 registered practitioners working in the UK.[37] By 1997 this figure had reached about 40 000, with aromatherapy, healing and reflexology accounting for over half of all registered

CAM practitioners. These people are therapists who have completed a course of training that may vary from a few days to several years. University degrees are also available in some disciplines. At present there are no statutory regulations or minimal education requirements for CAM practitioners (with the exception of chiropractic and osteopathy) and thus it is difficult to assess individuals' medical knowledge and limits of competence. Depending on the way in which the particular profession is organised, practitioners may or may not be registered with an appropriate professional body, which can act in a regulatory capacity.

There was a substantial use of practitioner-provided complementary therapies in England in 1998, with an estimated 22 million visits to practitioners of the main therapies being funded privately by users. Annual out-of-pocket expenditure on the six best-established therapies was estimated at £450 million. Further research into the cost-effectiveness of different CAM therapies for particular patient groups is now urgently needed to facilitate equal and appropriate access via the NHS.

The British Medical Association has published a report that highlights the need for good practice among what it terms 'discrete clinical disciplines', which include acupuncture, chiropractic, homeopathy, herbalism and osteopathy:[38]

> For all therapies, good practice would demand that each body representing a therapy demonstrate:
>
> - an organised structure
> - a single register of members
> - guidelines on relationships with medical practitioners
> - sound training at accredited institutions
> - an effective ethical code
> - agreed levels of competence
> - a proven commitment to research.

The National Association of Health Authorities and Trusts (NAHAT) has also addressed the problem. It has published a list of guidelines, stating that NMQPs should be selected from membership lists of professional bodies with codes of conduct, ethics and discipline, and should have appropriate indemnity insurance.[39]

Part of the problem that keeps health professionals and complementary practitioners apart concerns the approach to treatment. Health professionals see the advantage of using non-orthodox therapies to complement their extensive orthodox armamentarium, while complementary practitioners adopt an alternative approach using non-orthodox therapies alone, either by choice or because of a lack of training in orthodox techniques. There is always a suspicion that patients suffering from conditions that would benefit from orthodox treatments are not being offered this option. For example, with one or two notable exceptions, bacterial infections are not thought to respond to homeopathy alone, and homeopathy cannot be used alone to treat vitamin or hormone deficiencies. The British Medical Association report mentioned above reiterates the need for complementary practitioners to be well versed in medical sciences and to show an awareness of their limits of competence and the scope of their particular therapy so that they know when to refer cases to GPs. However, disquiet still exists and relationships between CAM practitioners and medically qualified practitioners, though improving, are often strained. The RPSGB supports the development of an ongoing and meaningful dialogue between the two groups.

In Canada it has been suggested that consultations with alternative care providers occur as an adjunct to, rather than a replacement of, visits to physicians. Particular types of medical conditions as well as psychosocial and spiritual factors are determinants of the concurrent use of physicians and alternative practitioners.[40]

In Germany there is a group of NMQPs known as *Heilpraktikers* or health practitioners.[41] These people are required to pass a test conducted by the local health authority, which puts emphasis on alternative diagnostic procedures. The *Heilpraktikers* are empowered to use injectables and tend to use several disciplines concurrently.

Lay practitioners

Certain individuals tend to act as a source of health advice more often than others:[42]

- those with first-hand knowledge of a long-standing chronic illness or different types of treatment
- those with considerable experience of certain life experiences, such as caring for elderly parents or raising children
- the organisers of self-help groups
- the members of certain healing cults or churches
- the spouses and staff of health professionals.

Any of these people, who are mainly self-taught through experience rather than formal study, may be viewed as lay practitioners, depending on the frequency with which they offer advice or treatment.

Self-treatment[43]

People who become ill typically follow a 'hierarchy of resort'[42] beginning with self-medication, leading on to consultation with relations, friends or lay practitioners in the groups outlined above, then perhaps more self-medication and finally consultation with a doctor or other health professional. However, people do not always follow this logical pathway. They may return to previous treatments if later ones fail, they may try different methods simultaneously or they may consult CAM practitioners along the way. This makes the assessment of certain treatment outcomes extremely difficult.

Self-treatment encompasses proprietary drugs, patent remedies, aromatherapy oils, herbal or homeopathic remedies as well as changes in diet or lifestyle. Increasingly, government policy is to drive patients away from the NHS for simple self-limiting conditions and encourage self-treatment. The switching of certain high-powered drugs from a prescription-only category to allow sale in a pharmacy has facilitated this. In the UK about 75% of abnormal symptoms are dealt with outside the NHS. The GP sees around 20% of patients, 16% of patients take no action, 63% self-medicate and 1% go directly to hospital. Thus the influence of the pharmacist or health-shop assistant is often important in recommending what remedies patients should purchase.

Integrating CAM into the UK healthcare system

Integrated medicine (or integrative medicine, as it is referred to in the USA) means practising medicine in a way that selectively incorporates elements of CAM into comprehensive treatment plans alongside solidly orthodox methods of diagnosis and treatment.[44] The term is not simply a synonym for complementary medicine. Integrated medicine has a larger meaning and mission, its focus being on health and healing rather than disease and treatment. It views patients as whole people with minds and spirits as well as bodies, and includes these dimensions in diagnosis and treatment. It also involves patients and practitioners in maintaining health by paying attention to environmental and lifestyle factors, such as quality of housing, diet, exercise, amount of rest and sleep, and the nature of relationships (Figure 3.2).

Homeopathy has been available theoretically under the NHS in both primary- and secondary-care environments since the service was set up in 1948. The remedies may be prescribed on standard prescription forms throughout the UK and are fully reimbursable. It has been

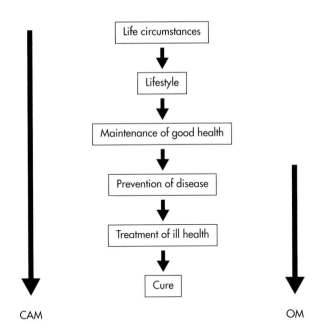

Figure 3.2 Representation of the factors involved in complementary and alternative medicine (CAM) and orthodox medicine (OM) healthcare systems.

suggested that integrating homeopathy into general practice, rather than pursuing it as a career in itself, is 'straightforward'.[45]

The Department of Health's stated aim was 'to give patients wherever they live in the UK better healthcare and greater choice of the services available'. The availability of other disciplines under the NHS has been limited and the provision of CAM and OM has largely developed along separate pathways. The call for integrating the two systems of medicine has grown considerably in recent years.

As long ago as 1989 a newspaper poll reported that almost three-quarters of the people questioned in a survey were in favour of CAM being more widely available under the NHS.[46] However, it is not always possible for patients to exercise their preference for a particular treatment. It is the purchasing agencies within the NHS who buy the services, not the consumers themselves. Choice is therefore limited to those treatments that are provided; for other treatments the patient is obliged to move to the private sector.

A second problem is that the patient must find a sympathetic GP trained in the particular CAM therapy required and this may not be easy, especially in rural areas. Currently some local health authorities (HAs) provide CAM on a limited scale under the NHS, while some do not provide it at all. The recent NHS reforms offered an environment for purchasers to reconsider the types of healthcare available. A study undertaken in the summer of 1994 examined the attitudes of HAs towards complementary therapies.[47] A questionnaire was sent to all 171 HAs throughout the UK to investigate whether or not they had a formal policy on CAM and how purchasing trends were likely to develop in the future: 57% of the HAs responded. The results showed that 67% of those HAs that responded were purchasing one or more complementary therapies. Only 10 HAs had an established policy on CAM, a further 10 were developing a policy and 77 had no formal policy. The survey suggested that a lack of information about the scientific evaluation of the therapies was the most frequent reason for having no formal policy. Of the HAs that did have a policy, four had decided to purchase CAM in limited and specific circumstances, three had agreed to purchase only those therapies they considered well established and the remaining three HAs had not yet purchased any CAM. Current HA purchasing varies greatly across individual therapies, with some considerably more popular than others. Whether this is due to the nature of the therapies or local availability is unclear.

Although formal policies on CAM were the exception and were fairly limited, it is significant that as many as 20 HAs were considering establishing a policy. Decisions are being made that are based on issues of scientific efficacy. This suggests that the potential for CAM to be made more widely available by HAs depends on resolving the problems of testing and evaluation.

A report on the future role of CAM and how therapies can be more fully integrated into the NHS was published in October 1997 by the Foundation for Integrated Medicine.[48] This 70-page document is entitled *Integrated Health Care – A Way Forward for the Next Five Years?* and summarises the conclusions of four working groups set up at the request of the Prince of Wales under the guidance of a steering committee. The culmination of 18 months' work, it was designed to stimulate debate on the possible role of CAM within the healthcare system. It contains 28 specific proposals and highlights research, professional regulation, education and training, and effective delivery of integrated healthcare as priority areas.[49] Speakers at a meeting held to discuss the proposals some months later identified a lack of both evidence-based material and good-quality research as being the main barriers to progress. The deans of all medical schools in the UK were asked to comment on the initial draft of this document, and those who responded highlighted the need for more research in association with an appropriate structure to carry such a policy forward. If the best of conventional medicine and CAM is to be combined in a truly integrative approach to healthcare, the CAM must be research-led and evidence-based.

The key issues involved in the provision of CAM have been studied in a survey of the 481 Primary-care Groups (PCGs) in England and Wales.[50] In 58% of the 60% of groups that responded, CAM was available through primary-care services. The most commonly used therapies were acupuncture (73%), osteopathy (43%), chiropractic (23%), homeopathy (38%) and hypnotherapy (12%).

A number of models exist of the provision of CAM in primary care in England,[51] including the Glastonbury Health Centre (acupuncture, osteopathy, herbalism and massage), St Margaret's surgery in Wiltshire (homeopathy), South Norfolk PCG (acupuncture) and Somerset Coast PCG (chiropractic). In London, the Marylebone Health Centre provides access to acupuncture, homeopathy, osteopathy, and massage for its 6000 patients. Secondary homeopathic care is provided by hospitals in London, Bristol and Tunbridge Wells.

The first phase of a new purpose-built homeopathic hospital – the first in the UK for more than 100 years – opened in Glasgow in January 1998, replacing an older facility that had served the west of Scotland for more than 50 years. The hospital seeks to integrate several complementary therapies into its portfolios of disease management. At the time of writing, the Royal London Homoeopathic Hospital is undergoing a major refurbishment.

Research into CAM

Importance of research

There is no doubt that many CAM disciplines suffer greatly from an inability to provide robust evidence acceptable to orthodox observers. In particular, homeopathy, which commonly uses dilutions of medicine that are well beyond Avogadro's number, is the subject of much scepticism. At this dilution level there are no molecules of drug left in solution – at least none that can be measured by the methods currently available.

It is important that CAM practitioners adopt the principle of evidence-based medicine sooner rather than later. This promotes the idea that for each form of treatment the evidence regarding clinical effectiveness should be systematically reviewed and the results implemented in practice.

Emphasis

Many of the studies demonstrating the clinical benefit of complementary techniques have reported improvements in subjective measures of disease activity. Subjective improvement in symptoms, or an increased sense of well-being, are valid therapeutic goals, just like objective improvements.[52] In fact, objective benefits might not actually be perceived by the patient. In a study of 82 asthmatics, 15% of patients were unable to perceive a 50% reduction in their capacity to exhale rapidly.[53] Notwithstanding this phenomenon, it is likely that until CAM therapies are able to show consistent objective benefits they will not achieve full promotion to mainstream medicine.

One possible way in which complementary therapies could produce an objective benefit is by first producing a subjective benefit. Such subjective perceptual improvements might promote objective improvements. Perception is an evaluative process involving a number of higher cognitive and limbic emotional centres of the brain. These centres are thought to be capable of regulating virtually all aspects of the immune system, with the involvement of neuropeptides and cytokines, which have a profound effect on health and illness.[54,55] Thus the immune system, perception and pathology are all closely interlinked.[56]

Quality

Much of the published research involves small numbers of patients and is of poor methodological quality but some high-quality systematic reviews of complementary medicine have been published recently which provide a reliable basis for making healthcare decisions. Specific areas of study will be dealt with under the appropriate section in this book. What follows is a general account of research activities common to CAM as a whole.

Inappropriate focus

It has been observed that currently much of the research effort in CAM looks at particular treatments for disease.[57] Almost no systematic research is taking place on the delivery, organisation and financing of different integrative healthcare models or on the appropriateness, quality, availability and cost of CAM modalities in the current healthcare system. At a time when there is much interest in marketing, to ignore this line of research will undoubtedly be counterproductive in the long run simply because money is easier to measure and relate to than healing. Only by combining both types of research, biomedical, which looks mainly at the mechanisms of effect, and health services, which looks mainly at modes of delivery, will true integration beyond the mere expansion of therapeutic tools be possible.

Problems in carrying out CAM research

Research into CAM is hampered by a number of factors.

Financial resources

Probably the most acute problem in CAM research is a lack of funding – at least in the UK.[58] Funding bodies are often unwilling to make grants in unorthodox areas. It has been claimed that only about 0.08% of NHS research funding goes to CAM.[59] Much CAM research originates from the UK but without appropriate support this embryonic academic discipline will certainly flounder.[60] It is claimed that public sources of funding should be responsive to patient need, and therefore with increasing use more should be made available to develop research structures within CAM.[60] British researchers cast their eyes enviously across the Atlantic, where funding in the USA is provided by the Office of Alternative and Complementary Medicine. This body, a department within the National Institutes of Health, has now become a centre in its own right, providing both a structure and appropriate annual funding to sustain a concerted programme of research. The centre's resources, although generous (amounting to $68.3m for fiscal year 2000), are not sufficient to study all CAM practices. The Office has therefore developed the following criteria to help prioritise the many possible research opportunities:[61]

* quantity and quality of available preliminary data to help determine the most appropriate type of research
* extent of use by the US public (greatest weight given to interventions in wide use)
* public health importance of disease being treated (greatest weight given to diseases associated with highest mortality or morbidity or for which conventional medicine has not proved optimal)
* feasibility of conducting the research
* cost of research.

A second problem with research into CAM in the UK is that much of it is performed without prioritising those projects with the best chance of success.

Lack of research skills

Many early clinical trials investigating CAM have had serious methodological flaws. Research is not included in many courses, although
attempts are being made by educationalists to interest students in this
aspect of CAM. In particular, the ability to critically assess evidence of
effectiveness is becoming increasingly important.

Research design   The design of research projects is often unsatisfactory
for a number of reasons, including the following:

- Lack of a suitable hypothesis to test. Most scientific research sets
  out to provide evidence for or against a hypothesis. Most CAM
  research does not usually have a formal hypothesis to test.
- Placebo design. There are difficulties in designing a placebo in
  many CAM disciplines to enable placebo-controlled trials. For
  example, sham acupuncture or sham reflexology is extremely difficult to achieve. Research design is further confounded by the wide
  variation in how many forms of CAM are practised. For instance,
  there are many different approaches to the practice of chiropractic
  and acupuncture.
- Inappropriate extrapolation of results. Despite the emphasis on
  multimodality treatment regimens in many CAM disciplines, most
  research has examined only one, or perhaps two, interventions
  taken from a whole treatment system. For instance, there are hundreds of small studies examining the efficacy of acupuncture
  needling alone for treating asthma, pain, hypertension or nausea.
  Yet in practice, acupuncture needling would be just one of a portfolio of interventions used by an acupuncturist, including herbal
  medicines, dietary changes, exercise therapy, etc. (Chapter 9). This
  makes forming an opinion of the effectiveness of a particular intervention in isolation difficult.
- Standardisation. The number and length of treatments and the
  specific treatment used may vary both between individuals and for
  an individual during the course of treatment. For example, when
  designing a randomised controlled trial for acupuncture, the
  investigator is faced with choices concerning the selection of points,
  the depth of needle insertion and the frequency and scheduling of
  treatment. Lack of standardisation of herbal medicines also makes
  comparisons between trials difficult.[61]

Lack of patients   There is an unfortunate Catch-22 situation in CAM: lack of evidence means lack of patients from the NHS, which means lack of evidence. Other problems include difficulties in retaining patients.

Despite these complexities, rigorously designed clinical trials are possible, including pragmatic studies of complete CAM systems. The quantity of applied health research on complementary medicine is growing rapidly, and the quality is improving. The number of randomised trials of complementary treatments has approximately doubled every 5 years,[62] and the Cochrane Library now includes nearly 50 systematic reviews of complementary medicine interventions.[63]

Main arguments used against CAM by sceptics

Bias   CAM practitioners often complain about bias against their research.[64] The effect of journal quality on published controlled clinical trials on CAM has been studied.[64] It was concluded that more positive than negative trials of CAM therapies are published except in high-impact mainstream medical journals. In CAM journals positive studies were of poorer methodological quality than in corresponding negative studies. The authors of this report stress that location of trials in terms of journal type and impact factor should be taken into account when the literature on CAM is being consulted.

Of the many explanations for a positive response to complementary medicine, perhaps the most acceptable in many sceptics' minds is that the patient was taking a conventional therapy at the same time, but did not mention it, underemphasised it, did not think it was important or perhaps did not realise what it was. Such circumstances will be very familiar to pharmacists interviewing patients prior to counter prescribing medicines for acute self-limiting complaints. Frequently, questions about specific drugs, for example oral contraceptives, need to be asked before the whole picture slowly emerges.

Penny Brohn, a co-founder of the Cancer Help Centre in Bristol, UK, wrote a book entitled *Gentle Giants* in which she described her experiences while suffering from breast cancer.[65] She found that a range of complementary therapies was successful in effecting a remission in her condition. In fact her cancer was found to be of a type that was likely to respond to hormone therapy and the drug tamoxifen was prescribed by orthodox doctors and indeed taken by Ms Brohn for 7 years. It is at least worth considering the fact that the orthodox drug, which has a high success rate when given for this type of cancer, was responsible.

Practitioner bias is another factor that can lead to credit for an apparently successful outcome being misplaced. It may be that practitioners can communicate to patients in some way a belief that one or other therapies is likely to be more successful in a given set of circumstances. For example, doctors' beliefs about treatment have been found to influence patients' experience of placebo-induced pain reduction.[66]

Placebo response   Sceptics consider the second probable reason for any success in certain complementary disciplines, notably homeopathy, to be 'the placebo response'.

In 1651 the English scholar Robert Burton wrote:

> An empiric oftentimes, and a silly chiurgeon, doth more strange cures than a rational physician – because the patient puts confidence in him.

Physicians have known for several centuries that patients often display marked improvement of symptoms when given a sugar pill or some other substance having no known medicinal properties, under the impression that it is an active drug. With the advent of large-scale clinical drug trials during the last 30–40 years, placebos have become an important way of eliminating investigator bias in medical research. As a result we have learnt much about the placebo and its effect. Unfortunately, researchers have not devoted much attention to rigorously defining what exactly is meant by the placebo effect, and to delineating the types of phenomenon to which it is intended the term should apply. What is known suggests that a patient's beliefs or expectations can influence the body state. This in turn appears to have implications for the interaction between mind and body.

The word 'placebo' is derived from the Latin, meaning 'I shall please'. From an original religious use the word acquired a medical and negative connotation. According to *Chambers Dictionary* (standard edition, 1993) placebo may be defined as:

> An inactive substance administered to a patient usually to compare its effects with those of a real drug, but sometimes for the psychological benefit to the patient through his believing he is receiving treatment.

A more comprehensive definition has also been provided:[67]

- A placebo is any therapeutic procedure (or the component of any therapeutic procedure) that is given deliberately to have an effect, or unknowingly has an effect, on a patient, symptoms or disease, but which is objectively without specific activity for the condition being treated.

- The therapeutic procedure may be given with or without conscious knowledge that the procedure is a placebo, and may be an active or non-inert or non-active (inert) procedure.
- The placebo must be differentiated from the placebo effect, which may or may not occur and which may be favourable or unfavourable.
- The placebo effect (or response) is defined as the changes produced by a placebo.

Placebo interventions may have an effect on most organ systems in the body. Benefits have been reported in postoperative pain, angina, cough, headache, peptic ulcer, hypertension, anxiety and arthritis.[68]

Studies have also shown that symptoms can change even when an active therapy expected to be present has in fact been withdrawn. A 1988 study investigated the outcome resulting from the application of ultrasound following the extraction of wisdom teeth.[69] Unknown to the therapist the machine was switched on and off without him knowing. Patients' symptoms improved in both cases. Sham surgery has also been used in investigating angina and improvements were noted in both the patients who had received a surgical intervention and those who thought they had been given an operation.[70,71] There is no doubt that physiological and psychological changes, both beneficial and non-beneficial, can result from the administration of a technically inert therapy.

The placebo effect is most powerful under the following conditions:[72]

- when the patient expects the symptoms to improve
- when the practitioner expects the patient's symptoms to improve
- when treatment is administered by someone considered by the patient to be of high status and authoritative
- when the treatment appears to be effective and credible to the patient
- when a positive practitioner/patient interaction is established.

None of the above factors exists in isolation. It is likely that a placebo effect results from the interaction of all of them. The placebo effect should be viewed as an interactive process in which the patient, treatment characteristics and practitioner all play an important part.

A general characteristic of the placebo effect is its relatively short duration – from 2 to 6 weeks is often quoted in the literature. In a two-part trial of patients with chronic rheumatoid arthritis in which separate groups of patients were treated with homeopathic remedies, salicylates and placebo, 60% of the patients receiving placebo withdrew from the study in 3 weeks because they were dissatisfied with their progress.[73] By 6 weeks all the placebo patients had withdrawn from the study, whereas after a year the homeopathic group still had 74% of its patients and the salicylate group 15% of its patients. Improvement in long-standing chronic conditions as a result of using homeopathy cannot therefore be due solely to a placebo effect.

Clinical studies – the importance of outcome measures and evidence base

A key element in promoting the use of CAM has been the rise of evidence-based medicine, which emphasises empirical data over theory, i.e. effectiveness rather than efficacy.[74] What happens in practice is the important issue – does the patient appear to get better?[75] However, impression and what might be called 'gut feeling' are not sufficient as evidence supporting widespread acceptance of CAM's ability to provide a positive outcome, nor is the 'art' or 'my philosophy' argument mentioned at the beginning of Chapter 1. Before any therapy can be fully integrated into clinical routine, a safe positive outcome must be demonstrated.

It has been suggested that complementary treatments which do not fulfil the basic requirements of providing a safe positive outcome do not make sense.[76] A similar statement was made forcefully by the UK Secretary of State for Health at a conference convened in London to discuss the Foundation for Integrated Medicine document.[77] He said that there was a critical need for evidence-based CAM and 'CAM therapies have no need to shy away from rigorous scrutiny'.

Clinical outcome may be defined as 'the attributable effect of intervention, or its lack, on a previous health state'. Ideally, outcome measures should be as robust as possible to ensure that reliance on subjective estimations of a patient's progress are minimised. This allows competing treatments to be compared and pharmacoeconomic considerations to be assessed.

A major criticism from OM is that most evidence-based research in the field of CAM does not meet the required methodological criteria. It has been made clear that claims of clinical effectiveness will only be universally accepted when interventions have been subjected to the same rigorous tests as those required in OM.

The stance of many orthodox practitioners is illustrated in the following:[78]

> If a claim of clinical efficacy cannot be put in a way that allows it to be corroborated or refuted, and its efficacy is challenged by a substantial group of well-informed observers, that claim belongs to the world of metaphysical discussion rather than medical practice.

The initial British Medical Association report on alternative therapy in 1986[79] dismissed alternatives to conventional medicine as flawed or fraudulent. Much of the criticism was based on the belief that the randomised double-blind clinical trial was the gold standard in demonstrating the value of a particular intervention. Indeed, there have been few innovations that have influenced clinical practice more than the development of such sophisticated methodology.

Yet the randomised clinical trial is far from being a gold standard. Most – but not all – results come from large groups of people and cannot easily be used to assist the prediction of an outcome in any given individual.[80] Others, including those for chemotherapeutic agents, may be $n = 1$ trials. There are few pediatric trials. It is difficult to design a suitable placebo for physical interventions such as exercise therapy, massage or acupuncture. Patient (and operator) blinding is difficult in such therapies. Studies involving relaxation or meditation provide similar difficulties.

In standardising a treatment to satisfy randomised clinical trial procedures, the trial may remove from the treatment some elements that are an essential part of it.[81] In a review of the use of acupuncture for the treatment of asthma, it was concluded that there is a disparity between the claims of acupuncturists of positive clinical benefits and the findings of clinical trials that demonstrate little objective change but emphasise subjective change.[82] It is argued that clinical trials have not investigated acupuncture as a therapy, but as a needling technique.

In some cases a placebo response to the administration of a placebo in a randomised clinical trial may mask the expected nil reaction. Another disadvantage of the randomised clinical trial is that it measures reaction under standard conditions, rather than under real or field conditions. The results produce statistical probabilities rather than an absolute prediction of what will happen with every patient. There are even examples of drugs being licensed on the basis of randomised clinical trial results, only to be withdrawn at a later date due to unacceptable adverse reactions.

It should be noted that bias in RCTs is an important possibility. Fifty-six known potential sources of bias in clinical research have been identified.[83]

In many instances, depending on the discipline involved, evaluation of CAM poses both paradigmatic and procedural difficulties. Manual therapies and herbalism are relatively easy to accept by OM and can be shown to be of benefit. Understanding acupuncture or homeopathy may involve changes to the conventional view of medicine. OM cannot easily make use of procedures that are seen to contradict its paradigmatic base. Despite this considerable hurdle, there is circumstantial evidence that change is occurring and that there is a will amongst regulatory authorities to allow limited claims of effectiveness, backed up with evidence of successful outcomes, to develop methods of measuring clinical outcomes based on patients' perceptions of success.

The House of Lords Report

In a letter dated 28 July 1999 the British House of Lords Science and Technology Committee (subcommittee 111) issued a call for evidence to numerous organisations and individuals involved in complementary medicine. The call related to six areas: evidence, information, research, training, regulation and risk, as well as provision within the NHS. The 140-page report was published in November 2000.[84] It set out major recommendations for action that will have a far-reaching impact in the development of integrated conventional and complementary health services in the UK. Some critics of the report argued that the House of Lords was calling for tougher regulation – a 'crackdown' – on alternative medicine. Others interpreted the report as an endorsement for complementary therapies. A *Lancet* editorial suggested that the report was 'thin on data, but replete with opinion – opinion that could be taken any way one wished'.[85] A CAM practitioner said that while the report was overall a good one, it did contain some 'sceptical and patronising turns of phrase'.[86] Despite these comments most CAM proponents thought the report provided a reasonable basis for future progress in integrating the major disciplines into mainstream medicine – an aim supported by the RPSGB in its response (see below).

The report included the recommendation that in the interests of public safety the complementary medicine sector should be properly regulated and more research carried out into its effectiveness. This was also supported by RSPGB. Fragmentation, disagreement between groups and concentration on differences rather than common aims have been identified as frequent problems with existing professional bodies for complementary medicine.[87] Fragmentation can be seen in such fields as aromatherapy, for example, where there are 12 professional member associations, each with a different training curriculum. Changes to the current situation would need to be phased in over a number of years, since much rationalisation is necessary.

The report found that complementary medicine suffered from a poor research infrastructure and a lack of high-quality work. The reasons given for this were a lack of understanding of research ethics and methodology, an unwillingness to evaluate evidence and a shortage of resources.

The committee recommended two strategies to address these issues. A central mechanism for coordinating, advising and training on research into CAM was suggested, using government and charitable resources. Secondly, the committee asked the NHS Research and Development Directorate and the Medical Research Council to provide dedicated research funding to create centres of excellence for complementary medicine research based on the National Center for Complementary and Alternative Medicine in the USA. The committee also stated that accredited training of complementary practitioners was vital to ensure consistently good standards.

Response to Lords' Report by the RPSGB

In its response to the Lords' Report, the RPSGB made a total of 15 recommendations, including the following:

- Patients should have ready access to professional help in case they require conventional medical management.
- The public should be protected from all forms of inappropriate claims and bogus therapies.
- There is a clear need for more objective and impartial advice to be available for the public and health professionals.
- Each therapy should be the responsibility of a registered professional body and all practitioners should be registered with their appropriate body.
- There should be a trend to increase funding to allow research that investigates the safety and efficacy of CAM.
- High-quality clinical trials should be set up to test the efficacy of selected CAM disciplines.
- There should be NHS research into the possible link between patient satisfaction and efficacy of therapies.
- There should be a registration system for suppliers of Chinese medicines.
- Herbal medicines should be licensed and prepared under good manufacturing procedures.
- CAM disciplines available under the NHS should be limited to those that are subject to formal regulatory approval.

The full response is available on the RPSGB website (www.rpsgb.org.uk).

Source of evidence on CAM

The CAM community accepted the House of Lords report's comments on research. In the past, available research data have been sparse. However, a review of recent advances in the status of CAM states that the quantity of applied health research is growing rapidly and the quality is also improving.[88] The number of randomised trials of CAM has approximately doubled every 5 years and the Cochrane Library now includes nearly 50 systematic reviews of CAM interventions.

The evidence available currently may be considered under three headings: clinical audit, anecdotal evidence and objective outcome measurements.

Clinical audit

This is the systematic evaluation of clinical activity, i.e. the effectiveness of a particular intervention. It involves the identification of a problem and its resolution as part of an audit cycle. Audit is about ultimately improving a procedure. Rarely is this work carried out as part of an audit cycle. Usually, practitioners conduct an uncontrolled observational study by recording an outcome in isolation without any recommendations or a commitment to improving clinical practice.

Three examples of good CAM audit studies have been quoted:[89]

- an audit of acupuncture practice in a rheumatology unit, which arose from a need to improve and standardise treatment, and to ensure that patient referrals were appropriate and measurements of outcome were sensitive and meaningful[90]
- a service offering osteopathy for back pain was rapidly adapted to meet the requirements of local GPs[91]
- an extensive audit of a German hospital specialising in Chinese medicine resulted in improvements in the hospital's efficiency.[92]

Anecdotal evidence

This type of evidence is the basis of many CAM procedures. It usually refers to a collection of single-episode reports collected in the literature over many years. This traditional bibliographical evidence is acceptable to regulatory authorities for certain licensing procedures. From an orthodox point of view such observations are interesting but do not necessarily mean that the next patient will respond in the same manner. To be acceptable to orthodox practitioners, anecdotal reports must be well documented and outline new findings in a defined setting. There is a requirement for information on the disease and its extent, and information about any other patients who did not recover after being administered similar treatment. Such detailed anecdotal reports are usually called case studies. In fact, several OMs, especially in the field of psychiatry, are administered on the basis of case studies, although the acceptability of this is often challenged by other orthodox practitioners.

CAM reports rarely include detailed information and tend to be statistically non-significant because of the small sample size. If there were enough anecdotal reports then the probability of success might be more predictable, but we would still be unable to answer the question: 'Would they have responded positively without treatment?' One often hears patients saying 'Yes, I got better, but I am unsure whether it was the treatment that did it or whether I got better on my own'.

Objective outcome measurements

These measurements have been developed to obtain some idea of the extent of positive or negative outcome. Examples include the visual analogue scale, the overall progress interactive chart and the Glasgow Homeopathic Hospital outcome scale. These measures were developed for studying outcomes resulting from homeopathic treatment and are dealt with in that chapter.

Safety

No formal dedicated system exists for health professionals to report adverse reactions to CAM, although in some instances orthodox reporting systems are available and can be amended as appropriate. The difficulty here is that mechanisms do not usually exist to act on these data. It is generally perceived by the public that CAM is entirely safe. In fact some disciplines, for example herbalism, have remedies which have a potential risk of toxicity if they are not used according to instructions. Contraindications and interactions with orthodox drugs which are being taken concurrently can be potentially dangerous.[93] Certain manipulative therapies can also cause damage if not performed correctly.

A study was conducted to explore UK community pharmacists' experiences with complementary remedies, in particular to determine if pharmacists identify or receive reports from patients/consumers of suspected adverse drug reactions (ADRs) to complementary remedies and if in the course of their work pharmacists routinely question patients/consumers specifically about their use of complementary remedies, for example when counter prescribing.[94] The study was a postal questionnaire survey of community pharmacists in six areas of England: Devon, Cornwall, Bradford, Leeds, Manchester and Stockport. Overall, 90 pharmacists (11% of respondents) provided 107 reports of suspected ADRs to complementary remedies where minimum details were provided. Where the source of the report was stated ($n = 99$), 25.3% were identified by pharmacists, and 72.7% were reported to pharmacists by patients/consumers. The majority of the reports were of non-serious suspected ADRs, but at least three reports could be considered serious.

The general dangers of using CAM may be categorised as direct or indirect risks.

Direct risks

- Allergic reactions or other adverse reactions to remedies or diagnostic agents used during the practice of CAM
- Use of adulterated or poor-quality preparations
- Interaction between CAM remedies and existing medication
- Manipulative or other damage caused by inexperienced practitioners.

Indirect risks

- Patient's condition deteriorates due to inaccurate diagnosis and/or inappropriate treatment
- Serious illness not detected through lack of knowledge or experience of practitioner
- Discontinuation of prescribed orthodox medication without permission (or knowledge) of patient's doctor
- Application of alternative approach to CAM prevents consideration of other orthodox procedures
- Patient attempts to self-treat in response to media pressure when professional advice should be sought.

To study the incidence of adverse effects, 1521 GPs were surveyed, of whom 45% responded.[95] A little over a third of these respondents reported a total of 291 non-serious adverse reactions. Eleven per cent of the respondents reported what they considered to be serious adverse effects, most of which involved damage during manipulative treatment and misadvice or misdiagnosis by homeopaths. In total, 12 different disciplines featured in the serious list; there were 52 serious direct effects and 44 serious indirect effects. The information in this paper is circumstantial and anecdotal, and suffers from similar limitations as the case studies referred to above. It does, however, give an indication of the sorts of problems that can arise. The need for proper training and control is substantial. A formal system for collecting reports on CAM should be established. Practitioners should be aware of their limits of competency and remain within them at all times. The public should be made aware of the potential dangers of using CAM.

Specific dangers are dealt with under each discipline.

UK pharmacists wishing to obtain information on matters of safety in CAM practice should contact their local medicines information service who will in turn consult specialist centres around the country if necessary.

Recent advances in CAM

The following advances in CAM have been noted:[88]

- The quantity of applied research in complementary medicine is growing rapidly and the quality is improving.
- There is good evidence supporting the use of some complementary medicine treatments.
- Guidelines and consensus statements have been issued by conventional medical bodies.
- Organisations have recommended some complementary medicine treatments.
- Complementary medicine is increasingly practised in conventional medical settings, particularly acupuncture for pain, and massage, music therapy and relaxation techniques for mild anxiety and depression.
- Osteopaths and chiropractors recently became the first complementary medicine practitioners in the UK to be regulated.
- There is a more open attitude to complementary medicine among conventional health professionals; this is partly explained by the rise of evidence-based research in CAM.

CAM and veterinary medicine

The Veterinary Surgeons Act 1966 states, subject to a number of exceptions, that only registered members of the Royal College of Veterinary Surgeons (RCVS) can practise veterinary surgery in the UK.

Veterinary surgery is defined in the Veterinary Surgeons Act as:

> encompassing the art and science of veterinary surgery and medicine, which includes the diagnosis of diseases and injuries in animals, tests performed on animals for diagnostic purposes, advice based upon a diagnosis . . .

The exceptions to providing veterinary treatment include:

- veterinary students and veterinary nurses, who are governed by various amendments to the Veterinary Surgeons Act
- farriers – whilst farriers have their own Farriers Registration Acts they are also governed by the Veterinary Surgeons Act and are not allowed to perform acts of veterinary surgery.

The other exceptions (including CAM) are governed by the Veterinary Surgery (Exemptions) Order 1962. With the movement of complementary therapies into the field of animal treatment, this order was introduced to amend the Veterinary Surgeons Act to take such legitimate therapies into account.

As far as complementary therapies are concerned, the order refers to four categories:

- **Manipulative therapies:** this covers only physiotherapy, osteopathy and chiropractic, and allows these therapies where a vet has diagnosed the condition and decided that this treatment would be appropriate.
- **Animal behaviourism:** behavioural treatment is exempt, unless medication is used, when permission must again be sought from the vet.
- **Faith healing:** according to the RCVS *Guide to Professional Conduct*,[96] faith healers have their own code of practice, which indicates that permission must be sought from a vet before healing is given by the laying-on of hands.
- **Other complementary therapies:** according to the *RCVS Guide to Professional Conduct 2000 – Treatment of animals by non-veterinary surgeons*, 'It is illegal, in terms of the Veterinary Surgeons Act 1966, for lay practitioners, however qualified in the human field, to treat animals. At the same time it is incumbent on veterinary

surgeons offering any complementary therapy to ensure that they are adequately trained in its application'.

Thus, apart from the manipulative therapies, behavioural treatment and faith healing, all other forms of complementary therapy are illegal in the treatment of animals in the UK when practised by non-vets.

More information

US National Center for CAM: www.nccam.nih.gov.
General CAM references: www.forthrt.com/~chronicl/archiv.htm.

References

1. Stone J, Matthews J. *Complementary Medicine and the Law*. Oxford: Oxford University Press, 1996.
2. Mills S Y. Regulation in complementary and alternative medicine. *BMJ* 2001; 322: 158–160.
3. Berman B M. Complementary medicine and medical education. *BMJ* 2001; 322: 121–122.
4. Owen D K, Lewith G, Stephens C R. Can doctors respond to patients' increasing interest in complementary and alternative medicine? *BMJ* 2001; 322: 154–158.
5. Bryden H. Commentary: Special study modules and complementary and alternative medicine – the Glasgow experience. *BMJ* 2001; 322: 158.
6. Wetzel M S, Eisenberg D M, Kaptchuk T J. Courses involving complementary and alternative medicine at US medical schools. *JAMA* 1998; 280: 784–787.
7. Kao F F, Kao J J (eds). *Recent Advances in Acupuncture Research*. New York: Institute for Advanced Research in Asian Science and Medicine, 1979.
8. Clark P A. The ethics of alternative medicine therapies. *J Public Health Policy* 2000; 21: 447–470.
9. Anon. The flight from science. *BMJ* 1980; 280: 1–2.
10. Anon. An ABC of complementary medicine: a new dawn. *BMJ* 1999; 319: ii.
11. Hunter A J. Attitudes to complementary medicine: a survey of general practitioners and medical students in the Tayside area. *Comm Br Homeopath Res Grp* 1988; 17: 34–44.
12. Reilly D T. Young doctors' views on alternative medicine. *BMJ* 1983; 287: 337–339.
13. Halliday J, Taylor M, Jenkins A, Reilly D T. Medical students and complementary medicine. *Complement Ther Med* 1993; 1 (suppl. 1): 32–33.
14. Ernst E, Resch K L, White A R. Complementary medicine. What physicians think of it: a meta-analysis. *Arch Intern Med* 1995; 155: 2405–2408.
15. White A R, Resch K L, Ernst E. Complementary medicine: use and attitudes among GPs. *Fam Pract* 1997; 14: 302–306.
16. Wharton R, Lewith G. Complementary medicine and the general practitioner. *BMJ* 1986; 292: 1498–1500.

17. Franklin D. Medical practitioners' attitudes to complementary medicine. *Complement Med Res* 1992; 6: 69–71.
18. Thomas K, Fall M, Parry G, Nichol J. *National Survey of Access to Complementary Health Care via General Practice*. Sheffield: University of Sheffield, 1995.
19. Barnes J. Can alternative medicine be integrated into mainstream care? Report on RCP/NCCM conference, London 23–24 Jan 2001. *Pharm J* 2001; 286: 367–369.
20. Akhtar S, van Haselen R. Why GPs refer or do not refer patients for homeopathy. In: *Proceedings of the 3rd International Conference on Homeopathy*. London: RLHH & Parkside Health, 2001: 62.
21. Treuhertz F. Homeopathy in general practice: a descriptive report of work with 500 consecutive patients. *Br Homeopath J* 2000; (suppl. S1): S43.
22. Borkan J, Neher J, Anson O, Smoker B. Referrals for alternative therapies. *J Fam Pract* 1994; 39: 545–550.
23. Verhoef M J, Sutherland L R. General practitioners' assessment of and interest in alternative medicine in Canada. *Soc Sci Med* 1995; 41: 511–515.
24. Marshall R J, Gee R, Dumble J *et al*. The use of alternative therapies by Auckland general practitioners. *NZ Med J* 1990; 103: 213–215.
25. Himmel W, Schulte M, Kochen M K. Complementary medicine: are patients' expectations being met by their general practitioners? *Br J Gen Pract* 1993; 43: 232–235.
26. Halliday J, Taylor M, Jenkins A, Reilly D. Medical students and complementary medicine. *Complement Ther Med* 1993; 1: 32–33.
27. Anon. News focus – bastions of tradition adapt to alternative medicine. *Science* 2000; 288: 1571.
28. Kayne S B. Demand and scepticism. *Pharm J* 1991; 247: 602–604.
29. Anon. The conference. *Pharm J* 2000; 265: 403.
30. Barnes J. Report – complementary medicine session, BPC Cardiff 1999. *Pharm J* 1999; 263: 644–646.
31. Barnes J. Report on complementary medicine session, BPC Birmingham 2000. *Pharm J* 2000; 265: 625–626.
32. Council statement. *Pharm J* 1986; June 14: 770.
33. Anon. Statement on Spagynk. *Pharm J* 1997; 259: 250–251.
34. Barnes J. *Uncovering Potential Problems Associated with Complementary Remedies: A Survey of Community Pharmacists*. London: Royal Pharmaceutical Society of Great Britain, 1999.
35. Kayne S B. Survey on the teaching of complementary medicine in British schools of pharmacy. *Br Homeopath J* 1993; 82: 172–173.
36. Fisher P, Ward A. Complementary medicine in Europe. *BMJ* 1994; 309: 107–111.
37. White A R, Resch K L, Ernst E. Methods of economic evaluation in complementary medicine. *Forsch Komplemenärmed* 1996; 3: 196–203.
38. British Medical Association. *Complementary Medicine: New Approaches to Good Practice*. Oxford: OUP, 1993.
39. NAHAT. *Guidelines to Employment of Complementary Therapists in the NHS*. London: NAHAT, 1995.
40. Muhajarine N, Neudorf C, Martin K. Concurrent consultations with physicians

and providers of alternative care: results from a population-based study. *Can J Public Health* 2000; 91: 449–453.

41. Ernst E. Towards quality in complementary health care: is the German 'Heilpraktiker' a model for complementary practitioners? *Int J Qual Health Care* 1996; 8: 187–190.
42. *The Patients' Charter*. London: HMSO, 1991.
43. Vincent C, Furnham A. *Complementary Medicine*. Chichester: Wiley, 1998: 29–30.
44. Rees L, Weil A. Integrated medicine. *BMJ* 2001; 322: 119–120.
45. Ryan K. Career focus. Medical homoeopathy. *BMJ* 1998; 316: 2.
46. MORI poll. *Times* 1989; 13 November.
47. Adams J. With complements. *Health Serv J* 1995; 105: 23.
48. Foundation for Integrated Medicine. *Integrated Health Care – A Way Forward for the next Five Years?* London: Foundation for Integrated Medicine, 1997.
49. Kmietowicz Z. Complementary medicine should be integrated into the NHS. *BMJ* 1997; 315: 1111–1116.
50. Bonnet J. *Complementary Medicine in Primary Care – What are the Key Issues?* London: NHS Executive, 2000.
51. *Complementary Medicine – Information Pack for Primary Care Groups.* London: Department of Health/NHS Alliance, 2000: 19–21.
52. Watkins A B. Contemporary context of complementary and alternative medicine. Integrated mind–body medicine. In: Micozzi M S, ed. *Fundamentals of Complementary and Alternative Medicine*. New York: Churchill Livingstone, 1996: 49–63.
53. Rubinfield A R, Pain M C F. Perception of asthma. *Lancet* 1976; i: 882–884.
54. Reichlin S. Neuroendocrine–immune interactions. *N Engl Med J* 1993; 329: 1246–1253.
55. Blalock J E. The immune system: our sixth sense. *Immunology* 1994; 2: 8–15.
56. Watkins A B. Perceptions, emotions and immunity: an integrated homeostatic network. *Q J Med* 1995; 88: 283–294.
57. Caspi O. Bringing complementary and alternative medicine (CAM) into mainstream is not integration. *BMJ* 2001; 322: 168.
58. Ernst E. Funding research into complementary medicine: the situation in Britain. *Complement Ther Med* 1999; 7: 250–253.
59. Ernst E. Regulating complementary medicine. *BMJ* 1996; 313: 882.
60. Lewith G T, Ernst E, Mills S *et al*. Complementary medicine must be research led and evidence based. *BMJ* 2000; 320: 188.
61. Nahin R, Straus S E. Research into complementary and alternative medicine: problems and potential. *BMJ* 2001; 322: 161–164.
62. Vickers A J. Bibliometric analysis of randomised controlled trials in complementary medicine. *Complement Ther Med* 1998; 6: 185–189.
63. Kayne S B, Reilly D, Smith M. *Herbal Medicine* (in preparation).
64. Pittler M H, Abbot N C, Harkness E F, Ernst E. Location bias in controlled clinical trials of complementary/alternative therapies. *J Clin Epidemiol* 2000; 53: 485–489.
65. Brohn P. *Gentle Giants: The Powerful Story of One Woman's Unconventional Struggle Against Cancer*. London: Century Hutchinson, 1986.

66. Gracely R H, Dubner R, Deeter W R, Wolskee P J. Clinical expectations influence placebo analgesia. *Lancet* 1985; i: 43.

67. Shapiro A K. A contribution to a history of the placebo effect. *Behav Sci* 1960; 5: 109–135.

68. Turner J A, Richard A D, Loeser J D *et al.* The importance of placebo effects in pain treatment and research. *JAMA* 1994; 271: 1609–1614.

69. Hashis I, Feinman C, Harvey W. Reduction of post operative pain and swelling by ultra sound: a placebo effect. *Pain* 1988; 83: 303–311.

70. Benson H, McCallie D P. Angina pectoris and the placebo effect. *N Engl J Med* 1979; 300: 1424–1428.

71. Diamond E G, Kittle C F, Crockett J F. Comparison of internal mammary artery ligation and sham operation for angina pectoris. *Am J Cardiol* 1960; 5: 483–486.

72. Mitchell A, Cormack M. *The Therapeutic Relationship in Complementary Health Care*. Edinburgh: Churchill Livingstone, 1998: 80.

73. Gibson R G, Gibson S I, MacNeill A D, Watson-Buchanan W. The place for non pharmaceutical therapy in chronic rheumatoid arthritis: a critical study of homoeopathy. *Br Homeopath J* 1980; 69: 121–133.

74. Haynes R B. A warning to complementary medicine practitioners: get empirical or else. *BMJ* 1999; 319: 1632.

75. Chalmers I. Evidence of the effects of health care. *Complement Ther Med* 1998; 6: 211–215.

76. Ernst E. Integrating complementary medicine? *J R Soc Health* 1997; 117: 285–286.

77. Barnes J. Integrated health care – the way forward. Report on FIM meeting. *Pharm J* 1998; 260: 919–920.

78. Micozzi M. *Fundamentals of Complementary and Alternative Medicine*. New York: Churchill Livingstone, 1996: 3.

79. *Alternative Therapy: Report of the Board of Science and Education*. London: British Medical Association, 1986.

80. Ernst E, Resch K L. The clinical trial – gold standard or naïve reductionism? *Eur Phys Med Rehabil* 1996; 1: 26–27.

81. Leibrich J. Measurement of efficacy: a case for holistic research. *Complement Med Res* 1990; 4: 21–25.

82. Aldridge D, Pietroni P C. Clinical assessment of acupuncture in asthma therapy: discussion paper. *J R Soc Med* 1997; 80: 222–224.

83. Sackett D L. Bias in analytical research. *J Chronic Dis* 1979; 32: 51–63.

84. Roach J O'N. News: Lords call for regulation of complementary medicine. *BMJ* 2000; 321: 1365.

85. Anon. Complementary medicine: time for critical engagement. *Lancet* 2000; 356: 2023.

86. Anon. Life after the Lords report on CAM – report on meeting London 29 Jan 2001. *Pharm J* 2001; 265: 808.

87. Mills S, Peacock W. *Professional Organisation of Complementary and Alternative Medicine in the United Kingdom: A Report to the Department of Health*. Exeter: University of Exeter, 1997.

88. Vickers A. Recent advances – complementary medicine. *BMJ* 2000; 321: 683–686.

89. Abbot N C, Ernst E. Clinical audit, outcomes and complementary medicine. *Res Complement Med* 1997; 4: 229–234.

90. Camp A V. Acupuncture audit in rheumatology. *Acupunct Med* 1994: 12: 47–50.

91. Peters D, Davies P. Audit of changes in the management of back pain in general practice resulting from access to osteopathy. Executive summary. *South and West RHA Report of Workshop on Research and Development in Complementary Medicine*. Winchester, UK: South and West RHA, 1994.

92. Melchart D, Linde K, Liao J Z *et al*. Systematic clinical auditing in complementary medicine: rationale, concept and a pilot study. *Altern Ther* 1997; 3: 33–39.

93. Brinker F. *Herb Contra-indications and Drug Interactions*, 2nd edn. Sandy, Oregon: Eclectic Medical Publications, 1998.

94. Barnes J, Abbot N C. Experiences with complementary remedies: a survey of community pharmacists. *Pharm J* 1999; 263: R37.

95. Abbot N C, Hill M, Barnes J *et al*. Uncovering suspected adverse effects of complementary and alternative medicine. *Int J Risk Safety Med* 1998; 11: 90–106.

96. Royal College of Veterinary Surgeons. *Guide to Professional Conduct*. London: RCVS, 2000.

Part Two

CAM in the pharmacy environment

4

Homeopathy and anthroposophy

Homeopathy, because of its availability under the UK National Health Service (NHS) since its inception in 1948, is often considered to be the most important of the complementary disciplines. In fact, it is not the UK's most popular therapy by total market value, and it is highly likely that herbal and perhaps also aromatherapy products will be fully reimbursable under the NHS in the foreseeable future. Notwithstanding this potential downgrading of status, homeopathy will be considered first.

Anthroposophical medicine is associated with homeopathy but has some important differences. This will be dealt with at the end of the chapter.

Definition

Homeopathy is a complementary discipline based on the law of similars, which involves the administration of ultra-dilute medicines prepared according to methods specified in various homeopathic pharmacopoeias with the aim of stimulating a person's own capacity to heal.

The terms 'law of similars' and 'homeopathic pharmacopoeias' will be further defined in the text.

History

The development of modern homeopathy

The practice of homeopathy has changed little in the last 200 years or so in the way its medicines have been used. In direct contrast to orthodox medicine (OM), only a handful of new remedies have joined the modern homeopath's armamentarium. For this reason, the founder of modern homeopathy, the German physician and apothecary Samuel Hahnemann, left a powerful legacy to successive generations. The remedies are largely prepared and administered as they were in the very early days of the discipline. Thus, the history of homeopathy, and especially that of its founder, occupies an important part in teachings on the subject.

Christian Friedrich Samuel Hahnemann was born just before midnight on 10 April 1755 in Meissen, the ancient town renowned for its porcelain and situated on the banks of the river Elbe, 100 miles or so south of Berlin. His parents were Johanna Christiane and Christian Gottfried Hahnemann. To avoid confusion with the many other family members with the same first name, the infant was known throughout his long and eventful life as Samuel. He qualified as a physician at the Frederick Alexander University in Erlangen in 1779. At this time disease was viewed as an invader to the body, to be fought with whatever chemical or other method that was in favour at the time. Blood letting, purgatives, emetics and leeches were all used, as was the administration of large quantities of chemicals, including arsenic and mercury.

Increasing frustration with such methods of treatment caused Hahnemann to withdraw from medical practice and concentrate on writing. In 1790 he translated and annotated a *Materia Medica* (Figure 4.1) written by the eminent Scottish physician William Cullen (1710–90), who practised in Edinburgh and was considered to be a medical guru by

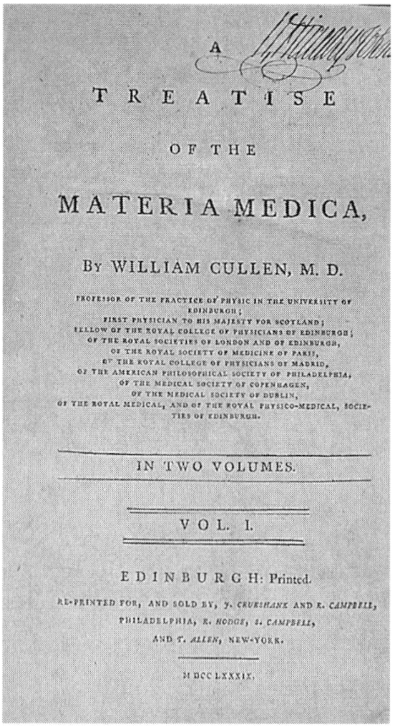

A

TREATISE

OF THE

MATERIA MEDICA,

BY WILLIAM CULLEN, M. D.

PROFESSOR OF THE PRACTICE OF PHYSIC IN THE UNIVERSITY OF EDINBURGH;
FIRST PHYSICIAN TO HIS MAJESTY FOR SCOTLAND;
FELLOW OF THE ROYAL COLLEGE OF PHYSICIANS OF EDINBURGH;
OF THE ROYAL SOCIETIES OF LONDON AND OF EDINBURGH,
OF THE ROYAL SOCIETY OF MEDICINE OF PARIS,
OF THE ROYAL COLLEGE OF PHYSICIANS OF MADRID,
OF THE AMERICAN PHILOSOPHICAL SOCIETY OF PHILADELPHIA,
OF THE MEDICAL SOCIETY OF COPENHAGEN,
OF THE MEDICAL SOCIETY OF DUBLIN,
OF THE ROYAL MEDICAL, AND OF THE ROYAL PHYSICO-MEDICAL, SOCIETIES OF EDINBURGH.

IN TWO VOLUMES.

VOL. I.

EDINBURGH: Printed.

RE-PRINTED FOR, AND SOLD BY, *J. CRUKSHANK* AND *R. CAMPBELL*, PHILADELPHIA, *R. HODGE*, *S. CAMPBELL*, AND *T. ALLEN*, NEW-YORK.

M DCC LXXXIX.

Figure 4.1 Cullen's *Materia Medica* – Hahnemann's inspiration for his involvement in homeopathy came while translating this book. (From the author's collection.)

many of his European colleagues during the second half of the eighteenth century.

Cullen had devoted 20 pages in his book to Cinchona (Peruvian bark), a drug that was administered widely for the treatment of malaria, then known as the ague or marsh fever. Hahnemann disagreed with Cullen's suggested mechanism of action as an astringent, and he decided to test the drug by taking relatively large doses himself. He found that the resulting toxic effects were very similar to the symptoms suffered by patients with marsh fever. Similar effects were witnessed for the use of Belladonna to treat scarlet fever, a disease with similar symptoms to those shown by people suffering from Belladonna poisoning.

Hahnemann then tried a number of other active substances on himself, his family and volunteers to obtain evidence to substantiate his findings. In each case he found that the remedies could bring on the symptoms of the diseases for which they were being used as a treatment. Thus he systematically built up considerable circumstantial evidence for the existence of a law of cure based on the concept of using 'like to treat like'. He called the systematic procedure of testing substances on healthy human beings in order to elucidate the symptoms reflecting the use of the medicine a *Prüfung*, which is translated into English as 'proving'.

Hahnemann returned to medicine in 1801, using his new homeopathic principles. Many colleagues viewed his methods with considerable scepticism despite a number of spectacular successes. In 1810 Hahnemann published his most famous work, the *Organon of the Rational Art of Healing*.[1] A total of five editions of this book appeared during Hahnemann's lifetime; the manuscipt for a sixth edition was not published for many years after his death. The subject matter in the sixth edition was set out in 291 numbered sections or aphorisms, usually denoted in the literature by the symbol § and the relevant section number.

Following the death of his first wife Johanna in 1830, Hahnemann married the Marquise Melanie D'Hervilly-Gohier, a colourful and eccentric companion many years his junior. The couple moved to Paris, where he died in 1843.

Theory

The vital force

The mechanisms of action of homeopathy are not understood, although many possible explanations for them have been put forward. There are claims that the apparent success of homeopathy is due solely to a placebo effect (Chapter 3). This may well be true to some extent, but this is only part of the story.

Homeopaths consider disease to be an expression of the vital force of each individual. Since all individuals are quite different in their expression of the vital force, patients are treated according to their idiosyncratic, rather than their common, symptoms. The symptoms are important only in that they act as an indicator for the selection of an appropriate remedy.

Hahnemann introduced the word 'dynamis' to describe the vital force indicating that life was dynamic and took an active part in organising biological activity. He called the process of potentisation 'dynamisation', a term that is still widely used by French and German homeopaths. Vitalists believe that the body is comprised of a hierarchy of parts (cells, tissues, organs and systems) that are all fully interdependent in both ascending and descending order, and whose relationship to one another is controlled by a vital force. Under normal conditions, the vital force is thought to be responsible for the orderly and harmonious running of the body, and for coordinating the body's defences against disease. However, if the force becomes disturbed by factors such as emotional stress, poor diet, environmental conditions or certain inappropriate allopathic drugs, then illness results.

It is believed that the vital force operates on three different vibratory levels:

- mental: changes in understanding and consciousness are recorded (e.g. confusion and lack of concentration)
- emotional: changes in emotional states are recorded (e.g. anxiety and irritability)
- physical: changes to the body's organs and systems are recorded (e.g. organ malfunction and disease).

Classical homeopaths consider the body's functions to be a *mélange* of all these levels when determining which homeopathic remedy is appropriate to restore the vital force to its normal levels. They consider the totality of symptoms rather than looking at individual planes in isolation. If only a partial image of the total symptom picture is acquired, they consider that the effect of the remedy will be limited to that vibrational level.

This comprehensive approach is not the only way homeopathic remedies can be used. It is possible to administer remedies chosen for their local effect in the physical plane alone. This approach is used especially for first aid and the treatment of many simple self-limiting situations.

The three principles of homeopathy

There are three important principles of homeopathy according to Hahnemann: like cures like, minimal dose and single remedy.

Like cures like

This principle first appeared in an article entitled 'Essay on a new principle for ascertaining the curative power of drugs'.[2] Hahnemann believed that in order to cure disease, one must seek medicines that can excite similar symptoms in the healthy human body. This idea is summarised in the phrase *similia similibus curentur*, often translated as 'let like be treated with like'.

Examples of such treatment might be the homeopathic use of:

- Apis (from the bee) to treat histamine-type reactions resulting from a sting
- Coffea (from the green coffee bean) to treat insomnia
- Urtica (from the nettle) to treat an urticarial rash.

At first sight, this method is rather different to the orthodox approach, in which the use of a laxative to treat diarrhoea might be viewed rather strangely! However, there are examples of this practice in orthodox pharmacy:

- Above a certain dose threshold digoxin causes many of the cardiac arrhythmias for which it is a treatment.
- Aspirin in large doses causes headaches.

It was this method of prescribing according to the matching of symptoms and drug pictures that prompted Hahnemann in 1807 to coin the term 'homeopathy' from the Greek words *homoios* (similar) and *pathos* (disease or suffering). He termed the more orthodox treatment by the law of contraries 'allopathy' from *alloios*, meaning contrary. This term is still widely used today.

Minimal dose

When Hahnemann carried out his original work he gave substantial doses of medicine to his patients, in keeping with contemporary practice. This often resulted in substantial toxic reactions; fatalities were not uncommon. He experimented to try and dilute out the unwanted toxicity while at the same time maintaining a therapeutic effect. There is much speculation as to how Hahnemann developed the method of serial diluting and agitating his remedies, which achieved his aim better than he could have hoped. To his surprise Hahnemann found that, as the remedies became more dilute, they became more potent therapeutically. To reflect this effect he called his new process 'potentisation'. The potentisation process is described in detail below.

Single remedy

Hahnemann believed that one should use a single remedy to treat a condition. Provings in all materia medicas relate to single remedies and there is no way of knowing whether or how individual remedy drug pictures are modified by combination with other ingredients. Classical homeopaths observe this rule carefully. In later life Hahnemann did use mixtures of two or three remedies and there are a limited number of such mixtures still used today, including Arsen iod, Gelsemium and Eupatorium (AGE, for colds and flu) and Aconite (or sometimes Arsen alb), Belladonna and Chamomilla (ABC, for teething).

Holistic approach

In addition to the three principles stated above, Hahnemann believed that homeopathy should be practised according to the holistic principles that are common to all complementary disciplines. Each patient should be treated as a complete individual. This means that remedies (or procedures) appropriate for one patient might be totally inappropriate for another even though the symptoms may be similar. Conversely, the same remedy may be used to treat very different conditions in different patients.

Homeopathic laws of cure

There are three laws of cure that may be applied to the practice of homeopathy: Hering's law, Arndt's law and the law of minimum action.

Hering's law

This law is attributed to the American homeopath Dr Constantine Hering. It states that cure takes place:

- from the top to the bottom of the body
- from the inside to the outside

- from the most important organs to the least important
- in reverse order of the onset of symptoms.

Hence mental symptoms (emotions) might be expected to improve before physical symptoms are resolved, and recent symptoms will subside before long-standing chronic symptoms. A good example of this law in practice is the resolution of asthma, which is often associated with skin conditions. It is not uncommon to see the physical symptoms of asthma improving only to find an underlying skin condition becoming more pronounced.

Arndt's law

This is a general pharmaceutical law that states:

- Weak stimuli encourage living systems (e.g. homeopathy).
- Medium-strength stimuli impede living systems (e.g. biochemical pathway blockers).
- Strong stimuli tend to destroy living systems (e.g. chemotherapy).

It is suggested that small quantities of homeopathic medicine administered to an individual stimulate the body's own defence mechanisms to deal with disease. In fact, the situation is probably much more complicated than this simplistic explanation suggests, and is not as yet understood (see below).

Law of minimum action

The third law is associated with the minute doses administered in homeopathy:

- A change in nature is effected by the least possible action.
- The decisive amount of action needed to produce change is always the minimum.

Clinical experience suggests that the minute amounts of active ingredients administered by homeopaths are still sufficient to produce a therapeutic effect. It is generally accepted that the frequency of administration is more significant than the size of dose.

Proving homeopathic remedies

All remedies have a 'drug picture', a written survey of the symptoms noted when the drug was given to healthy volunteers, a process known as 'proving the drug'. Hahnemann defined very precisely guidelines for carrying out provings.

Theoretically, the proving of a substance refers to all the symptoms induced by the substance in healthy people, according to Hahnemann's original instructions. However, drug pictures may also contain symptoms derived from the following sources.[3]

- observations of toxological effects arising from therapeutic, deliberate or accidental administration
- observations of pathological symptoms regularly cured by the remedy in clinical practice: this is the source of many seemingly strange symptoms that occur in some drug pictures.

In some instances the complete drug picture may be derived from toxicological or clinical observations and not from a true proving at all.

The drug pictures are collected together in materia medica, many of which have been computerised. These are usually consulted when an appropriate remedy is being chosen to treat a patient (see below).

Nomenclature of homeopathic remedies

Homeopathic products are traditionally called remedies, although the term 'medicine' is preferred by many people. The existing nomenclature of homeopathic remedies and the connected abbreviation system by which remedies are identified have evolved over 200 years and are full of irregularities and mistakes. Traditionally remedies are described by an abbreviation of the Latin name together with an indication of the potency. There are so many synonyms, different spellings, different abbreviations and differences in the source material used for the remedy preparation that confusion is difficult to avoid. However, within a particular country it is unlikely that any conflict will arise. Patients are well advised to take any prescribed medication with them when they travel because the remedy obtained abroad may be different to the remedy they are used to buying in their own country.

Some examples that illustrate sources of potential confusion have been highlighted in a report prepared under the auspices of the European Committee for Homeopathy.[4] Most botanical names currently used in homeopathy are still similar to the current botanical nomenclature used for the source material. However, other remedies have other synonyms that do not correspond with either the pharmacopoeias or the current botanical names. For example, Belladonna (*Atropa belladonna*), Cactus grandiflorus (*Cercus grandiflorus*) and Chamomilla (*Matricaria chamomilla*) all have commonly used homeopathic names that are not correct. Further, the botanical nomenclature used in homeopathy does not indicate the part of the plant that has been used. In some countries the whole plant is used; in other countries it can be the root, the seeds, the leaves, the flower or the fruits.

Most zoological names currently used in homeopathy are still similar to the current zoological nomenclature, such as *Apis mellifica* (bee), *Latrodectus mactans* (spider) and *Vespa cabro* (wasp). Some, however, are not. For example, Cantharis would be more correctly called *Lytta vesicatoria*. Remedies from chemical sources have their problems too. Compounds with F, Ca, Br, I, O and S ions are usually called fluoratums, bromatums, iodatums, sulphuratums, etc., but calcium fluoride is called Calcarea fluorica in some countries and Calcium fluoricum in others, which is not consistent (Calcium fluoratum would be more logical).

Many of the nosode names currently used in homeopathy are insufficiently specified names, e.g. Psorinum, Carcinosinum, Tuberculinum and Medorrhinum. The nosodes often show different starting materials and manufacturing methods in different communities.

Homeopathy needs a consistent international nomenclature system to ensure the accurate supply of currently available remedies and the logical incorporation of new remedies in the future. The European Committee on Homeopathy has made proposals for the development of a more logical system of abbreviations that will ensure international standardisation.

Difficulties with nomenclature are not confined to naming remedies. A group of Latin American and European authors have pointed out that international confusion also exists as to the exact meaning of many words used routinely in homeopathy and they suggest that many inaccurate or imprecise terms should be replaced.[5]

The manufacture of homeopathic remedies

The homeopathic pharmacopoeias

Homeopathic medicines are prepared in accordance with the methods described in various national homeopathic pharmacopoeias. For many years British manufacturers have relied on a selection of foreign reference works, principally the *German Homeopathic Pharmacopoeia* (GHP, or HAB in the German abbreviation) with its various supplements, together with the *French Pharmacopoeia* and the *Homeopathic Pharmacopoeia of the US*, for most of their information, particularly with regard to the analysis of starting materials. After an interval of almost 100 years a new edition of the *British Homeopathic Pharmacopoeia* (BHomP) was published by the British Association of Homeopathic Manufacturers (BAHM) in 1993[6] and this is used alongside the GHP, although the BHomP has not been formally adopted as a national pharmacopoeia by the Medicines Control Agency and has no status under European legislation (see the section on regulatory affairs, below). A second edition of this text was published in 1999.[7]

The source materials

Plant material

Well over half of all homeopathic remedies are prepared from extracts of plant materials, and because of this homeopathy is often confused with herbalism. However, the ways of producing the two types of medicines are quite different. Herbal products are generally the result of an aqueous or alcoholic extraction alone, whereas in homeopathy an additional dilution process is involved. Either the whole plant may be used or only selected parts, as specified in the pharmacopoeia monographs. The specimens are collected in dry sunny weather and cleaned by careful shaking, brushing and rinsing with distilled water. They are then examined to ensure the absence of moulds and other imperfections. Fresh plant material is desirable, but for a variety of reasons dried specimens are sometimes used. Arnica, for example, grows best above 3000 m and is often subject to conservation orders at certain times of the year, while Nux vomica is readily available in relatively large amounts, but is difficult to obtain in the very small quantities required by homeopathic pharmacists. Soil differences may mean that the most easily accessible plants are not the most suitable. Crataegus, the hawthorn, varies in quality from country to country. These difficulties may be appreciated if one considers the analogy of wines: grapes grown in different soil and climatic conditions, even if adjacent to each other, produce wines with different characteristics. Calendula, which is used for the treatment of superficial abrasions, is illustrated in Figure 4.2.

Animal and insect material

This material must be obtained from healthy specimens. The bee yields Apis, a remedy used to treat peripheral oedematous conditions and the

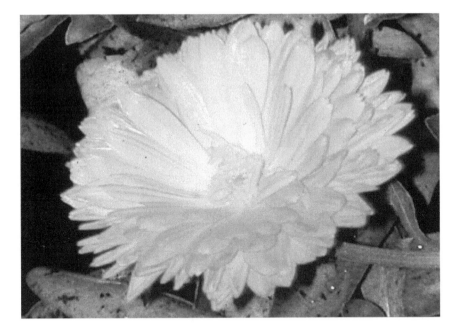

Figure 4.2 *Calendula officinalis* (marigold). This plant has wide oral and topical applications in homeopathy.

effects of stings. Other examples are remedies made from snake and spider venoms, musk oil and the juice of the cuttlefish (Sepia). Musk is obtained from the African cevit, a fox-like animal kept in battery accommodation, mainly in Ethiopia. There have been calls recently for the practice of milking animals to be discontinued in favour of synthetic production.

Biological material

Material may be used from bacterial cultures, pathological samples or healthy animal secretions. These materials are known as 'isopathics'.

Chemical material

Highly purified chemical material is rarely used in the preparation of remedies. For example, Calcium carbonicum is obtained from the interspaces of oyster shells and is not prepared in the laboratory. Sulphur is obtained from a naturally occurring source (e.g. a geothermal area) and is not precipitated in the laboratory.

Chemical material and drugs may also be used in the preparation of isopathic preparations, when they are said to be 'tautopathic' (see below).

Miscellaneous

Isopathic source material is used to prepare allergodes (e.g. grass pollens, flowers, animal hair, feathers, foods, etc.), sarcodes (e.g. bacterial cultures or healthy secretions), nosodes (pathological samples) and tautopathics (chemicals, drugs, vaccines, etc.). See section on isopathic remedies below.

Preparation of remedies

Extraction procedure

Mother tinctures are liquid preparations resulting from the extraction of suitable vegetable source material with, usually, alcohol/water mixtures. They form the starting point for the production of most homeopathic medicines, although some are used orally (e.g. Crataegus) or topically (e.g. Arnica). The resulting extract solutions contain on average one part drug to three parts mother tincture, although this strength can vary depending on the species and type of extraction process. The solutions are strained to remove any extraneous pieces of debris.

Insoluble chemicals such as Aurum (gold), Graphites (graphite or lead) and Sulphur (and most isopathic preparations) must be processed differently. The solid material is triturated with lactose in a pestle and mortar. The resulting triturate may be compressed directly into trituration tablets or administered as a powder. More usually, however, trituration continues until the particle size has been reduced sufficiently to facilitate the preparation of a solution, usually achieved after three to six serial dilutions depending on the scale being used. From this point the standard potentisation procedure described below can be followed.

In the case of soluble chemicals, solutions of known concentration in distilled water or alcohol can be prepared initially as the starting solution.

International variations

The methods of preparing remedies differ between the various pharmacopoeias and this introduces an international variable. For example, the

German text states that to make a mother tincture the source material must be macerated for at least 10 days at a temperature not exceeding 30°C, while the French publication specifies a period of 3 weeks. Little research has been carried out to quantify the variance in active principles that may occur, although nuclear magnetic resonance techniques exist for testing different source materials.[8] These differences mean that remedies may well differ from country to country even though the potencies appear to be equivalent.

The potentisation process

With some remedies, for example Arnica or Calendula, the mother tincture may be applied directly to the skin, or it may be diluted and used as a gargle; Crataegus mother tincture is often administered as five drops in water. Most mother tinctures, however, are diluted in a special manner. Because this dilution increases the homeopathic strength (although the chemical concentration decreases), the process is known as potentisation (Figure 4.3).

The Hahnemannian method   The Hahnemannian method of potentisation has two scales of dilution: centesimal and decimal. In the former,

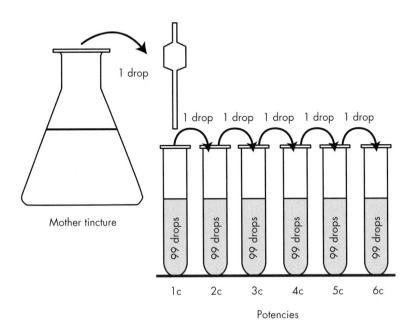

Figure 4.3 The homeopathic potentisation process.

one drop of mother tincture is added to 99 drops of diluent in a new clean screw-cap glass vial. The diluent is a triple-distilled alcohol and water system, the strength of which varies from 20 to 60%. The solution resulting from admixture of the two liquids is subjected to a vigorous shaking with impact, known as succussion. The extent to which the vials are shaken depends on the individual concerned, but within each manufacturing process the number of succussions remains constant. Hahnemann's ideas on how often to succuss the vial varied widely from once or twice right up to 100 times. After the initial process, successive serial dilutions are made, using fresh glass vials at each stage until the solution reaches 12c, 30c, 200c and so on (the number refers to the number of successive 1 in 100 dilutions and 'c' indicates the centesimal method). The stages are summarised in Table 4.1. In the decimal scale, one drop of mother tincture is added to nine drops of diluent. This is indicated by a number and 'x' (e.g. 6x). At the higher centesimal dilutions, letters are normally used. The 1000 dilution level is therefore M, and 10 000 is CM (Table 4.2).

Potencies up to 200c are still made by hand by skilled operators agitating the container between each serial dilution stage by striking it on the heel of the hand. Most large manufacturers have small mechanical shakers that perform the task with rather less effort.

The Korsakovian method   There is some doubt concerning how M and 10M potencies are made. These are often described as being 1000 and 10 000 centesimal dilutions. Although it is still possible to prepare potencies of this magnitude according to Hahnemann's original instructions using special machinery, many of these remedies are prepared robotically using a method described in 1832 by the Russian homeopath Nicolaevich Korsakov, although they are seldom correctly labelled to show this.

Table 4.1 Centesimal potencies

Centesimal potency	Concentration	Dilution
1 (1c or 1cH)	10^{-2}	$1{:}100$
6 (6c or 6cH)	10^{-12}	$1{:}10^{12}$
12 (12c or 12cH)	10^{-24}	$1{:}10^{24}$
30 (30c or 30cH)	10^{-60}	$1{:}10^{60}$
200 (200c or 200cH)	10^{-400}	$1{:}10^{400}$
M[a]	10^{-2000}	$1{:}10^{2000}$
10M[a]	$10^{-20\,000}$	$1{:}10^{20\,000}$

[a]Korsakovian dilutions.

Table 4.2 Decimal potencies

Decimal potency	Concentration	Dilution
1x (D1)	10^{-1}	1:10
6x (D6)	10^{-6}	$1:10^6$
12x (D12)	10^{-12}	$1:10^{12}$
30x (D30)	10^{-30}	$1:10^{30}$

A first dilution known as 1K or 1cK is prepared by adding a measured volume of mother tincture to an appropriate volume of diluent and the resulting solution succussed thoroughly. Liquid is then removed from the vial by suction or inversion, leaving droplets of solution adhering to the container wall. New solvent is then added, the vial is agitated vigorously and the process is repeated. Korsakovian potencies are usually denoted by a number denoting the number of serial dilutions followed by the letter 'K' (e.g. 1000K).

The LM method   In later life Hahnemann began using potencies based on serial dilutions of 1:50 000 at each level. These are called LM (or occasionally Q) potencies. Remedies are triturated to the third centesimal level with lactose before being diluted according to the scale described above. Homeopaths often instruct patients to success LM potencies prior to taking each dose to minimise the possibility of developing the symptoms of the remedy.

The effects of potentisation   One of the fundamental tenets of homeopathy is the concept of potentisation, and yet it continues to be one of the major stumbling blocks to its widespread acceptance, with many sceptics claiming that it is just a myth.[9] It is not known how Hahnemann came upon the procedure of potentisation; most likely it arose from his knowledge of chemistry and alchemy. Over the past two decades research into structure formation and structure conservation in water systems has created significant interest in the homeopathic community. Geometric and dynamic models have been constructed to try and explain how remedies can be therapeutically active at such extreme dilutions.[10]

There is some evidence to indicate that the structure of solvent molecules may be electrochemically changed by succussion, enabling it to acquire an ability to 'memorise' an imprint of the original remedy. It is acknowledged that this concept is difficult for many highly trained personnel with scientific backgrounds to accept. The simplest suggestion is that succussion may merely facilitate a complete mixing.

The dose forms

Solid dose forms in allopathic medicine tablets and capsules are made in different forms to control the speed at which the active ingredient is delivered. In homeopathy one is not faced with this necessity, so the choice of carrier is governed by convenience rather than therapeutic efficiency.

Tablets are similar to the classical biconvex plain white tablets used widely in conventional medicine. The size is about the same as a 75 mg dispersible aspirin tablet. The tablets are manufactured commercially from lactose and appropriate excipients. On an industrial scale blank lactose tablets and granules, or sucrose pills, can be surface-inoculated by spraying on the liquid potency in alcoholic tincture or as a syrup in a revolving pan, rather like the old method of sugar coating. The exact amount of remedy to be applied to ensure an even covering is determined using dyes. Pills are similarly prepared.

On a small scale in the pharmacy, the solid dose forms may be placed in glass vials and medicated by placing drops of liquid potency in strong alcohol on the surface; the number of drops used depends on the amount of solid dose form being medicated (Figure 4.4). The container is agitated in a manner similar to succussion to disperse the remedy throughout the dose form.

Granules are mainly made from lactose, and are about the size of the 'hundreds and thousands' used as cake decorations. They can be useful for infants and animals.

Crystals are made from sucrose and have the appearance of granulated sugar.

Individual powders are made from lactose impregnated with liquid potency and are useful where small numbers of doses are required.

Liquid potencies, prepared from the mother tinctures by serial dilution as described above, may be administered directly, in water or on a sugar cube.

Mother tinctures may also be given orally (e.g. Crataegus), usually in water. They are more often applied topically, either singly (e.g. Arnica for bruising, Thuja for warts or Tamus for chilblains) or in mixtures (e.g. Hypericum and Calendula).

Ointments, creams, lotions and **liniments** (generic and patent) usually contain between 5 and 10% of mother tincture, or in a few cases where no mother tincture exists, liquid potency (e.g. Graphites or Sulphur) incorporated in a suitable vehicle. Absorption of homeopathic substances applied to the skin varies greatly depending on their physical and chemical properties. The skin's structure is especially suited to the

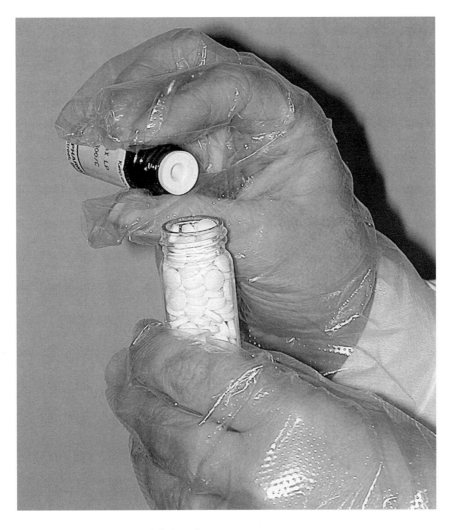

Figure 4.4 Medicating solid dose forms.

absorption of lipophilic compounds into deeper-lying tissues. Using a flat-bed electrophoresis device and thin-layer chromatography it was shown that Hamamelis and Hypericum moved more quickly than Arnica and Calendula.[11]

Eyedrops have caused manufacturers licensing difficulties and at the time of writing are restricted in the UK to prescription on a named-patient basis. However, Calendula, Cineraria and particularly Euphrasia eyedrops are all extremely useful and are likely to prove very popular if and when they become more widely available.

Containers

There has been much discussion as to whether plastic or glass containers are appropriate for solid dose forms. The traditionalists still favour neutral glass containers, suggesting that there is a possibility of chemicals leeching out from the plastic. Little work has been done to investigate whether the fears of those eschewing plastic have a firm foundation.

There have also been suggestions that the glass may play some part in 'holding' the potency. Again, these have not been substantiated.

Liquids are packed in glass dropper bottles. The major suppliers use amber screw-cap bottles with a plug in the neck with a channel that facilitates the delivery of one measured drop (0.05 ml). Silicone rubber teat droppers are also used.

Regulatory affairs – the licensing of remedies

Manufactured homeopathic remedies are subject to careful scrutiny to ensure that they are of the highest quality and safety. In the UK they have been treated as medicines since the inception of the NHS in 1948 and are available on medical prescription just as orthodox medicines are. As a result, they are subject to rules governing their manufacture and supply.

During the late 1950s and early 1960s a number of babies were born with deformed limbs as a direct result of their mothers taking the drug thalidomide during pregnancy. Unfortunately it was not the practice in those days to test new drugs for adverse reactions prior to marketing. Following these tragic consequences, the Medicines Act 1968 was implemented to protect the public. Thereafter, manufacturers wishing to bring a new medicine to the market were obliged to demonstrate safety, quality and, in the case of OM, efficacy before their product could be licensed for any given application. In addition, premises used for manufacturing medicines became subject to inspection and approval on a regular basis. About 3000–4000 homeopathic medicines were already on the market prior to the Medicines Act coming into force and these were granted product licences of right (PLRs) and allowed to remain on sale.

On 22 September 1992 the European Parliament adopted directive number 92/73/EEC, which was designed to establish regulations for homeopathic medicinal products throughout what was then called the European Economic Community (EEC), but which is now known as the European Union (EU). The directive is divided into four chapters and 11 articles covering scope, manufacture, control and inspection, placing on the market and final provisions. It passed into UK law on 1 January 1994 and defines the term 'homeopathic medicine' as being 'any medicinal product prepared from products, substances or compositions called homeopathic stocks in accordance with procedures described in any recognised pharmacopoeia'.

The labelling requirements for homeopathic medicinal products and the provisions for controlling the import, export and manufacture of homeopathic medicinal products are specified in the European directive. In addition, member states are obliged to discuss with each other all the information necessary to guarantee the quality and safety of homeopathic medicinal products within the EU. The directive acknowledges the difficulty in applying established scientific methods of demonstrating efficacy to homeopathy by adopting a special licensing scheme for homeopathic medicines based on safety and quality only.

The main provisions of this scheme are:

- The remedies must be intended for oral or external use only (i.e. not injections).
- The remedies must be sufficiently dilute to guarantee safety. A minimum dilution of 4x (a homeopathic dilution made by serially diluting a mother tincture 1:10 four times) is specified for most remedies. Mother tinctures are covered by other means.
- No claims for therapeutic efficacy can be made. The remedy must be sold without specific indications (e.g. 'for backache' or 'for colds and flu'). Despite this requirement, when seeking a licence manufacturers are obliged to submit evidence from authoritative repertories and textbooks that the remedy has been recommended for a particular use in the past. The customer is obliged to choose the correct product, by whatever method he or she can. Advice from health professionals, from the media or from leaflets in the retail outlet are the main sources of information.
- The words 'Homeopathic medicinal product without approved therapeutic indications' and 'Consult your doctor if symptoms persist' must be on the label.
- Brand names, and names that indicate possible uses (sometimes called fantasy names), are officially banned, but there appear to be areas where the licensing authorities will allow some latitude in the regulations with respect to the naming of homeopathic products containing a number of different remedies. Following representations from some manufacturers on the basis of safety, some complex remedies containing several ingredients are being licensed

with names of the type 'Remedy X Co' to obviate the necessity of attempting to remember a long list of ingredients when requesting a remedy over-the-counter (OTC) or writing a prescription. There is a potential source of confusion here, for some products that were on the market prior to the new legislation being adopted are still allowed to use brand names and even make limited claims of effectiveness. The authorities have not announced a date by which the products licensed under the old regulations have to be relicensed under the new EU regulations. Until this happens, the two types of medicine will exist side by side, although many manufacturers are beginning to register their products voluntarily. There is provision for one other national route of registration under the directive. Individual member states can introduce a set of national rules. Sets of national rules, allowing limited claims of effectiveness to be made (based on bibliographic evidence), are under construction in several countries at the time of writing.

A multidisciplinary expert committee, known as the Advisory Board on the Registration of Homeopathic Products, was established in the UK in 1993 to give advice to the Medicines Control Agency, the government body responsible for assessing the safety and quality of homeopathic remedies prior to licensing. The Committee comprises a number of practising doctors, pharmacists and vets as well as academics. Similar bodies exist in other EU countries.

The directive has been implemented across EU member states to varying degrees. It is generally accepted that the UK interprets the directive strictly and this has traditionally presented a barrier to foreign companies wishing to bring their products to this country. In particular, the inclusion of certain nosodes and other biological material, the purity of which is thought difficult to prove, has not been viewed favourably by the Advisory Board in the UK. A few foreign remedies have been licensed, however, and it is likely that this trend will continue in the future.

None of the above precludes experienced homeopathic practitioners and pharmacists from continuing to recommend and supply remedies compounded for individual needs.

The practice of homeopathy

Types of homeopathic remedy

The general types of homeopathic remedies that are used most widely in pharmacy practice are likely to be either polychrests or isopathics. Many of the polychrests are also constitutional remedies prescribed according to individual patients' characteristics rather than their symptoms directly. This rather specialised application is not described in this basic introduction to homeopathic practice.

Polychrests

OTC prescribing in pharmacies is generally, but not exclusively, based on polychrests. Polychrests are remedies whose drug pictures show a very wide spectrum of activity and therefore have a broad range of applications. The term 'polychrest', meaning 'many uses', was taken from the Greek by Hahnemann and was first used by him in an 1817 article on Nux vomica. This group of 20–30 remedies forms the basis of most commercially available homeopathic ranges as they lend themselves to prescribing based on abbreviated drug pictures (Table 4.3) without protracted consultations. Although they are used mainly for first aid and acute situations, polychrests are also often indicated in chronic disease because they affect so many body tissues.

Isopathic remedies

In general, modern isopathic remedies are administered on the basis of the principle *aequalia aequalibus curentur* (let same be treated by same) rather than the classical *similia similibus curentur* (let like be treated by like). Most have not been subjected to provings and therefore do not appear in the materia medica. Some of the older nosodes and sarcodes do have drug pictures, although their use is limited to rather specialised circumstances. Examples include Bacillinum, Medorrhinum and Psorinum (nosodes) and Lachesis (sarcodes).

Isopathic remedies may be classified as allergodes, nosodes, sarcodes or tautopathics, according to the origin of the source materials.

Allergodes These are potentised allergens derived from many sources (e.g. grass and flower pollens, moulds, house dust mites, animal hair, chocolate, milk, shellfish, wheat, etc.). Several companies produce OTC packs of allergodes, specifically mixed pollens and mixed grasses. These can be used effectively, providing the patient knows that he or she is allergic to that substance. There are geographic variations that need to be considered. Allergodes have been shown to be effective in the treatment of a range of allergic reactions.[12]

Table 4.3 List of common polychrest remedies

Polychrest	Main feature of drug picture
Aconite	Fear, first signs of cold
Allium cepa	Allergies and colds
Arnica	Mental and physical tiredness
Arsen alb	Diarrhoea (food)
Belladonna	Sudden-onset bursting headache
Bryonia	Productive cough, arthritic pain (better from cold, worse with movement)
Calc carb	Abdominal pains, swelling of joints, sweating
Calc phos	Forgetfulness, restlessness, catarrh
Cantharis	Burns, frequent urination with burning sensation
Carbo veg	Wind; collapse accompanied by 'blueness'
Chamomilla	Teething and colic
Euphrasia	Allergies accompanied by eye symptoms; acid lacrimation
Gelsemium	Colds and flu; anxiety about failing
Hypericum	Painful injuries, especially of digits – blood and crush remedy
Ignatia	Effects of grief
Ipecac	Wheezing cough
Ledum	Puncture wounds
Natrum mur	Sneezing, cold sores
Nux vom	Effects of overeating, constipation
Pulsatilla	Premenstrual syndrome; catarrh (bland, yellow or green in colour)
Rhus tox	Arthritic pain (better from heat, movement), strains
Ruta	Soft-tissue injuries; sprains
Sepia	Premenstrual syndrome
Symphytum	Assists healing of fractures

Nosodes These are prepared from diseased plant, animal or viral material (e.g. fluid from an arthritic joint, bowel tissue and vesicles). Autoisopathics are similar to nosodes but are prepared from an individual patient's own products (e.g. blood, pustules, urine, warts and verrucae) or milk from a cow or sheep suffering from mastitis. There are various childhood illnesses represented amongst the nosodes, for example, whooping cough (Pertussin) and German measles (Rubella). There are also tropical nosodes, such as cholera and malaria.

Sarcodes These are generally obtained from bacterial cultures or healthy secretions, such as Lac can (dog's milk) or Moschus (musk oil). Amongst the sarcodes, Lachesis, from bushmaster snake venom, is a remedy that has a comprehensive drug picture.

Tautopathics These are derived from drugs (e.g. chloramphenicol, diazepam, nitrazepam, penicillin, etc.) chemicals (e.g. pesticides, industrial fluids and biological washing powders) or synthetic products (e.g. nylon, plastics and rubber latex). One of the first tautopathic preparations was made during the Second World War from mustard gas. Most tautopathic remedies are administered on the basis that they cause the condition for which they are being used therapeutically, but there are a few, mainly derived from allopathic drugs, that have a drug picture and can be used classically.[13] Attempts to use homeopathic dilutions of certain drugs of abuse to wean patients off their habit have met with partial success.

Isopathic remedies as 'vaccines'

The word 'vaccine' is sometimes used erroneously by homeopaths to describe sarcodes, nosodes and tautopathics when used to stimulate the autoimmune response.

As a general rule sarcodes are used prophylactically, nosodes are used to treat the symptoms of a disease and tautopathics (made from orthodox vaccines) to treat adverse reactions resulting from immunisation.

Unfortunately the exact source of the material used to manufacture the remedy is seldom stated on the label. There could conceivably be three variants of each so-called vaccine.

It should be noted that none of these remedies are true vaccines and there is little scientific evidence as to whether or not they can confer any protection against a disease when given prophylactically, although an interesting randomised study has demonstrated that a nosode made from infected tissue could confer some protection on laboratory mice subjected to bacterial challenges.[14] High-potency remedies prepared from tissue infected with *Francisella tularensis* were administered to the test animals. It was found that 75% of the untreated controls died while only 53% of the isopathically treated group succumbed.

Because of the implications for public health, pharmacists are normally best advised to refer requests for these so-called vaccines to a registered medical practitioner. In the case of the nosode Pertussin, specific instructions to this effect were circulated by the health authorities some years ago. It may be considered that a prescription, although not legally necessary, would provide appropriate evidence that this advice has been followed. Nosodes are also used by homeopathic veterinarians against a variety of conditions, including kennel cough, leptospirosis and parvo.

Similar advice should be given to owners who seek to protect their animals from disease by using homeopathic nosodes without professional advice.

Homeopathic practitioners

In the UK, Ireland and many other English-speaking countries, most health professionals have responded reactively to a demand for homeopathy from clients, rather than encouraging its use proactively, although with improved access to training this position is changing. In these countries homeopathy may be practised not only by statutorily registered qualified health professionals but, under common law, also by non-medically qualified practitioners (NMQPs) and by lay homeopaths with no formal training. The NMQPs, and to an increasing extent lay homeopaths, are recognised by the NHS in the UK. Common law permits freedom of choice of patients to choose the healthcare provision they feel appropriate, and the freedom of people to practise homeopathy if they so wish. The main drawback of such a liberal system is that it allows a person to set up as a homeopath with little or no training.

Medical homeopathy, together with veterinary homeopathy and other professions allied to medicine, and the NMQPs have quite separate educational facilities and governing bodies. Practice by the former is supervised by the Faculty of Homeopathy, which was founded in 1950 by an act of parliament. The Faculty accredits training courses for health professionals, awarding the qualification of Licentiate (LFHom with appropriate professional suffix) as a basic qualification for all health professionals and Membership (MFHom) and Fellowship (FFHom) for medical and veterinary practitioners. The postgraduate courses in medical homeopathy are claimed to be the fastest growing of any speciality and currently more than 300 doctors hold the MFHom qualification. In addition there are 350 with the LFHom and an unspecified number of prescribers occasionally prescribing homeopathy but who do not have a formal qualification. Dental and pharmacy diplomas are also available.

Training for NQMPs is offered by a number of colleges, each giving their own qualification. Homeopaths registered with the Society of Homoeopaths in Northampton may use the letters RSH (or FSH) after having followed a course of instruction and a period of clinical supervision. Another professional body is the UK Homeopathic Medical Association, whose full members must complete similar requirements. These practitioners use the initials MHMA.

Despite their substantial training in well-established colleges, the professional NMQPs were formerly regarded with disdain by medical homeopaths, an opinion that continued into the 1980s. However, discussions are now proceeding on an amicable basis and the two groups are moving together slowly. There are NHS homeopathic hospitals in Bristol, Glasgow, London and Tunbridge Wells, and other facilities in Manchester and Liverpool.

Interestingly, Germany also has two classes of practitioners: doctors (95% of whom practise some form of complementary medicine) and *Heilpraktikers*. The latter group, translated as 'health practitioners', developed in the years prior to the Second World War, when doctors did not have a monopoly on the delivery of healthcare. At present the ratio of practising *Heilpraktikers* to physicians is about 1:4. *Heilpraktikers* are not obliged to undertake formal medical training, but are obliged to take a test administered by the local health authority. If a candidate fails, he or she may continue to resit until successful. The *Heilpraktiker*'s activities are comparable to those of NMQPs in the UK, except that the former tend to use several different therapies concurrently and place more emphasis on diagnostic procedures.[15]

Approaches to the practice of homeopathy

There are many schools of thought around the world as to how homeopathy should be practised with respect to the choice of remedy and the potency and frequency with which remedies should be administered. There is no establishd norm. Writers on homeopathy frequently refer to classical or European homeopathy, usually with the implication that this is the most complete and authoritative version of Hahnemann's views and most nearly represents his methods. However, such claims do not correspond with the historical facts. The influence of the great American homeopaths has also been significant in shaping current practice. The notion that there is a standard or pure form of homeopathic practice has been criticised, with the argument that instead the so-called classical homeopathy is really a complex mixture of ideas drawn from a variety of sources.[16]

There are broadly three ways in which homeopathic remedies are administered in Europe and in other countries where European influence is strong:

- One remedy at a time in a single dose or repeated doses is prescribed by those claiming to be classical or unicist homeopaths. This approach is generally favoured by homeopaths in the UK. However, Hahnemann changed his ideas several times, especially towards the end of his life, and so the term 'classical' could be applied to several different methods of using remedies and not just unicist prescribing. The influence of the great American homeopaths has also been significant in shaping current practice. There is no standard or pure form of homeopathy, rather the so-called classical homeopathy is a complex mixture of ideas drawn from a variety of sources, some of which are unconnected with homeopathy.[16]

- More than one remedy at a time, given simultaneously in alternation or concurrently. This is called pluralist prescribing and claims to treat more than one aspect of a patient's condition. It is common in France, Germany and Italy, and where remedies from these countries are available.

- Mixtures in one container of different remedies and different potencies, selected and combined for their combined effect on particular diseased states. This method is known as complex prescribing and is very popular in France and Germany where it is not uncommon to have 15–20 remedies ranging from very low to high potencies in the same preparation. It is likely that many of these complex mixtures will appear in the UK market within the foreseeable future. They do have some advantages for the OTC environment, as Table 4.4 shows. Classical homeopaths claim that this is not true homeopathy as there is no individual matching of the symptom and drug picture. Furthermore, no provings exist of the

Table 4.4 Comparison of single (simplex) and combination (complex) remedies

Single-remedy prescribing	*Combination-remedy prescribing*
More difficult to pick remedy – needs time to repertorise	Easier to prescribe – covers number of indications
Carefully targeted to patients' requirements – more precise	'Blunderbuss' approach
Provings available	No provings available for combination remedies
Outcome clearly attributable to remedy	Doubt as to which remedy is working
No problems with interactions	No knowledge of how remedies might interact with each other
Favoured by classical prescribers	Resistance amongst classical prescribers

mixtures. Interestingly, this complex approach to prescribing is being adopted in modern OM as an element of care plans involving the treatment of various diseases, including diabetes.

Homeopathy in the pharmacy

Supply of a named homeopathic remedy

Almost all homeopathic remedies are classified as part of the general sales list (GSL) in the UK and may be sold without restriction in a wide range of retail outlets. Exceptions include very low potencies of traditional poisons (e.g. Aconite and Belladonna), which have little if any use in homeopathy, and certain formulations such as eyedrops and injections that are presently unlicensed. It is appropriate to exert some voluntary control when certain nosodes are being used as human or veterinary vaccines (see previous section).

Interpreting a written or verbal request for a homeopathic medicine

The request for supply may be by prescription signed by either a medical practitioner or an NMQP or an OTC request from a client. Vets and dental surgeons may also issue private prescriptions. Thus, the stimulus prompting the purchase of a remedy may come from the practitioner, who may issue a formal prescription or give verbal instructions on what to buy. Other prospective purchasers are influenced by friends, family and the media. In order to comply with a request the following information is required:

- **Name of remedy**. Care should be taken to ensure that the abbreviations used are correctly interpreted, for example *Staph*. could be *Staphylococcus* or *Staphisagria*. If in doubt, revert back to the practitioner.
- **Potency**. Normally in the UK the potency will be on the centesimal scale (6c or 30c) or the decimal scale (6x). Very high potencies such as M and 10M may also be requested. Some pharmacists believe that high potencies should not be used to self-treat and may only sell these remedies in small quantities to ensure that they are not being misused.
- **Dose form**. Ideally the dose form should be specified. Therapeutically the carrier is thought to be insignificant (although this has not

been proven experimentally) but there may be other reasons why one or other form is preferred.

- **Quantity.** Solid dose forms in the UK are often made available in 7, 14 or 25 g glass vials, indicating the capacity of the container. These correspond to approximately 55, 125 and 250 tablets respectively, depending on the physical characteristics of the tablet. Tablets may also be available in quantities of 100 or 125. Liquid potencies and mother tinctures are supplied in 10, 20 and 50 ml dropper bottles that can deliver their contents dropwise.
- **Dose.** It is necessary to specify the dose required on prescriptions, rather than state 'as directed'. Some of the homeopathic dose regimes are complicated and easy to forget, especially by older patients.

Dispensing the remedy

Endorsing the prescription

To avoid contaminating the remedy, especially in the early days of dealing with homeopathic prescriptions, it is probably wise to issue an original pack as near as possible to the amount specified. Homeopathic remedies have been available under the UK NHS since its inception in 1948 and the prescription form (or, in Scotland, the doctor's stock order) should be endorsed with the amount supplied and the supplier's name if not given by the prescriber. Adding the trade price will be helpful to the pricing bureau. If in doubt, suppliers are usually very willing to give advice. If the bulk is broken then solid dose forms should not be handled or tablets counted in a tablet counter but instead transferred by first shaking them into the lid.

Increasingly, the costs of private homeopathic treatment are being met by health insurance schemes but as the situation is changing from month to month patients should be advised to check with their own insurer prior to presenting their prescription.

Labelling

Dispensed remedies should be labelled in the normal way and a clear indication given of the name and potency. Occasionally it may be necessary to reinforce complicated instructions with a separate sheet of written instructions.

Counselling

Most patients will know that they are likely to receive a homeopathic prescription if they attend a suitably qualified practitioner, but some may not. There may be evidence of some anxieties about the validity of the therapy and it may be considered necessary to say a few words about the general features of homeopathy so that the patient is aware of the type of treatment being given. It can be said that it is safe, will not interfere with other medicines and is tailored to the patient's particular requirements. It is difficult to give exact guidelines because each individual situation is different. However, something appropriate should be said.

The other important information concerns taking the remedy. Because the active ingredient is placed on the surface of the dose form and is absorbed through the oral mucous membranes, a number of precautions should be taken:

- The solid dose forms should not be handled to prevent deterioration due to bacterial or chemical contamination. They should be transferred to the mouth by way of the container cap. If dropped on the floor they should be discarded.
- The solid dose forms should be allowed to dissolve in the mouth rather than being chewed and/or swallowed.
- Liquid remedies should be held in the mouth for 20–30 s before swallowing.
- Remedies should be taken half an hour before or after food, drink, tobacco or sweets. Aromatic flavours are thought to inactivate homeopathic remedies. Ideally, peppermint-flavoured toothpaste should be avoided, but if it is being used then at least 1 h should be allowed between cleaning the teeth and taking the remedy and the mouth should be rinsed out thoroughly with water prior to taking the remedy.
- Remedies should be kept in the original container and stored in a cool dry place.
- Existing allopathic medication should not be stopped without the permission of the original prescriber.

Safety

Potential sources of concern on safety issues include inappropriate treatment, toxicity, aggravation and interactions.

Inappropriate treatment

Most ranges of homeopathic remedies available for sale commercially OTC are designed to be used for the treatment of simple self-limiting conditions. Some may also be used for ongoing conditions such as back pain or soft-tissue injuries. Clients who request unusual remedies or who return repeatedly to purchase the same remedy on several occasions should be gently reminded that advice from a physician or registered homeopath might be appropriate to confirm that their condition lends itself to self-treatment.

It is vital that all practitioners only offer advice and treatment according to their levels of competency. Patients whose problems fall outwith these boundaries should be referred to suitably qualified colleagues. Generally pharmacists should use homeopathy to deal with conditions they would normally treat OTC and not seek to widen their portfolio.

Toxicity

Adverse reactions have been investigated using electronic databases, hand-searching, searching reference lists, reviewing the bibliography of trials and other relevant articles, contacting homeopathic pharmaceutical companies and drug regulatory agencies in the UK and USA, and by communicating with experts in homeopathy.[17] The authors, Dantas and Rampes, reported that the mean incidence of adverse effects of homeopathic medicines was approximately 2.5 times greater than for placebo in controlled clinical trials but effects were minor, transient and comparable. There was a large incidence of pathogenetic effects in healthy volunteers taking homeopathic medicines but the methodological quality of these studies was generally low. It was found that anecdotal reports of adverse effects in homeopathic publications were not well documented and mainly reported aggravation of current symptoms. Case reports in conventional medical journals pointed more to adverse effects of mislabelled homeopathic products than of true homeopathic medicines. It was concluded that homeopathic medicines in high dilutions, prescribed by trained professionals, were probably safe and unlikely to provoke severe adverse reactions. Once again it is difficult to draw definite conclusions because of the low methodological quality of reports claiming possible adverse effects of homeopathic medicines.

Some isolated cases of adverse reactions in the literature have also been highlighted.[18] Two dermatological problems were reported after the use of a remedy containing mercury in low potency.[19,20] However, another more recent paper concluded that the dosage of arsenic, mercury and lead in homeopathic medications manufactured under good manufacturing practices and following the US Pharmacopoeia guidelines are generally below detection level and are not thought to be a risk to health.[21]

From time to time lactose sensitivity is encountered. This can be overcome by using a sucrose-based carrier or a liquid potency.

Aggravation

In about 10% of chronic cases the patient's condition may be exacerbated within 2–5 days of taking a remedy. Typically, a skin condition may become worse after taking a low-potency remedy. Such a reaction usually only occurs the first time the remedy is used. This reaction, known as an aggravation, has been described as an adverse drug reaction, and in the sense that it is unwanted by the patient it might be considered thus. When told of the possibility of aggravation many patients will say that they expect to get worse before they get better. Far from being upset by the apparent adverse drug reaction they consider an aggravation as a sign that the medicine is working.

If an aggravation appears, the patient should be instructed to cease taking the remedy until the symptoms subside and then recommence taking the remedy at a lower frequency. If the symptoms continue to get worse when the remedy has been temporarily suspended, then it is likely that the wrong remedy is being taken. Patients who are receiving prescribed medication should be advised to consult their practitioner for ways of dealing with aggravations.

Interactions

There is no evidence that homeopathic remedies interfere with any concurrent allopathic medicines and indeed they are particularly useful for treating trivial conditions in people who are taking several orthodox medications. It is thought that steroids may inactivate homeopathic remedies to some extent and while this potential interaction is certainly not dangerous, it could reduce their expected effectiveness. Some homeopathic remedies are considered to antidote or inactivate other remedies in some circumstances, for example, Camphor, Aconite and Nux vom. Traditionally, homeopaths usually advise patients to refrain from taking coffee, tea, chocolate and spicy food when taking homeopathic medication, but in fact there is little evidence that such abstinence is necessary.

Supply of homeopathic remedies by counter prescribing

Counter prescribing may be summarised by the following six steps:

- taking a decision on whether to treat in the pharmacy or to refer
- obtaining the necessary information
- deciding on a particular remedy
- establishing a dose regime
- providing the remedy
- follow-up.

Step 1: deciding whether to treat or refer

The problem of whether to treat or refer is one with which the pharmacist is entirely familiar. Working within the bounds of competency is implied in the codes of ethics of all health professionals. The decision, which with experience can be taken without an indepth investigation, is based on the severity and type of symptoms being presented, the length of time during which symptoms have been experienced, etc. Having decided to treat, the next question is whether to treat with homeopathy or allopathy. Normally the pharmacist would not seek to widen his or her portfolio of conditions treated with homeopathy, but rather would endeavour to complement existing methods of responding to requests for advice. There are one or two exceptions to this. Requests for help with examination nerves can be effectively met with Arsenicum album or Gelsemium, and Cocculus may be suggested with confidence to women suffering from nausea during the first trimester of pregnancy. In neither case do suitable OTC allopathic products exist. Homeopathy might also be indicated for patients with an existing extensive portfolio of medication where adding extra drugs might cause worries about interaction.

There is an increasing demand from the public for homeopathic medicines to treat animals. Under the Veterinary Surgeons Act 1966, diagnosis and treatment of animals are restricted to veterinarians and owners. Pharmacists are able to advise on the availability of different items but the final choice of remedy must always rest with the owner. If in doubt, the case should be referred to a veterinary practitioner. Potential problems are illustrated by pharmacists' involvement in supplying Borax to farmers during a foot and mouth epidemic (see below).

Borax and foot and mouth disease   In 2001 the UK was in the grip of a major epidemic of foot and mouth disease, with approximately 4 million animals being slaughtered throughout the country. The disease started at a pig farm in north-east England and spread quickly through-out the country. Farmers desperate to provide protection for their animals from foot and mouth turned to homeopathy for help, placing extreme pressure on many pharmacies to supply them with the appro-priate remedy. Demand for the remedy Borax 30c increased rapidly as the knowledge of its existence spread amongst the farming community. There was some anecdotal evidence of its beneficial use during the last foot and mouth epidemic which hit the UK in the 1960s but the Faculty of Homeopathy, the governing body for medical and veterinary home-opathy, felt that this was insufficient to claim its effectiveness in pre-venting the disease.

The eradication scheme being followed by the government relied on a wholly susceptible animal population in order to be able to detect the disease signs promptly. According to Chris Day, Veterinary Dean to the Faculty, the danger of using any potentially prophylactic medicine was that, if it was effective, it may render the animals unsusceptible. This could theoretically result in animals being able to harbour the virus and shed it while remaining symptom-free themselves. It is recommended that pharmacists direct enquiries for homeopathic Borax to a suitably qualified veterinary surgeon.

Step 2: obtaining the necessary information

Before choosing an appropriate remedy to counter prescribe, infor-mation is required from:

- the patient: signs and symptoms, both observed and reported
- the practitioner's observational and listening skills
- the practitioner's own knowledge and limits of competency
- sources of reference, including materia medicas and repertories.

A useful acronym to use when assessing a case is provided by the letters LOAD, standing for listen, observe, ask and decide:

- Listen to what the patient tells you about his or her symptoms.
- Observe the patient's general demeanour, appearance, tempera-ment, etc.
- Ask the patient appropriate questions to learn more about the con-dition.
- Decide what to do next after assessing the information provided.

Given the restrictions on resources in most pharmacies it is not possible to pursue the extended consultations felt necessary by most complementary practitioners. This means that the conditions being treated are likely to be restricted to simple self-limiting conditions using polychrests.

Step 3: deciding on a particular remedy

If all the preparatory work in step 2 has been carried out assiduously, then the choice of remedy is not as daunting as it might appear. Another acronym may be useful: ACT stands for assess, confirm and talk.

Assess   Having gathered all the requisite information, an appropriate remedy can be chosen. Most practitioners keep the drug pictures of 20–30 simple remedies in their memory and can often prescribe a polychrest quickly without reference to the repertory. For most of us it is necessary to use the repertory, a textbook that lists diseased states and gives remedies in whose drug picture the various symptoms appear. An appropriate remedy may be chosen by using a repertory to identify one or more remedies that might fit the symptom picture and then using the materia medica to see which drug picture fits best. There are several materia medica and repertories available. Boericke's *Materia Medica and Repertory* has both texts in the same book and is probably the easiest for the beginner to use. It has the disadvantage that the language is rather old-fashioned and written in patient's terminology, hence the appearance of words like 'brain-fag'. In some instances lateral thinking must be used to navigate through the index. The repertory gives remedies in normal type and italics: italics indicates a higher importance of remedy than normal type.

Probably the most widely used text is the *Repertory of the Homeopathic Materia Medica* by Kent, the great American homeopath.[22] This text gives three grades of remedy, indicated by plain, italic and bold text. Other examples of repertory include texts by Murphy,[23] Phatak[24] and Schroyens.[25] In some cases the drug picture may be very extensive. Arnica, for example, extends over several pages and it would be impossible to identify a complete match. When used for acute conditions the polychrests can be prescribed on the basis of an abbreviated drug picture, picking out just a handful of the most important symptoms. These symptoms, known as keynotes, are considered to be important because they have been reported more often by volunteers taking part in provings than have other symptoms. Examples of keynotes are given for some common polychrests at the end of this chapter. When starting out it is perfectly possible to counter prescribe using keynotes, providing only acute self-limiting conditions are prescribed for.

Computerised repertories are increasing in popularity but tend to be rather complicated for most beginners. RADAR and Cara are the programs most frequently used by professionals; other less extensive programs are available.

Confirm   Having chosen the remedies most likely to be of assistance the final decision must be made. This can be achieved by checking the materia medica drug picture and asking a few confirmatory questions, particularly about modalities and what makes the condition better or worse.

Examples of modalities are that the condition is made better or worse by:

• the application of heat or cold to the affected part
• movement
• exposure to warm or wet weather.

For example, the remedies Rhus tox and Bryonia are both indicated for the treatment of rheumatic pain. Patients who find that they are stiff first thing in the morning but improve as the day proceeds and for whom the application of heat is beneficial respond well to Rhus tox. Patients who find any movement painful and for whom the application of cold is beneficial respond well to Bryonia.

Talk   It might also be appropriate to give the patient some general information on homeopathy, especially if the pharmacist is acting proactively rather than reactively to a request for homeopathic remedies from the client.

Step 4: establishing a dose regime

In first-aid situations the remedy is given frequently – up to every 10–15 min for 6–8 doses in some cases. Here the term 'first aid' refers to a suggested initial treatment for any condition being treated, not just for an injury, as in OM.

With acute prescribing the dose should be taken three times daily for 7–10 days.

In chronic conditions frequencies of once or twice a day (or even once a month) are more appropriate.

By convention it is generally stated that the dose for a child under 12 years should be half that of an adult (i.e. one tablet instead of two).

Step 5: providing the remedy

Having chosen the remedy, the patient should be given information on how to take the medicine.

Step 6: follow-up

After the dose regime periods stated above the treatment should be reviewed. A number of responses are possible:

- The medicine has proved successful and may be discontinued.
- The outcome is not satisfactory, but the client has not been taking the medication according to instructions – instructions should be given to restart the course of treatment.
- The outcome is unsatisfactory, but the client has returned too soon – the course should be completed before further action is taken.
- The client appears to have completed the treatment but the outcome is unsatisfactory – consider changing the remedy or referring.

User characteristics

In order to study the characteristics of users of homeopathic medicine, a four-part questionnaire was distributed by Furnham and Bond.[26] Respondents were required to read eight vignettes (each about 70 words long) describing a British male patient who visits either a homeopath or general practitioner with specific and different medical problems. In each vignette the patient gets better after treatment or remains unwell; he is described as being either emotionally balanced (stable) or slightly neurotic in character. Participants were required to rate each vignette on criteria such as did they think the treatment was effective, and did they think the person would remain feeling better. A total of 165 people completed the questionnaire. Homeopathy was perceived as more effective for treating patients with unstable psychological characteristics and OM was seen as more effective for treating patients with stable psychological characteristics. Homeopathy was perceived as more effective by participants who themselves used complementary medicine. Participants who had visited a complementary therapist felt more strongly that psychological factors were important in illness than participants who had never consulted a complementary practitioner. Non-complementary medicine users perceived OM to be more effective than complementary medicine users.

Because homeopathic remedies are readily available at a number of outlets (pharmacies, health stores, etc.), they provide consumers with an attractive option for self-treating. The buyer characteristics of the British homeopathic OTC market have been investigated.[27] In a questionnaire-based study of 407 purchasers in 109 pharmacies it was found that very few people under 25 bought OTC homeopathic medicines, and only 12% of buyers aged 25–35 years were male. Most respondents bought the remedy for themselves rather than for other members of their family, emphasising the individualistic nature of homeopathic medicines. As regards the main remedy grouping of the homeopathic medicines bought, the most popular were polychrests (remedies with a wide spectrum of activity, making them well suited to the OTC environment) and complex remedies (mixtures of remedies usually with specific uses). There were a small number of branded medicines. The most frequently purchased polychrests were Arnica (6.3% of all purchases), Pulsatilla (3.0%) and Rhus tox (2.3%). The predominance of polychrest homeopathic medicines is understandable, as this is the type that is best suited to the OTC environment. With polychrests buyers can readily equate remedies with ailments and so buy the medicine most likely to be effective for their particular condition. Retailers also benefit by not having to offer what can be lengthy and complex advice to buyers, given that current legislation precludes giving uses on the label.

The ailments for which OTC homeopathic medicines were bought were very wide-ranging. Many were acute self-limiting ailments such as coughs and colds and minor injuries; others included digestive complaints, skin conditions and anxiety. In most of these categories, with the exception of anxiety, orthodox OTC products were also available.

Most respondents (60%) reported that they took the homeopathic medicine as sole medication for their problem; others (27%) used more than one homeopathic medicine at a time or combined homeopathic and allopathic medicines (13%).

Concern should be expressed at the excessive length of time for which some respondents took their remedies. Most homeopathic remedies offered for sale OTC are designed for short-term administration. Long-term chronic conditions are best treated under the guidance of a practitioner; this should ensure the choice of appropriate therapy, as well as minimising the possibility of provings. Although taking homeopathic medicines for long periods should not cause any irreversible harm, since the medicines are not in themselves toxic, patients may suffer because they may not be receiving appropriate treatment for their condition.

A similar study in New Zealand produced comparable results.[28] There was a high degree of awareness of homeopathy in New Zealand, with 92% of a sample of 503 pharmacy clients claiming to have heard of homeopathy. Sixty-seven per cent said they had used the therapy.

Evidence

It is beyond the scope of this chapter to look at the research carried out in homeopathy in great detail, particularly that associated with evidence on effectiveness. The reader is referred to specialist texts on this subject for such information.[29,30] The library at Hom-Inform (see below) is able to locate appropriate books and papers. In this section a flavour of the topics available is offered.

There is much circumstantial evidence from case studies that homeopathy is effective, both from patients and practitioners. Scientific evidence is rather sparse and much of what is available suffers from poor methodology.[31] Examples of poor methodology include dubious accuracy of test materials, inappropriate measurements and poor randomisation techniques. This is unfortunate, to say the least, because increasingly, decisions on whether or not to use or purchase homeopathic services require evidence of positive outcomes and value for money. The availability of funds for research is limited. Organisations such as the Homeopathic Trust (now merged with the British Homeopathic Association) and the Scottish Homeopathic Research and Education Trust have generously supported workers over many years but the sums available are modest. The relatively small value of the market means that manufacturers have little to invest in research outwith their own commercial requirements.

Broadly, homeopathic research falls into five main categories:

- placebo studies designed to demonstrate that homeopathy is not merely a placebo response and satisfy criticism from sceptics
- clinical trials to establish efficacy
- physicochemical studies on mechanisms of action
- audit and case study collection to establish effectiveness and improve the use of homeopathy
- attitudes and awareness studies and sociological research to determine why and how homeopathy is used.

Placebo studies

The first investigation of the placebo effect used the hypothesis that homeopathy was due to a placebo response rather than the converse.

Following a pilot trial in 1983 with 35 patients,[32] the hypothesis was tested in a double-blind placebo-controlled trial, using a model based on the use of mixed grass pollens to treat 144 hayfever patients.[33] The authors concluded that homeopathy appeared to be effective in its own right, i.e. they disproved their original hypothesis. This result was reinforced by further work in this area.[34]

It has been suggested that the evidence supporting the hypothesis that homeopathy may be solely a placebo response can be considered under a number of headings:[35]

- theoretical evidence – immunological-type responses to minute quantities of stimulant are well documented
- practical evidence – outcome measures based on patient-oriented methods demonstrate an improvement in both overall well-being and clinical symptoms
- laboratory research – difficult to replicate and apply to in vivo situations
- the self-healing response – in assembling the varying sources of evidence for the existence of a placebo response to homeopathy, the interesting idea is introduced of replacing the term 'placebo' with 'intention-modified self-healing response', which is affected by the circumstances of the healing encounter. Reilly[35] suggests that the intention-modified self-healing response may exist alone or be combined with an intervention to give a therapeutic intention-modified self-healing response.

A meta-analysis on 89 randomised clinical trials (RCTs) assessed whether or not the clinical effect reported in RCTs of homeopathic remedies was equivalent to that reported for placebo.[36] The results of the meta-analysis were not compatible with this hypothesis, but insufficient evidence was found from these studies that homeopathy was clearly efficacious for any single clinical condition.

Randomised clinical trials – meta-analyses

It used to be said that constructing RCTs for homeopathic medicines was impossible because of the individualisation required in prescribing. Over the years various techniques have been developed for RCTs, but most of these set out to test homeopathy as an intervention versus placebo, rather than to test a specific remedy.

Homeopathic RCTs are always scrutinised very carefully by the scientific community, so their quality needs to be extremely high for the outcomes to be accepted. The objective of one of the most frequently cited papers on homeopathic clinical trials[37] was to establish whether or not there was any firm evidence of the effectiveness of homeopathy from all the many controlled trials that have been carried out in recent years. The methodological quality of 107 controlled trials published in 96 journals worldwide was assessed. The trials were scored using a list of predefined good criteria. A total of 81 positive trials were recorded. The five allergic trials included in the analysis were all positive: the next most successful therapeutic group, with 90% of its 20 trials positive, was trauma and pain. The authors acknowledge that the weight of presented evidence was probably not sufficient for most people to make a decision on whether homeopathy works or not, but that there would probably be enough evidence to support several common applications if it were an orthodox therapy.

A systematic review has been carried out of 32 trials (28 placebo-controlled, two comparing homeopathy and another treatment, two comparing both, i.e. comparing outcomes from trials comparing homeopathy with a placebo with outcomes from trials comparing homoeopathy with another non-homeopathic treatment) involving a total of 1778 patients.[38] The methodological quality of the trials was highly variable. In the 19 placebo-controlled trials providing sufficient data for meta-analysis, individualised homeopathy was significantly more effective than the placebo effect but when the analysis was restricted to the methodologically best trials, no significant effect was seen. The results of the available randomised trials suggest that individualised homeopathy had a greater effect than placebo. The evidence was not convincing because of methodological shortcomings and inconsistencies.

Several individual trials have yielded negative results.[39–41] A high-quality randomised double-blind placebo-controlled trial was conducted involving 63 patients on the homeopathic prophylaxis of migraine using a technique approved by the International Headache Society under good clinical practice.[42] The authors concluded that homeopathy could not be recommended for migraine prophylaxis.

The results from a German randomised double-blind placebo-controlled trial were presented at the 6th Annual Symposium on Complementary Medicine at Exeter in December 1999. The clinical efficacy and tolerance of Caulophyllum D4 was investigated using 40 pregnant women with premature amnion rupture.[43] The effect of the remedy in D4–D18 on smooth muscle was also investigated in vitro. Patients between the 38th and 42nd gestational weeks with premature amnion rupture, no regular contractions and cervix dilation of less than 3 cm were randomised. Appropriate tests were used to measure outcomes. In the second experiment the effect of the homeopathic remedies was measured on the spontaneous contraction activity of smooth muscle obtained from the uterus and stomach of guinea pig and rats. It was concluded that the remedy was tolerated without adverse reactions, and had no myogene effects.

The influence of indicators of methodological quality on study outcome in a set of 89 placebo-controlled clinical trials of homeopathy has been investigated.[44] It was concluded that in the set studied there was clear evidence that studies with better methodological quality tended to yield less positive results.

A great deal more work is necessary to prove the efficacy of homeopathy to the satisfaction of sceptical colleagues.

Studies on mechanisms of action

Usually patients are not worried about – or in many cases are not even interested in – how a remedy works. Their main concern is safety and a positive outcome. The emphasis on proving that homeopathy works has been overtaken by a wish to improve its use. However, there is no doubt that homeopathy would benefit from a plausible explanation of its mechanisms of action.

Where there are material doses of remedy present, generally below the 12c potency, it is easier to accept a pharmacological response, albeit not one that can necessarily be explained in standard pharmacological terms. Once the remedy has been diluted beyond Avogadro's number, theoretically there are no molecules of the drug present, therefore how can the potentisation process possibly give a therapeutic result? How, indeed! It has to be said that we are not even close to finding out. There has not been much progress since George Vithoulkas wrote in 1985 'as far as is yet known, there is no available explanation in modern physics or chemistry for the phenomenon of potentisation'.[45] The literature contains numerous hypotheses that seek to explain how homeopathic remedies might work – some are so plausible that they are as difficult to disprove as to prove!

There are three main diluents used during the potentisation process: water, alcohol and, in the case of non-soluble source materials, lactose. All of these are thought to play an important part in the mode of action.[46]

It is possible to construct a mathematical model for the potentisation process, identifying a relationship between the dilution factor, the number of succussions and the oscillatory function, which is said to contribute to a biological effect. Amongst the simpler explanations are those based on molecular geometries or shapes and a concept of hydration shells formed by the close association of water molecules with the ions of remedy molecules.

Audit, perception of benefit studies and case study collection

In the current climate of audit collection it is not surprising that homeopathy has begun to get its act together with respect to gathering data on outcomes. Proposals have been presented for Europe-wide data collection.[47] Data-gathering schemes have also been suggested in Germany.[48] There is now an impressive amount of information about the effectiveness of many remedies.

A typical perception outcome study has been reported.[49] It involved patients being treated by homeopathic medicine at the Tunbridge Wells Homeopathic Hospital in England during 1997. The study aimed to assess firstly, the range of diagnoses presented by patients and secondly, patients' own impressions of benefit. A total of 1372 questionnaires were completed by patients, after their consultations, to record their impressions of the effects of homeopathic treatment. Patients were asked to score their responses on a $+3$ to -3 scale. The three main diagnostic groups were dermatology, musculoskeletal disorders and malignant disease, especially carcinoma of the breast. Overall, 74% of patients recorded positive benefits, with 55% recording scores of $+3$ or $+2$.

The collection of case studies has always been an important aspect of homeopathic practice. Several publications accept these, including the Faculty of Homeopathy Newsletter *Simile*.

Attitude and awareness studies

These studies provide important information on topics such as why people turn to homeopathy and how they obtain the necessary guidance on which remedies to purchase. The attitudes of providers of homeopathy are also important. Examples of such studies in the pharmacy environment have been provided.[50,51]

Materia medica

Examples of common remedies to counter prescribe

In this abbreviated materia medica section some useful remedies are given with indications. The details given are not meant to be comprehensive.

Aconite   Anxiety, distress, fear – almost terror – before and after receiving bad news. Aconite is also given at the first sign of a sneeze. It may be combined with other remedies in mixtures like ABC (Aconite, Belladonna and Chamomilla).

Arnica   Mental and physical fatigue. Bruises, sprains and after accidents. Pre- and postoperatively. Pre- and post-childbirth.

Argent nit   Feelings of fear and nervousness (but not terror), especially of an anticipatory nature. Exam nerves with gastrointestinal symptoms (often diarrhoea) and insomnia.

Arsen alb   Effective for simultaneous diarrhoea and vomiting; when patient is chilly and restless.

Belladonna   Burning, hot, flushed appearance. Tonsillitis, sore throat, earache. Generalised effects of sunstroke. Bursting headache. Sudden onset of symptoms.

Bryonia   Joint pains that are worse on movement and with warmth (cf. Rhus tox), better for pressure. Dry hacking cough.

Cantharis   Burns, scalds, sunburn. Cystitis with burning feeling and frequent desire to urinate, often drop by drop; hot, scalding urine. Gnat bites.

Euphrasia   Allergic symptoms, especially red weepy eyes.

Ferrum phos   First stage of head cold, croup, stiff neck.

Gelsemium   Useful for influenza. Pre-exam nerves, when the mind goes blank.

Hamamelis   Blood and crush injuries, especially those involving digits.

Ignatia   Stress, especially following bereavement, nervous headaches.

Ipecacuanha   Constant nausea not relieved by vomiting. Unproductive cough, with loose chesty rattle. Infantile diarrhoea with green-coloured stools.

Nux vomica   Ill effects of overeating and overdrinking. Indigestion, nausea and constipation.

Pulsatilla   Non-corrosive thick coloured catarrh that is better in the open air.

Rhus tox   Rheumatic and arthritic conditions where symptoms are made worse by initial movement but improved with gentle continuing movement and the application of heat.

Ruta   Soft-tissue injuries. May be combined with Rhus tox or Arnica.

Specialities   In addition to the complexes for internal use, there are remedies on the market that might be called specialities – products that are usually produced by one manufacturer alone. Examples are Weleda's Combudoron gel for burns, scalds, sunburn, bites and skin rashes and Nelson's insomnia remedy, Noctura.

Repertory

In this section the process of counter prescribing has been greatly simplified: this will upset purists who resist the shortening of drug pictures in this way. However, this pragmatic approach, using polychrests, enables a relatively quick response to an OTC request for treatment. Using a repertory style of presentation, appropriate choices can be made from Tables 4.5–4.14.

Homeopathy has applications in:

- the initial treatment for simple self-limiting conditions (coughs, colds and flu) and for injuries (abrasions and soft-tissue injuries) and allergies (Tables 4.5–4.10)

- allergies (Table 4.11)
- dental surgery – before and after treatment (Arnica) and for anxiety (Aconite or Argent nit: Table 4.12)
- conditions associated with women (Table 4.13)
- sports care – treating simple conditions and injuries in athletes (Arnica, Ruta: Table 4.14)
- veterinary medicine (pets and farm animals) notwithstanding the limits on counter prescribing afforded by the Veterinary Surgeons Act 1961, which restricts diagnosis and treatment to veterinarians and owners (as there are no provings on animals, despite anatomical variances veterinary uses generally mirror human applications).

Tables 4.5–4.14 offer guidance on how to respond to requests for assistance in treating a number of common conditions. They are not meant to be comprehensive – there are many excellent repertories available – but will serve to illustrate what can be treated in the pharmacy environment. The indications represent a highly abbreviated drug picture that highlights the most common uses for each of the remedies.

The biochemic tissue salts

The tissue salts are often included under the homeopathic umbrella, although their inventor insisted that they were quite separate from homeopathy.

Dr Wilhelm Heinrich Schüssler, a German homeopathic physician from Oldenburg, introduced a number of inorganic substances in low potency to his practice in 1872, and developed the idea of biochemic tissue salts. Proponents cite unhealthy eating practices that could lead to deficiencies of various salts considered to be vital for the healthy functioning of the body. It is argued that this situation may be corrected by taking tissue salts.

There are 12 single biochemic tissue salt remedies, together with some 18 different combinations. They are made by a process of trituration, each salt being ground down with lactose sequentially up to the sixth decimal potency (6x) level. The resulting triturate is then compressed directly into a soft tablet. Although most of the salts are soluble, there is no intermediate liquid stage, and surface inoculation is not used as it is thought to render the tissue salts ineffective. The tablet readily

Table 4.5 Remedies used for colds and flu

Nasal symptoms	Other symptoms	Modalities	Comments	Remedy
Sneezing, congestion	Thirst	Worse in stuffy atmosphere	Initial stages of colds and flu	Aconite
Runny nose, sore nostrils	Streaming eyes – lacrimation bland	Better wrapped up	Treatment of colds	AGE[a]
Streaming coryza, sneezing	Streaming eyes, hot, thirsty, sore throat	Better for fresh air		Allium cepa
Sore red nostrils	Sore eyes 'aching bones'	Better for warmth	Treatment of flu	Gelsemium
Right nostril congested	Yellow nasal discharge, neuralgia	Better in open air		Pulsatilla

[a]AGE is a combination of three remedies – Arsen iod, Gelsemium and Eupatorium.

dissolves in the mouth, releasing fine particles of mineral material that can be absorbed into the blood stream through the mucosa.

The salts are often referred to by a number, from 1 to 12 in order of their names. They are listed in Table 4.15.

For many ailments, more than one tissue salt is required. In order to simplify treatment there are a number of combination remedies containing three, four or five different salts, usually referred to by the letters A–S and given specific indications. For example, combination A contains Ferr phos, Kali phos and Mag phos, and is used for sciatica and neuralgia, and combination S contains Kali mur, Nat phos and Nat sulph, and is used for stomach upsets.

Anthroposophy

Echoing the ancient Greek axiom 'Man, know thyself', Rudolf Steiner, the founder of anthroposophy, described it as 'awareness of one's humanity'. The Austrian-born Steiner (1861–1925) was the head of the German Theosophical Society from 1902 until 1912, at which time he broke away and formed his Anthroposophical Society. One of his main motives for leaving the theosophists was that they did not consider Christian teachings as special.[52]

Table 4.6 Remedies used for gastrointestinal problems

Condition	Symptoms	Modalities	Comments	Remedy
Colic	Severe abdominal cramps	Better from drawing up knees or bending double	May be associated with diarrhoea	Colocynth
Colic	Abdominal pain, distension, wind		Infant colic and discomfort from teething	Chamomilla
Constipation	Stools hard, dry, thick and brown; nausea and thirst	Worse in the morning		Bryonia
Constipation	Frequent ineffectual straining; patient cold and irritable	Worse in the morning		Nux vomica
Diarrhoea	Colic, watery stool, flatulence, trembling	Better from warmth	Anxiety-related ('exam nerves') Worried about failing exam	Argent nit Gelsemium
Diarrhoea	Rectal pain, small dark stools	Worse from cold	Food-related	Arsen alb
Diarrhoea	Explosive frequent diarrhoea with flatulence	Better with gentle rubbing over hepatic region	With indigestion; common in children	Podophyllum
Indigestion	Belching and flatulence; cold sweat; nausea in morning	Worse in evening and from cold air	May be combined with Belladonna for irritable bowel syndrome	Carbo veg
Nausea	Accompanied by abdominal pain; retching	Better after stool passed	Associated with overeating	Nux vomica
Nausea	Accompanied by vomiting		Morning sickness in pregnancy; also for motion sickness	Cocculus (Tabacum specific for sea sickness)

Table 4.7 Remedies used for coughs

Speed of onset	Symptoms	Modalities	Comments	Remedy
Slow	Hacking productive cough	Worse with change of atmosphere and after food	Best as cough mixture sipped slowly in warm water	Bryonia
Slow	Dry; long-lasting	Worse at night and with exertion	Often after flu	Phosphorus
Steady	Spasmodic, dry and irritating	Worse at night in bed	Said to be associated with whooping cough	Drosera
Sudden	Wheezing cough with shortness of breath, nasal coryza	Worse at night, especially when lying down		Ipecac
Sudden	Dry 'bark', headache	Worse with excitement and cold air Better from lying down		Spongia

Steiner's most lasting and significant influence has been in the field of education. In 1913 at Dornach, near Basel, Switzerland, Steiner built his Goetheanum, a 'school of spiritual science'.

Steiner designed the curriculum of his schools around his spiritual ideas and ascribed the following qualities to the living body:

- a life force that maintains the physical body functions
- an etheric body of non-physical formative forces, particularly active in growth and nutrition
- an astral body, particularly active in the nervous system
- a spiritual core or ego, reflected in a person's ability to change him- or herself inwardly

Anthroposophical practitioners seek to understand illness in terms of the way in which these four elements interact. Anthroposophy embraces a spiritual view of the human being and the cosmos, but its emphasis is on knowing, not purely faith.

Steiner's early experiments in Switzerland finally led to the founding of the Waldorf School Movement, which by 1969 had 80 schools

Table 4.8 Remedies used for headaches

Speed of onset	Symptoms	Modalities	Comments	Remedy
Sudden	Bursting pain with flushed appearance	Beter for lying down in dark room	May be caused by exposing head to cold	Belladonna
Gradual	'Blinding' headache	Better in open air	May follow eye strain and emotional stress – students?	Natrum mur
Gradual	Splitting or crushing pain in occiput	Worse with warmth and motion	Patient irritable	Bryonia
Occasional	Throbbing pain	Worse when standing	May result from lack of food	Sulphur

Table 4.9 Remedies used for mental states

Condition	Symptoms	Modalities	Comments	Remedy
Fear, terror	Bursting sensation in head	Worse in warm room	Will not go to the dentist; will not fly	Aconite
Anticipatory anxiety of event to come	Headache	Better for fresh air	Will do both of above but extremely unhappy	Argent nit
Worry about not performing well; failure of exams	Dry mouth, tremble	Worse when weather wet	Desire to be left alone	Gelsemium (also for agitated pets)
Grief	Crying; mood swings, headache	Worse from open air	Used for recent bereavement	Ignatia
Grief	Irritable, depressed Headache	Better from open air	Ongoing effects of grief	Natrum mur

Table 4.10 Remedies used for skin conditions

Condition	Symptoms	Modalities	Comments	Remedy
Abrasions – superficial	Cuts, grazes, nappy rash		Topical application	Calendula Hypercal[a]
	Cold sores		Painful abrasions, especially on fingers or toes	Hypericum
Acne, eczema	Rough dry skin, oozing sores	Worse with warmth and at night	Topical or oral if skin broken	Graphites
	Abscesses, suppurating and unhealthy skin	Worse from exposure to cold winds		Hepar sulph
	Dry, scaly, itching and burning	Worse with scratching and washing with warm water		Sulphur
Allergic response	Urticarial-type skin rash	Worse from touch and scratching		Urtica
Boils	Abscesses, boils, cracks at the end of fingers; coldness in extremities	Worse from washing	Has 'drawing' effect: expels foriegn bodies from wounds	Silica
Burns	Burns and scalds	Better with rubbing Worse with touch		Cantharis
	Throbbing red rash		Sunburn	Belladonna
Chilblains			Topical (ointment, cream or mother tincture) if skin unbroken; if skin broken oral as tablets, etc.	Tamus
Insect bites	Puncture wound – cold to the touch	Better with cold	Also for rheumatism in feet	Ledum
Insect stings	Histamine reaction		Also for oedema in extremities	Apis
Warts		Worse with heat and touch	As with Tamus above	Thuja

[a]Hypercal is a mixture of the remedies Hypericum and Calendula.

Table 4.11 Remedies used for allergies

Condition	Symptoms	Modalities	Remedy
Bland lacrimation	Watery bland coryza	Worse in cold air – causes cough	Allium cepa
Acid burning lacrimation	Fluid watery coryza	Worse indoors and at night	Euphrasia
Heavy swollen eyes	Sneezing, watery coryza, sore throat	Worse in damp weather and with excitement	Gelsemium
Urticarial rash on skin	Profuse discharge	Worse from touch	Urtica

Isopathic remedies – allergodes and tautopathics – may also be considered for the treatment of allergies and contact dermatitis.

attended by more than 25 000 children in the USA and Europe. Many other projects grew out of Steiner's work, including centres for handicapped children, schools of art, sculpture and drama, and research centres.

People who follow an anthroposophic way of life use antibiotics restrictively, have few vaccinations and their diet usually contains live lactobacilli, which may affect the intestinal microflora. In a cross-sectional study, 295 children aged 5–13 years at two anthroposophic (Steiner) schools near Stockholm, Sweden, were compared with 380 children of the same age at two neighbouring schools in terms of history of atopic and infectious diseases, use of antibiotics and vaccinations, and social and environmental variables.[53] Prevalence of atopy was found to be lower in children from anthroposophic families than in children from other families. It was concluded that lifestyle factors associated with anthroposophy may lessen the risk of atopy in childhood.

Table 4.12 Remedies used in dentistry

Condition	Remedies to be considered
Anxiety, fear of dentist	Aconite, Argent nit
Preoperative	Arnica
Postoperative	Arnica, Calendula, Hypercal
Gum disorders	Merc sol
Mouth ulcers	Borax orally or Calendula mouthwash

Table 4.13 Remedies used for treating women

Condition	Symptoms	Modalities	Comments	Remedy to consider
Cystitis	Burning pains, frequent urge to urinate	Worse in the morning		Cantharsis
	Constant involuntary 'dribble', especially when coughing or sneezing	Worse in cool dry weather		Causticum
Premenstrual syndrome	Breasts painful, irregular scanty periods, weepy	Worse from heat and after eating	Best in short and stoutish fair-skinned women who are affectionate	Pulsatilla
	Abdominal pain, cystitis, flatulence	Better by going to bed	Best for tall slim women with waxy skin who are not affectionate	Sepia
Heartburn	Indigestion and wind			Carbo veg
Insomnia	Difficulty in getting to sleep	Worse from cold and excitement	May be associated with toothache	Coffea
Morning sickness	Nausea with fainting and vomiting	Worse with food or smoking		Cocculus
	Nausea, heartburn and sore breasts	Worse lying down		Conium
Pregnancy: Prior to delivery	Anxiety To help recovery To help delivery		Commence at around 35 weeks	Argent nit Arnica Caulophyllum
After delivery	To reduce bruising			Arnica

Table 4.14 Examples of remedies useful for sportspersons

Condition	Symptoms	Modalities	Comments	Remedy to consider
Anxiety prior to competition	Worry, diarrhoea, sweating, dry mouth			Argent nit
Diarrhoea			From anxiety From excess or rich food	Argent nit Arsen alb
Muscle tiredness	Delayed-onset muscle soreness		May be combined with Rhus tox	Arnica
Sprain	Ligament damage causing impaired movement	Better for warmth Better for cold		Rhus tox Bryonia
Strain	Soft-tissue injury, pain		May be combined with Rhus tox and/or Arnica	Ruta
Tennis elbow	Painful elbow; detachment of muscular and tendinous fibres			Argent met

Anthroposophical medicines

Great care is taken in collecting raw materials for preparing anthroposophical medicines.[54] Vegetable material is grown using methods of biodynamic farming, a development of organic practice in which the soil is fed to improve its structure and fertility. Soil additives are restricted to homeopathic remedies; all other hormones and chemicals are excluded. Due cognisance is taken of the natural cycles of the moon, sun and seasons. The first growth of plants is harvested and composted, and a second crop grown on the composted material. The process is repeated, and the third generation of plants is used to prepare the medicine. Manufacturers prefer to produce their own source material whenever possible. Weleda of Ilkeston, Debyshire, one of 26 Weleda companies worldwide, grows many medicinal plants in its extensive herb gardens. Anthroposophical pharmacy uses different temperatures during the manufacturing process according to the particular remedy involved. Aconite, said

Table 4.15 Tissue salts and examples of their indications for use

Number	Tissue salt	Indication
1	Calc fluor	Maintain elasticity of tissues, for impaired circulation
2	Calc phos	Impaired digestion and teething
3	Calc sulph	Acne, pimples, sore lips
4	Ferr phos	Coughs, colds, chills
5	Kali mur	Respiratory ailments, children's fevers
6	Kali phos	Nervous exhaustion
7	Kali sulph	Catarrh, skin eruptions
8	Mag phos	Antispasmodic, neuralgia, flatulence
9	Nat mur	Watery colds, flow of tears, loss of smell or taste
10	Nat phos	Gastric disorders, heartburn
11	Nat sulph	Bilious attacks, flu. 'The liver salt'
12	Silica	Boils, brittle nails

to exhibit the properties of coolness, is prepared at a lower temperature than Crataegus, a remedy acting on heart muscle and therefore active at body temperature. Anthroposophical practitioners believe that there is a link between warmth and the ego. Paying attention to temperature during preparation can be seen as helping to relate the remedies to human use. The remedies are extracted, diluted and used without potentisation, or prepared using the homeopathic process of serial dilution and succussion. Iscador, marketed by Weleda in the UK, is a mistletoe preparation used for cancer care. Its complex method of extraction involves mixing winter and summer sap. Drops of winter sap are added to a fine film of summer sap on a rapidly spinning disc; there is also a controlled fermentation process.

Although an anthroposophical prescription is often highly individualised, taking into account the physical and spiritual features of a patient, there are specifics, usually mixtures of several potentised remedies, that can be used in all patients to alleviate certain symptoms. There are treatments for bruises and sprains, burns, chilblains, constipation, indigestion and many other common ailments. Some examples are:

- *Formica* (red ant juice) and Bambusa (bamboo nodes), combined with either silver or tin, is indicated for a variety of acute or chronic back pain problems.
- *Silicea comp.* contains potencies of Silica (quartz), Belladonna (deadly nightshade) and Argent nit (silver nitrate) and is used to treat sinusitis.

Evidence

Evidence of successful outcome of treatment for anthroposophical medicine is sparse, although there is considerable anecdotal data. In a German study 18 unselected patients with chronic inflammatory rheumatic conditions, including 10 with confirmed rheumatoid arthritis, were treated according to anthroposophical principles in an open prospective uncontrolled pilot study with a mean follow-up period of 12 months.[55] Main outcome targets were local and systematic inflammation, subjective status and functional capacity. Treatment comprised a combination of Bryonia, Rhus tox, Apis, Formica and Vespa, individualised to each patient's requirements. There appeared to be a definite reduction in local and systemic inflammatory activity and an improvement in mental symptoms. These results must be considered to be of limited validity because the patients were self-selected, in that they asked to be treated using anthroposophical medicine, the numbers of patients were low and there was no double-blinding.

More information

Homeopathy

Faculty of Homeopathy &
British Homeopathic Association (Administration)
15 Clerkenwell Close
London
EC1R 0AA
Tel: 020 7566 7810
Fax: 020 7566 7815
E-mail: info@trusthomeopathy.org/faculty
www.trusthomeopathy.org/faculty

Society of Homoeopaths
2 Artizan Road
Northampton
NN1 4HU
Tel: 01604 621400
Fax: 01604 622622
E-mail: info@homeopathy-soh.org
www.homeopathy-soh.org

Hom-Inform, British Homeopathic Library
Glasgow Homeopathic Hospital
1053 Great Western Road
Glasgow
G12 0XQ
Tel: 0141 211 1617
Fax: 0141 211 1610
E-mail: hom-inform@dial.pipex.com
www.hom-inform.org

Academic Department (AdHom) and
Faculty of Homeopathy in Scotland
Glasgow Homeopathic Hospital
1053 Great Western Road
Glasgow
G12 0XQ
Tel: 0141 337 1824
Fax: 0141 211 1610
E-mail: carolanderson@dial.pipex.com
www.adhom.org

Anthroposophy

Anthroposophical Society of America
1923 Geddes Ave
Ann Arbor
MI 48104-1797
USA
Tel: 734 662 9355
Fax: 734 662 1727
E-mail: Information@anthroposophy.org
www.anthroposophy.org

Allgemeine Anthroposophische Gesellschaft
Goetheanum Postfach 134
CH-4143 Dornach
Switzerland
Tel: 61 706 42 42
Fax: 61 706 43 14
E-mail: wochenschrift@goetheanum.ch
www.goetheanum.ch

Rudolf Steiner Library
65 Fern Hill Rd
Ghent
NY 12075
USA
Tel: 518 672 7690
Fax: 518 672 5827
E-mail: rsteinerlibrary@taconic.net
http://rslibrary.elib.com

References

1. Hahnemann C S. *Organon of the Rational Art of Healing*. Dresden: Arnold, 1810.
2. Hahnemann C S. Versuch uber ein neues Prinzip zur Auffindung der Heilkerafte der Arzneisubstanzen. *Hufland's J* 1796; 2: 2, 3. Translated into English by Dudgeon R E. London: Lesser Writings, 1852: 295–352.
3. Belon P. Provings. Concept and methodology. *Br Homeopath J* 1995; 84: 213–217.
4. Dellmour F, Jansen J, Nicolai T *et al*. *The Proposal for a Revised International Nomenclature System of Homeopathic Remedies and their Abbreviations*. Brussels: European Committee for Homeopathy, 1999.
5. Guajardo G, Bellavite P, Wynn S *et al*. Homeopathic terminology: a consensus quest. *Br Homeopath J* 1999; 88: 135–141.
6. *British Homeopathic Pharmacopoeia* (BHomP), vol. 1. Ilkeston, Derbyshire: BAHM, 1993.
7. *British Homeopathic Pharmacopoeia* (BHomP), vol. 1. Ilkeston, Derbyshire: BAHM, 1999.
8. Kayne S B. *Homeopathic Pharmacy – An Introduction and Handbook*. Edinburgh: Churchill Livingstone, 1997: 57.
9. Isbell W, Kayne S B. Potentization – just a myth? *Br Homeopath J* 1997; 86: 156–160.
10. Schulte J. Effects of potentisation in aqueous solutions. *Br Homeopath J* 1999; 88: 155–160.
11. Schmolz M. Thin-layer chromatography in electrophoresis of homeopathic single remedies. *Biomed Ther* 2000; 18: 202–203.
12. Beattie N, Kayne S B. The treatment of allergies with isopathy. *Br Homeopath J* (in press).
13. Julian O. *Materia Medica of New Homoeopathic Remedies*. Beaconsfield: Beaconsfield Publishers, 1979.
14. Jonas W B. Do homeopathic nosodes protect against infection? An experimental test. *Altern Ther Health Med* 1999; 5: 36–40.
15. Ernst E. Towards quality in complementary health care: is the German 'Heilpraktiker' a model for complementary practitioners? *Int J Qual Health Care* 1996; 8: 187–190.

16. Campbell A. The origins of classical homeopathy? *Complement Ther Med* 1999; 7: 76–82.

17. Dantas F, Rampes H. Do homeopathic medicines provoke adverse effects? A systematic review. *Br Homeopath J* 2000; 89 (suppl. 1): S35–S38.

18. Barnes J. Complementary medicine: homoeopathy. *Pharm J* 1998; 260: 492–497.

19. Montoya-Cabrera M A, Rubio-Rodriguez S, Velazquez-Gonzalez E, Montoya S A. Intoxicacion mercurial causada por un medicamento homeopatico. *Gac Med Mex* 1991; 127: 267–270.

20. Wehner-Caroli J, Scherwitz C, Schweinsberg F, Fierbleck G. Exazerbation einer Psoriasis pustulosa bei Quecksilber-intoxikation. (Pustular psoriasis with exacerbation from mercury toxicity.) *Hautarzt* 1994; 45: 708–710.

21. Clement R T. Lead, mercury, and arsenic in complex homeopathic remedies and child safety. *Townsend Lett* 1998; 176: 102–103.

22. Kent J T. *Repertory of the Homeopathic Materia Medica*, 2nd edn. London: Homeopathic Book Service, 1986.

23. Murphy R. *Homeopathic Medical Repertory*, 2nd edn. Pagosa Springs, CO: Hahnemann Academy of North America, 1998.

24. Phatak S R. *Concise Repertory of Homeopathic Remedies*, 2nd edn. Bombay: Homeopathic Medical Publishers, 1977.

25. Schroyens F. *Synthesis*, 7th edn. London: Homeopathic Book Publishers, 1998.

26. Furnham A, Bond C. The perceived efficacy of homeopathy and orthodox medicine: a vignette-based study. *Complement Ther Med* 2000; 8: 193–201.

27. Kayne S B, Beattie N, Reeves A. Self-treatment using homeopathic remedies bought over-the-counter (OTC) in a sample of British pharmacies. *Br Homeopath J* 2000; 89 (suppl. 1): S50.

28. Kayne S B, Usher W. Homeopathy – attitudes and awareness amongst pharmacy clients and staff in New Zealand. *NZ Pharm* 1999; 19: 32–33.

29. Bellavite P, Signorini A. Is homeopathy effective? In: *Homeopathy. A Frontier in Medical Science*. Berkeley, CA: North Atlantic Books, 1995: 37–55.

30. Ernst E, Hahn E G (eds) *Homeopathy. A Critical Approach*. Oxford: Butterworth-Heinemann, 1998.

31. Kayne S B. *Homeopathic Pharmacy – An Introduction and Handbook*. Edinburgh: Churchill Livingstone, 1997: 164–167.

32. Reilly D T, Taylor M A. Potent placebo or potency? A proposed study model with initial findings using homeopathically prepared pollens in hayfever. *Br Homeopath J* 1985; 74: 65–75.

33. Reilly D T, Taylor M A, McSharrry C, Aitchison T C. Is homeopathy a placebo response? Controlled trial of homeopathic potency with pollen in hayfever as model. *Lancet* 1986; ii: 881–888.

34. Taylor M A, Reilly D, Llewellyn-Jones R H *et al*. Randomised controlled trial of homoeopathy versus placebo in perennial allergic rhinitis with overview of four trial series. *BMJ* 2000; 321: 471–476.

35. Reilly D. Is homeopathy a placebo response? What if it is? What if it is not? In: Ernst E, Hahn E G, eds. *Homeopathy – A Critical Approach*. Oxford: Butterworth-Heinemann, 1998: chapter 8.

36. Linde K, Clausius N, Ramirez G *et al*. Are the clinical effects of homoeopathy placebo effects? A meta-analysis of placebo-controlled trials. *Lancet* 1997; 350: 834–843.

37. Kleijnen J, Knipschild J, ter Riet G. Clinical trials of homoeopathy. *BMJ* 1991; 302: 316–323.

38. Linde K, Melchart D. Randomized controlled trials of individualized homeopathy: a state-of-the-art review. *J Altern Complement Med* 1998; 4: 371–388.

39. Walach H, Haeusler W, Lowes T *et al*. Classical homeopathic treatment of chronic headaches. *Cephalalgia* 1997; 17: 119–126.

40. Hart O, Mullee M A, Lewith G, Miller J. Double blind placebo-controlled randomised clinical trial of homeopathic arnica C30 for pain and infection after total abdominal hysterectomy. *J R Soc Med* 1997; 90: 73–78.

41. Ernst E, Barnes J. Are homeopathic remedies effective for delayed-onset muscle soreness? A systematic review of placebo-controlled trials. *Perfusion* 1998; 1: 4–8.

42. Whitmarsh T, Coleston-Shields D M, Steiner T J. Double blind randomised placebo-controlled trial of homeopathic prophylaxis of migraine. *Cephalalgia* 1997; 17: 600–604.

43. Beer A-M, Heiliger F, Lukanov J. Caulophyllum D4 to introduction of labour in premature rupture of membranes – a double blind study confirmed by an investigation into the contraction activity of smooth muscles. *FACT* 2000; 5: 84–85.

44. Linde K, Scholz M, Ramirez G *et al*. Impact of study quality on outcome in placebo-controlled trials of homeopathy. *J Clin Epidemiol* 1999; 52: 631–636.

45. Vithoulkas G. Homeopathic experimentation: the problem of double blind trials and some suggestions. *J Complement Med* 1985; 1: 10–15.

46. Singh P P P, Chabra H L. Topological investigation of the ethanol/water system and its implications for the mode of action of homeopathic medicines. *Br Homeopath J* 1993; 82: 164–171.

47. Haselen van R, Fisher P. Describing and improving homeopathy. *Br Homeopath J* 1994; 83: 135–141.

48. Heger M. Prospective documentation in homoeopathic practice – an essential contribution to quality assurance. *HomInt Res Dev NewsLett* 1998; 2: 3–18.

49. Clover A. Patient benefit survey: Tunbridge Wells Homoeopathic Hospital. *Br Homeopath J* 2000; 89: 68–72.

50. Alton S, Kayne S B. A pilot study of the attitudes and awareness of homeopathy shown by patients in three Manchester pharmacies. *Br Homeopath J* 1992; 81: 189–193.

51. Davies M, Kayne S B. Homeopathy – a pilot study of the attitudes and awareness of pharmacy staff in the Stoke-on-Trent area. *Br Homeopath J* 1992; 81: 194–198.

52. *The Skeptics Dictionary*. http://skepdic.com/steiner.html.

53. Alm J S, Swartz J, Lilja G *et al*. Atopy in children of families with an anthroposophic lifestyle. *Lancet* 1999; 353: 1485–1488.

54. Evans M, Rodger I. *Anthroposophical Medicines*. London: Thorson's, 1992.

55. Simon L, Schietzel T, Artner C G *et al*. An anthroposophical treatment design for inflammatory rheumatic conditions. *J Anthroposoph Med* 1997; 14: 22–40.

5

Medical herbalism

Plants, medicines and environmental awareness[1]

Environmental awareness

The World Health Organization has estimated that an impressive 80% of the world's population relies mainly on 'natural' medicines in one form or another, while up to 40% of all pharmaceuticals in industrialised countries are derived from natural sources.[2] In the USA about 2% of prescriptions are for drugs that have natural ingredients, are synthetic copies or have artificially modified forms of natural chemicals. The search continues for more therapeutically active plant-sourced materials, not always with the approval of resident communities in whose areas the investigations are being conducted.

Two centuries ago, all orthodox medicine (OM) had to offer was digitalis and laudanum, but now there are thousands of powerful, efficacious drugs that save lives somewhere almost every second of the day.[3] However, modern drugs struggle to make much impact on the rise in cancer, heart disease and other afflictions of the industrialised world. This lack of efficacy, together with patients' growing unease over the side-effects of synthetic drugs, has coincided with an international growth in environmental awareness, particularly concern about the depletion of natural resources. In turn, this has led to a greater sensitivity to the delicate symbiotic balance that exists in nature.

Disappearing rainforests

It is likely that rainforests offer the greatest chance of discovering new potent drugs. Unfortunately, the rainforest is being destroyed at such a rate that thousands of species may become extinct before their medicinal potential can be examined. Five thousand years ago the rainforest covered two billion hectares, or 14% of the earth's land surface. Now only half remains, but it is inhabited by 50% of all the plants and animals found on the globe.[4] The human race is continuing to destroy an area of rainforest equivalent to 20 football fields every day, a rate that if maintained will cause the rainforest to vanish by the year 2030. Slash-and-burn agriculture accounts for 50% of the annual loss. This is a primitive system that involves cutting down a patch of forest and setting the timber alight to release phosphorus, nitrogen, potassium and other nutrients. The resulting ash fertilises the soil, which will then support crops for 2 or 3 years. After this time the land becomes barren, necessitating the clearing of another patch of forest. Logging is the second major cause of forest destruction. In 1990, 3.5 billion cubic metres of tropical wood were felled throughout the world, more than half for fuel sources.

Trees are also consumed for their important products. For example, India earns $125m annually from its production of perfumes, essential oils, flavourings, resins and pharmaceuticals. The petroleum nut tree yields an oil that can power engines as well as provide a homeopathic remedy. Another example is the bark of the cinchona tree, which provides the antimalarial quinine (also known as *china*), a product of immense historical significance to homeopathy. In Madagascar, common Cantharanthus (Vinca) species are exploited for the anticancer drugs vinblastine and vincristine, two naturally occurring alkaloids isolated in the early 1960s by the pharmaceutical company Eli Lilly. Although there is no fear of these particular plants becoming extinct, serious damage has been done to the ecosystem of which they are a part.

Curare, a South American poisonous vine extract, is a muscle relaxant. In fact, the Amazon Indians use at least 1000 plants medicinally. In Malaysia and Indonesia more than twice this number of plant materials are used to make jamu, the traditional medicine.

Growing demand

It is not only in the developing world that there are demands for herbal plant sources. Germany, the largest European medicinal plant importer, is also a major exporter of finished herbal products, accounting for at least 70% of the European market.

A patent taken out by a US company in 1999 angered Indian scientists and ecology experts greatly; they were furious at what they considered to be the raiding of their country's storehouse of traditional knowledge.[5] The Americans were granted a patent on a composition of bitter gourd, eggplant (aubergine) and jamun, the fruit of the rose-apple tree, which is abundant all over India during the summer months. The use of these substances to treat diabetes dates back many centuries and is mentioned in many ancient texts on healing. Other indigenous Indian herbal products on which patents have been taken out include mustard seeds (used for bronchial and rheumatic complaints), Indian gooseberry (used for coughs, asthma, jaundice and wounds) and neem (which has pesticidal, dermatological and antibacterial properties). Neem has attracted dozens of patent applications and is probably the most celebrated medicinal tree in India.

A Worldwide Fund for Nature (WWF) report has warned that the enormous market demand could have an irreversible impact on many species unless action is taken to regulate trade.[6] For example, *Taxus baccata*, a yew tree which grows among pine forests at around 3000 m in the Himalayas, contains the terpenoid taxol, believed to be of use in the treatment of ovarian, and perhaps breast, cancer. Pharmaceutical companies have stripped forest areas of this species and available trees are now insufficient to meet the demand for this new drug. One cause of this problem is an earlier unconsidered arbitrary decimation of the yew tree population. In 1977 the plant was not considered important enough even to be included in a book on trees, but within 15 years it had become an endangered species.

The WWF report reviews the data available on the medicinal plant trade and cites the urgent need for further investigation. One problem is that it is often difficult to decide whether the medicinal plant imports are derived from cultivated or wild specimens. Brazil, China and Nepal have conservation programmes, but India and Pakistan still harvest from the wild, and little is known of the ecological impact of such trade.

Climatic changes

As well as the direct threat to plants through human actions on the habitat or by exhausting the plant stock, there are other more natural problems, such as climate, although it has to be said that this may well also have been changed due to human actions. Scientific tests at Canberra's Australian National University have proved a link between stunted plant growth and higher ultraviolet radiation caused by depletion of the earth's protective ozone layer. This depletion is being caused by synthetic chemicals, especially chlorofluorocarbons, which are found in products such as air-conditioners and foam packaging.[7] Changes in climate from global warming as a result of the greenhouse effect are also important. However, we cannot be sure how long-term changes in the composition of the mix of atmospheric gases, soil structure or pest and disease patterns are going to affect the capacity of plants to manufacture the important active principals for which we presently want them.

Arnica montana usually grows in alpine regions, but has been known to flourish in milder climates too. Following the increased use of natural gas and low sulphur fuels, the amount of sulphur dioxide in the atmosphere has fallen. At the same time, ammonia concentrations have risen, which has the effect of changing the pH of rootwater and directly affecting the chances of survival of this charming plant.[8]

Tackling the problem

In the UK, John Evelyn (1620–1706) was the first person to warn about the fact that native trees were disappearing faster than they could grow. Evelyn's *Sylva*, published in 1664, was the tree growers' handbook for two centuries.[9] Collecting is a threat to some rare plants; other plant species on the sea coast and hilly areas are affected by the trampling feet of hikers or climbers. The greatest number of endangered species (38) are those of lowland pasture, open grassland and other natural open habitats.[10] Examples of UK endangered or vulnerable species with herbal or homeopathic applications include species of rock cinquefoil (*Potentilla*), Jersey cudweed (*Gnaphalium*), gentians (*Gentiana* spp.), rough marshmallow (*Althaea*) and purple spurge (*Euphorbia*). There are several ways of tackling the problem of endangered species.[3] Perhaps the most important way of conserving resources is to work closely with the people who live in and use the forest, the indigenous population, rubber tappers, ranchers, loggers and so on, to strike a balance between the extremes of conservation and exploitation that will protect species and threatened environments while still fostering economic development and reducing poverty. Finding alternative uses for crops is one solution; the town of Aukre in Brazil is making money harvesting Brazil nut oil for the Body Shop.

Another solution is to find a use for the deforested areas. The return of large-scale cattle ranching is a possibility, providing grass can be grown for fodder. Programmes of continuing education to encourage better forestry management and appropriate legislation, such as the British Wildlife and Countryside Act or the US Endangered Species Act, are also necessary. A total of 332 plants were either listed or proposed for listing under the US act from 1985 to 1991. It has been suggested that companies should fund forest protection schemes by putting up cash in exchange for exploitation rights. One million dollars has been invested by an American drug company in a pilot scheme in Costa Rica. However, the costs are enormous, running into billions of dollars just to preserve resources solely for the pharmaceutical industry. Some of the

UK's rarest wild flowers are likely to be encouraged to make a return as a result of a European Union (EU) set-aside scheme in which 15% of arable land will be taken out of production.[11] Arrangements for the scheme are still to be finalised.

Plant alternatives

Chemical synthesis would reduce the amount of plant material consumed in extraction processes. Ideally, pharmaceutical companies require novel, single active molecules that can be made in a laboratory. While this may be possible for some allopathic drugs, the activity of most crude extracts can seldom be attributed to a single molecule but is usually the result of several compounds acting in synergy, making production of synthetic copies extremely difficult. Medical herbalists are obliged to use the original source material to protect this unique mix of active principals. Furthermore, the holistic principles of herbal medicine suggest that the relative concentrations of useful plant chemicals achieved by mixing different species together in individualised prescriptions are important in treating patients, despite the general lack of standardisation. We know little about the interactive abilities of naturally occurring chemicals, much to the consternation of our orthodox colleagues, whose demands are for purified, fully characterised medicines given in regulated doses. Homeopaths need to use naturally occurring source materials too, complete with any inherent impurities, so that modern drug pictures can be exactly matched with Hahnemann's own work.

There is also the possibility of creating a problem of another kind by following a die synthesis strategy. The isolation of the chemical diosgenin from the Mexican *Dioscorea* species in the 1940s led to a booming steroid industry in that country. As sophisticated isolation, separation and elucidation techniques developed, the requirement for this particular raw material fell away completely and with it went the accompanying industry, causing widespread local social deprivation. *Dioscorea* continues to be used by homeopaths. There is some irony in the fact that the largest pharmaceutical companies in the world are scouring the South American rainforests increasingly, seeking natural sources for drug products.[12] Estimates of the hit rate from random screening programmes in the rainforests vary widely, but are put between 1 in 1000 and 1 in 10 000. The chances of finding active plant extracts is greatly increased by studying the use of plants by various cultures, and the discipline of ethnobotany is growing slowly. There are 119 drugs still extracted commercially from higher plants, of which 74% were obtained as a result of ethnobotanical information.[13] Table 5.1 lists a number of common drugs that came to scientific attention as a result of ethnobotany.

Success story

Certainly it is not all doom and gloom. There have been successes, for example Ginkgo biloba (Figure 5.1). It is the only survivor from the Jurassic dinosaur era some 190 million years ago, all of its related species having long since died out. The tree survived in cultivation because of its valuable fruit and wood, and possibly because of temple plantings. It was introduced to Europe from its native China in 1730. Ginkgo biloba was heading for extinction until fortuitous intervention saved it. Its extracts are used in Chinese herbalism under the name baguo to treat hypertension.

It is some consolation that complementary practitioners are not the cause of endangering species, for their uses are but a fraction of the total requirements. It would be unforgivable if future generations were to suffer because remedies disappeared due to the actions of others. We must work out a compromise in plenty of time.

Introduction to medical herbalism

Only the medical aspects of herbalism are considered here; the cosmetic applications, for example creams, bath additives and haircare products, are not covered. Some authorities would say that the inherent feel-good factor associated with the use of such products could be considered to be a positive activity that promotes a significant health benefit and there

Table 5.1 Common orthodox drugs derived from plants

Medicine	Plant
Atropine	Atropa belladonna
Cocaine	Erythoxylum coca
Colchicine	Colchicum autumnale
Digoxin	Digitalis purpurea
Ephedrine	Ephedra sinica
Hyoscymine	Hyoscymus niger
Morphine	Papaver somniferum
Pilocarpine	Pilocarpus jaborandi
Quinine	Cinchona legeriana
Strychnine	Strychnos nux vomica
Theobromine	Theobroma cacao

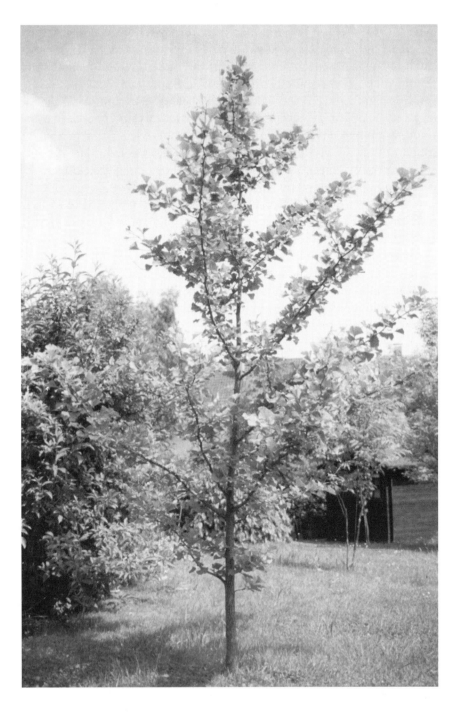

Figure 5.1 Young Ginkgo biloba tree growing in Germany.

may be some merit in this argument. Another psychological benefit may accrue from the process of growing herbs, as well as taking them medicinally or using them to make food more interesting and palatable. In his book *The Therapeutic Garden*, Donald Norfolk, an osteopath, suggests that gardening is the oldest of the healing arts and says that the high-tech medical profession recognises that the sick and despairing respond to gardens.[14] The fact that postoperative patients recover sooner if they are given a view of grass and trees has led to demands to revive the old tradition of hospital gardens. Such a facility exists at the new Glasgow Homeopathic Hospital.

The body of knowledge about plants, herbs and spices and their respective and collective roles in promoting human health is modest.[15] Flavonoids in tea and anthocyanins in tart cherries have been cited as examples of how to move forward our understanding of active compounds. Dietary compounds, their roles in maintaining human health and their interactions with established nutrients, require much investigation.

Herbal remedies are becoming increasingly popular with the public for the following reasons:

- They are readily available from health stores and pharmacies, as well as from other specialist outlets.
- They are often highly effective.
- They provide clients with the means to self-treat a range of conditions for which orthodox over-the-counter (OTC) medicines are limited or unavailable.
- As they are naturally occurring, herbal medicines are perceived as being free of side-effects, and in some cases to be complementary to western medicine or OM – unfortunately this is not entirely true, as there is evidence to the contrary in a number of well-researched circumstances, necessitating caution, particularly when self-treating.

Definition

Quite simply, medical herbalism may be defined as the practice of treating the sick using products in which all active ingredients are of herbal origin. In practice, rather more detail is required. Herbal medicines may be described thus:[16]

> finished, labelled products that contain as active ingredients aerial or underground parts of plants, or other plant material, or combinations thereof, whether in the crude state or as plant preparations. Plant material contains

juices, gums, fatty oils, essential oils and any other substances of this nature. Herbal medicines may contain excipients in addition to the active ingredients.

The European directive EC 65/65 defines a herbal medicine thus:[17]

> A substance or combination of substances presented for treating or preventing disease or with a view to making a medical diagnosis or to restoring, correcting or modifying physiological functions.

Yet another definition is provided by the UK Medicines Act 1968 (Section 132), much of which has now been superseded by pan EU legislation:

> A 'herbal remedy' is a medicinal product consisting of a substance produced by subjecting a plant or plants to drying, crushing or any other process, or of a mixture whose sole ingredients are two or more substances so produced, or of a mixture whose sole ingredients are one or more substances so produced and water or some other inert substances.

This definition underlines the belief that products comprising both herbal and non-herbal ingredients (e.g. minerals) are generally not considered to be herbal medicines.

The term 'phytotherapy' is generally attributed to the Frenchman Henri Leclerc (1870–1955).

History

The exact origins of herbalism are unknown. Probably several different groups of prehistoric people discovered that some herbs were good to eat, while others had curative powers. Humans also discovered plants with peculiar, reality-altering, stimulating and inebriating effects. In ancient cultures these were considered to be the plants of the gods. Ingesting them could lead to contact with the realms of the gods and demons, their ancestors or various other forces of nature not normally visible. Some of these plants had interesting side-effects – many were considered to be aphrodisiacs, awakening sexual desire and increasing pleasure.[18]

The opium poppy, *Papaver somniferum*, is perhaps the earliest medicinal plant, being well known in ancient Greece.[19] Hippocrates mentions the use of poppy juice as a cantharic, hypnotic, narcotic and styptic. Pliny the Elder indicates the use of the seed as a hypnotic and the latex as an effective treatment for headaches, arthritis and curing wounds. The smoking of opium was not noted until much later; it was extensive in China and the Far East in the later part of the eighteenth century.

The mechanism of action remained a mystery for centuries, and in some cases it still remains a mystery. Only the development of sophisticated techniques of chemical analysis in the last century has begun to provide some of the answers. Those who took a special interest in the healing powers of herbs, acquiring a special knowledge and skill, came to enjoy an honoured place in society. The earliest medicine men assumed a link with religion, believing that their powers were divinely granted. The first medical records date from ancient Assyria, China, Egypt and India.

William Turner was the first person to study plants scientifically, in the sixteenth century. He travelled widely throughout Europe and grew plants in his gardens in south-west London (later the Royal Botanical Gardens, Kew). At this time the doctrine of similars promoted by Paracelcus (1493–1541), determined how plants were used. According to this paradigm every plant acted in effect as its own definition of its medical application, resembling either the part of the body afflicted or the cause of the affliction. Nicholas Culpepper (1616–54) was an influential proponent of the doctrine of signatures as well as various astrological theories by which herbs were set under the domination of the sun, moon or one of the five planets then known. His herbal, published in 1652, was extremely successful, being reprinted many times.

Subsequently the apothecaries, who had acquired healing skills in addition to selling herbs, took over. A number of physic gardens were set up to produce important medicinal herbs under controlled conditions and ensure an uninterrupted supply.

By the end of the eighteenth century the heyday of herbalism was passing, but an interest was still maintained. Plants were classified and studied carefully. Expeditions were mounted to uncharted territories to collect new species that could be used medicinally. Several important discoveries were made, for example, digoxin from the foxglove and quinine from cinchona bark. They were all used until wars in the nineteenth and twentieth centuries caused shortages of naturally occurring materials, necessitating the development of synthetic processes.

In the USA the name of Samuel Thomson (1769–1843) deserves attention.[20] Samuel is usually referred to in the literature as being a medical doctor. This does considerable credit to the man who enjoyed but one month's schooling in his life. Thomson's practice involved using simple herbs for bodily correction. He was so successful that opposition from the medical profession was strong and uncompromising. They succeeded in prosecuting him, but his name was cleared and he became universally recognised as an outstanding figure in the medical world. His fame spread to England where thanks to promotion by George Lees, the Thomsonian system was embraced by Jesse Boot when he opened the first of what was to become the UK's biggest multiple pharmacy chain, in Goose Gate, Nottingham in 1872 (Figure 5.2).

Renewed interest in natural medicines has led to a resurgence of demand for herbal remedies in the last 20 years.

Theory[21]

Traditionally, the herbalist has recognised four clear stages when offering treatment for any particular condition, individualising the prescription according to holistic methodology to take account of patients' particular needs. These four stages are:

- Cleansing the body – removal of toxins and other noxious influences, real or imagined, that might cause a physical or mental barrier to treatment. Diuretics, expectorants and laxatives are involved here.

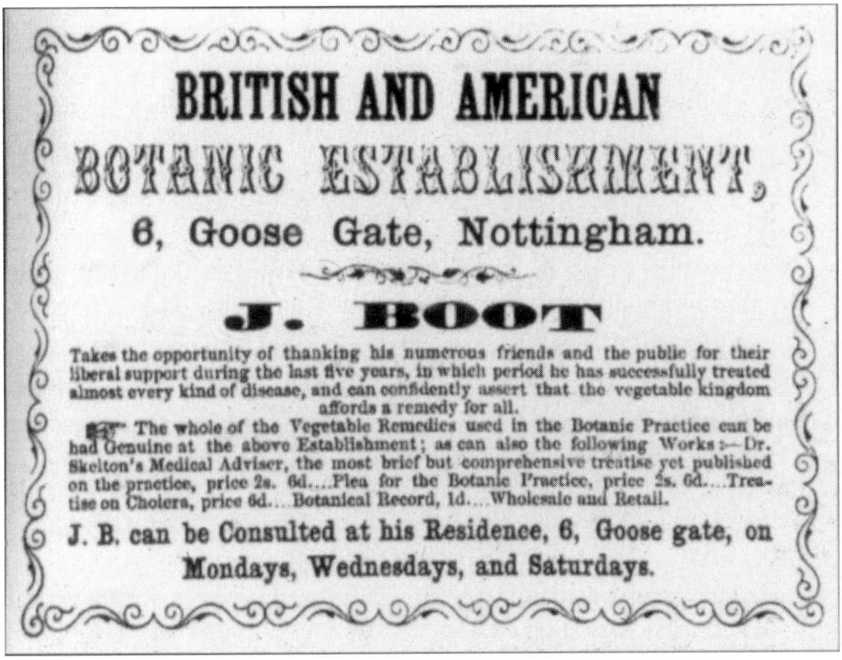

Figure 5.2 Advertisement for early herbal remedies by well-known high-street pharmacy. Courtesy of Boots Company.

- Mobilising the circulation – traditionally disease was seen as a 'cold' influence on the body and before any other treatment the body had to be comforted by heating agents. Hot spices and pungent remedies (e.g. ginger) and more gentle warming remedies are used for this purpose. Hot spicy food (curries) prompts gastric defence against enteric infections in the tropics.
- Stimulating digestion – inappropriate or too much heat in the body manifests itself as fevers and inflammatory conditions. Thus, the so-called 'cooling remedies' are used to treat these circumstances, leading to improved digestion. Anti-inflammatories, antiallergics and sedatives are examples of the therapeutic classes of drugs that fall into this category.
- Nourishment and repair – in this phase the herbalist deals with the debility arising from disease in the body. The term 'tonic' covers a wide range of medicines used to support the body. Examples include hawthorn (Crataegus), milk thistle (Silybum) and St John's wort (Hypericum).

There is a tendency in modern herbalism (as in homeopathy) to skip this measured approach and seek a remedy that deals with local problems rather than the body as a whole. This has been called, perhaps unkindly, a fire-fighting approach. In part this has been fuelled by the growing OTC market, which has produced a number of remedies labelled for use in specific conditions, making it easy for the seller and buyer alike. Therapists claim that this approach goes against the principles of complementary practice. On the other hand the public seem to be satisfied that the medicines they buy work in many situations, otherwise they would have voted with their feet long ago. There is no doubt that long-term chronic conditions do need the considered approach offered by qualified practitioners.

Sources of reference

Having carried out an extended consultation, in common with all complementary disciplines, the following texts are used routinely by herbal practitioners to facilitate the choice of remedy:

- materia medica: a comprehensive list detailing the main characteristics and uses of remedies, e.g. *Potter's New Cyclopaedia of Botanical Drugs and Preparations*[22]
- repertory: a comprehensive list of medical conditions with suggested remedies for treatment e.g. *Herbal Medicine* by Weiss[23]

- the *British Herbal Pharmacopoeia* 1996 gives identification and usage information as well as providing instructions on how remedies should be prepared.[24]

Herbal medicines

The use of herbals as a source for drugs

Many of the plants used in modern herbal preparations contain active ingredients whose effects can be pharmacologically demonstrated. For some OTC products the situation is complicated by the frequent use of drugs in polypharmaceutical combinations. In these circumstances prescriptions are often empirical, resulting from clinical observation and experience rather than scientific deduction.

The main reasons for the attraction of using herbal source material are:

- long periods of experience with traditional remedies
- many isolated constituents are to be found in modern drugs
- large pool of plant material is available; this is particularly important in developing countries
- profit for pharmaceutical companies – a wish for part of the action in many cases in response to customer demand.

Differences between herbal and orthodox medicine

- Use of whole plant: herbalists believe that giving an extract from a whole plant rather than using active principals in isolation (when known) allows them to take advantage of a synergism that is believed to exist between the various constituents. There are some cases where the synergistic effect of the herb might be more helpful than giving an isolated agent. There is also some evidence that the active ingredients in certain whole herbs (glycyrrhizic acid from liquorice, for example) are absorbed differently than when extracted in pure form, and thus the whole herb might be less dangerous than a particular extract.
- Combination of medicinal herbs: herbalists tend to use mixtures of herbs to treat different aspects of a disease in order to exhibit the individualistic therapy demanded by using a holistic approach to medicine. It is true to say that in OM it is usual for patients to be given extra drugs during the progression of their disease (e.g.

diabetes patients may be given antihypertensives and diuretics in addition to hypoglycaemic drugs) but initially polypharmacy is not viewed sympathetically.

- While orthodox drugs are synthetic, homogeneous and standardised, herbals are naturally occurring and extracted, heterogeneous and in many cases non-standardised.
- Diagnosis: herbal treatments are often symptomatic in their approach, whereas most orthodox practitioners tend to seek a diagnosis on the basis that if the cause of a disease can be treated then the symptoms will resolve naturally.

General types of medicinal herbs used

Practitioners use medicinal plants with:

- powerful actions, e.g. liquid extracts of Foxglove and Belladonna, with substantial toxic risk
- intermediate actions, e.g. tinctures of Arnica and Khella, with some adverse drug reactions
- gentle actions, e.g. infusions of German Chamomilla and Peppppermint, with less risk of adverse drug reactions.

In many instances conditions can be treated by drugs in each of these three categories. For example, cardiac disease responds to Foxglove in the powerful group, Arnica in the intermediate group and Hawthorn in the gentle group. Herbal medicines for nervous diseases include opium in the powerful group, St John's wort in the intermediate group and Valerian in the gentle group. Examples of the main therapeutic groups of herbal remedies are summarised in Table 5.2. Some remedies (including garlic and ginger) have wide spectra of activity and may be considered as being equivalent in some respects to the homeopathic polychrests.

Active constituents in herbal medicines[25,26]

Herbal medicines contain a bewildering array of chemicals. In this section the most frequently occurring types found in common herbs are mentioned.

General classes of constituents

Bitters Traditionally, these were used extensively to stimulate appetite (i.e. in the final fourth stage of the healing process outlined above). It is

Table 5.2 Examples of the therapeutic use of herbal remedies

Therapeutic group	Example of herbal remedy
Anticoagulants	Alfalfa, arnica, fucus, garlic, ginger
Coagulant	Mistletoe
Cardioactive	Coltsfoot, devil's claw, ginger, ginseng, parsley, wild carrot
Diuretic	Burdock, dandelion, elder, juniper, pokeroot, squill
Hyperglycaemic	Devil's claw, ginseng, liquorice
Hypoglycaemic	Alfalfa, garlic, ginger, juniper, marshmallow, myrrh
Hypolipidaemic	Alfalfa, garlic, ginger
Hypertensive	Blue cohosh, coltsfoot, gentian, ginger, liquorice
Hypotensive	Celery, devil's claw, fucus, garlic, ginger, St John's wort
Sedative	Camomile, hops, passionflower, St John's wort, valerian

now thought that they will only be effective if a malnourished state exists. The bitter constituents simulate the bitter receptors in the taste buds at the back of the mouth and give rise to an increase in the psychic secretion of gastric juice. The most effective chemicals are the monoterpene seecoiridoid glycosides of gentian. Other extracts that have been used as bitters include quassia, quinine (Cinchona) and strychnine (Nux vomica).

Resins   The term 'resin' is applied to the sticky, water-insoluble substance with a complex chemical nature often exuded by a plant, which soon hardens to protect an injury. Its consitituents include resin acids, resinols, resintannols, esters and chemically inert compounds known as resenes. On heating resins soften and eventually melt. Resins are usually produced by the plant in ducts or cavities, but may also be found in special cells elsewhere, for example in elements of the heartwood of guaiacum and the internal cells of the male fern. The term may also be applied to that part of a plant that is soluble in ether or alcohol (e.g. guaiacum resin and kava resin).

Resins are used as astringents and antiseptics of the mouth and throat, and have also been applied to inflammatory conditions of the upper digestive tract.

Propolis, a product collected by bees from resinous plants, is used in herbal medicine, although it is not strictly herbal in nature. The product is also used in homeopathy.

A balsam, for example balsam of Peru and balsam of Tolu, is an oleoresin containing a high proportion of aromatic balsamic acid.

Saponins   Saponins are glycosides that produce frothy aqueous solutions. Plants containing these compounds (e.g. *Quillaia saponaria*) have been used for centuries as gentle detergents. Decoctions of soap-wort (*Saponaria*) have been used to wash and restore ancient fabrics. They also have haemolytic properties and when injected into the blood stream are highly toxic. When taken by mouth saponins appear to be comparatively harmless. Sarsaparilla is rich in saponins but is widely used in the preparation of non-alcoholic drinks.

Two distinct types of saponins may be recognised. The steroidal saponins are of great pharmaceutical importance because of their relationship to compounds such as the sex hormones, cortisone and the cardiac glycosides. Some species of the yam (*Dioscorea* spp.) and potato (*Solanum* spp.) contain steroidal saponins.

The second group of saponins are known as the pentacyclic triter-penoid saponins. This includes quillaia bark and liquorice root (gly-cyrrhiza). The former is used as an emulsifying agent, the latter as a flavouring agent, demulcent and mild expectorant.

Tannins This is not a specific phytochemical group but a name for a group of chemicals that have a particular characteristic. The term 'tannin' was first applied by Seguin in 1796 to denote substances present in plant extracts that were able to combine with animal proteins in the hides, preventing putrefaction, and converting them to leather. Most tannins have molecular weights of about 1000–5000 and many are glycosides.

Tannin-producing drugs will precipitate protein and have been used traditionally externally as styptics and for burns and weeping eczema, and internally for the protection of the inflamed surface of the mouth and throat. They are also claimed to be antioxidants. Witch-hazel (*Hamamelis virginiana*) is a tannin-containing drug used principally for its astringent properties.

Volatile oils Volatile oils are dealt with in greater detail in Chapter 6, which covers the medical use of aromatherapy.

As the name suggests, volatile oils are volatile in steam. They differ widely in both chemical and physical properties from fixed oils. They are secreted in oil cells, in secretion ducts or cavities, or in glandular hairs, and are frequently associated with gums and resins.

With the exception of oils derived from glycosides (e.g. bitter almonds and mustard oil), volatile oils are generally mixtures of hydro-carbons and oxygenated derivatives, and are mainly responsible for odour and taste. In some oils (e.g. oil of turpentine) the hydrocarbon portion dominates while in others (e.g. oil of cloves) the opposite is true.

Volatile oils are used in perfumery, cosmetics (e.g. oil of rose, oil of bergamot) and in food flavourings (e.g. oil of lemon) as well as in medicine.

Many oils with a high phenolic content (e.g. clove and thyme) have antiseptic properties, whereas others are used as carminatives. Oils showing antispasmodic activity include peppermint (*Mentha piperita*) and camomile (*Matricaria chamomilla*).

Phytochemical groups of constituents

Alkaloids Alkaloids show great variation in their botanical and biochemical origin, chemical structure and pharmacological action. Consequently a precise definition is difficult. Typical alkaloids are basic, contain one or more nitrogen atoms and have a marked physiological action on humans and animals.

Coumarins Coumarins are benzo-alpha-pyrones, generally with a hydroxyl or methoxy group in position 7. They are often associated with glycosides. Simple coumarins have a pleasant odour, variously described as new-mown hay or vanilla. The widespread nature of coumarins – they have been found in about 150 different species – means that they are consumed by humans via many routes, e.g. carrots, celery and parsnips. Simple substituted coumarins are used as pigments in sunscreens.

Flavonoids Flavonoids consist of a single benzene ring joined to a benzo-gamma-pyrone structure. They are widespread in herbal material, functioning as plant pigments and being responsible for the colours of flowers and fruits. Although the name is derived from 'flavus', meaning yellow, many of the pigments are in fact blue, purple, red and white.

About three-quarters of the 2000 types known are glycosides, the balance being aglycones. According to the state of oxygenation, derivatives include flavones, flavonols and flavonones.

Glycosides Glycoside is a term that covers many different combinations comprising a monosaccharide part (e.g. fructose or glucose) and a non-sugar part, which may be a simple phenol, flavonoid, anthraquinone, triterpenoid or other structure, known as the aglycone. It is this latter part that determines the therapeutic characteristics.

Some glycosides may occur as reduced derivatives, anthroquinones, anthranols and anthrones. Anthrones can exist either free or combined as glycosides.

Cardiac glycosides contain deoxysugars (e.g. cyamarose) as the sugar part of their molecules. Cardiac glycosides from the foxglove (*Digitalis purpurea*) and lily of the valley (*Covalleria majalis*) both act on the heart, increasing the contractile force and speed of the cardiac muscle.

Polysaccharides Polysaccharides are polymers based on sugars and uronic acid. They are found in all plants, especially as a component of the cell wall. Some plants accumulate polysaccharides (e.g. Aloe vera).

Polysaccharides are thought to have an important role as immunoenhancing agents (e.g. Echinacea).

The preparation and presentation of herbal medicines

Herbal medicines are made according to standards quoted in the appropriate pharmacopoeias, e.g. *British Herbal Pharmacopoeia*. There are a number of ways in which herbal extracts may be presented. Infusions, decoctions and macerates may be freshly prepared by the consumer, while extracts and tinctures are industrially produced. There are also ranges of solid dose forms and topical preparations available.

Crude drugs – infusions and decoctions

Crude drugs are still widely available both commercially and from professional medical herbalists. They are extracted by the consumer as an infusion if the herbs are of a light fleshy nature or as a decoction if fibrous and woody (roots and barks). The extraction process is outlined below. The advantage is that the extraction is freshly prepared and therefore this method is particularly appropriate for herbs whose active constituents need to be given hot.

Infusions This is the preferred method of extracting fresh active ingredients from light leafy herbs and teas. The drug may be extracted alone or in the form of a herbal tea, of which there are simple (e.g. camomile, peppermint, etc.) and more complex varieties with more than one active principal and a number of excipients. They are convenient when the active constituents are water-soluble.

Instructions for preparing an infusion are as follows:

- Plants containing aromatic oils, e.g. anise, fennel and juniper fruits, should be crushed or bruised; other plants should be finely chopped or minced.

- Pour 150–200 ml boiling water over the herbal material and allow to stand for 10–30 min. If the material contains volatile oils it should not be boiled. Infusions made from drug material that does not include volatile oils (e.g. hawthorn) may be simmered on a low flame for an additional 5 min or so.
- Strain and take in divided doses during the day of preparation.

Commercially available medicinal teas are ready formulated for the consumer and are usually prepared freshly as an infusion prior to taking. They contain the following constituents:[27]

- the remedium cardinale – one or more basic medicinal agents, for example a laxative tea may contain senna leaves and frangula bark
- the adjuvans – one or more auxiliary remedies that enhance the action of the basic remedy or reduce undesirable side-effects, for example, drugs with carminative (anise, caraway or fennel) and/or spasmolytic (camomile flowers, silverweed) properties may reduce unwanted side-effects of senna
- the constituens, corrigens and colourants – fillers and aesthetic agents to improve aroma, appearance, colour or texture. Up to 20% of the tea may be a filler (e.g. raspberry leaves) that prevents it from separating into its components. To ensure concordance, herbal teas must be reasonably palatable; this is especially important in pediatrics. Widely used excipients include bitter orange peel, orange blossom, hibiscus flowers and peppermint leaves. Colourants such as cornflower, mallow and marigold are also used.

Decoctions   Roots and barks may be extracted using a decoction method:

- Pour about 200 ml cold water over the prescribed amount of finely divided botanical material and allow to simmer at around 30°C for about 30 min.
- Cool, strain and take on day of preparation.

Liquid extracts

Strengths   Traditionally, practitioners have used liquid extracts as the preferred method of administering herbal medicines, despite their unpalatable bitter taste in many instances. The strength of a liquid is usually expressed as a ratio, for example a 1:5 ratio means that 5 ml of the final liquid preparation is equivalent to 1 g of original dried herb.

Liquid preparations weaker than 1:2 are usually called tinctures, while 1:1 and 1:2 preparations are called extracts. Tinctures are usually made by maceration and extracts by percolation.

Use of liquids Although liquid extracts are still used widely and are relatively easy to make, because of worries over inconsistent quality there has been a move towards 1:5 tinctures, with doses of 2.5–5 ml three times daily. In other countries herbalists use much smaller doses – 15–20 drops of a diluted tincture is not uncommon in the USA. The manufacturing process for tinctures and liquid extracts differs, principally in that no heat and stronger alcohol are involved in the preparation of the former. Calculating an equivalent dose may be difficult because it is likely that there could be some variance in the active constituents.

The extraction processes

Macerates Occasionally extracts are made at room temperature because of a high starch content (e.g. marshmallow root) or to improve tolerance (e.g. bearberry leaves).

- Place minced material in cold water and leave to stand for 8 h with occasional stirring.
- Strain and bring to the boil briefly to kill any bacterial contamination before allowing to cool and taking.

Extraction with solvent under vacuum

- Percolate or macerate chopped-up drug using appropriate solvent.
- Evaporate under vacuum.
- More permanent preparation.

Alcoholic tinctures: used for resins and volatile oils

- Extract material with varying strengths of alcohol solvent.
- Strain and adjust strength.
- Alcoholic tinctures are elegant and long-lasting preparations.

The strength of alcohol used for the extraction process is important. An investigation into the extraction of volatile oil from camomile plants found that 55% alcohol (ethanol) was the optimum strength.[28] Another worker has found that 40–60% alcohol provided the best range for extracting a range of different herbs.[29]

Other extracts   The following extracts are occasionally seen:

- Solid extracts are pastes made by evaporating expressed juice or liquid extract.
- Dry extracts are solid extract dried under vacuum.

Legal issues – the regulation of herbal medicines

Europe

The question as to whether herbal products should be licensed as medicines has been debated for some time, especially as homeopathic remedies are subject to controls.[30]

The Medicines Control Agency in the UK has reached a wide measure of agreement with the natural health sector on the need to improve the regulatory position of herbal products, and is engaged in ongoing dialogue with around 40 interest groups. The European Commission has recognised that a number of member states have difficulties with the current European framework of law in this area. Unfortunately, the drawing of sharp borderlines is difficult. Many medicine-like products on the British herbal market remain unregistered because acceptable data on efficacy, safety and quality are not available, and the licensing fee is comparatively high. Making substantial alterations to the requirements for registration to accommodate requests from herbal (and homeopathic) manufacturers because of the 'special' nature of their products is likely to introduce double standards. On the one hand, a single protocol for all medicinal products ensures that the same high standards and close control apply equally to all kinds of medicines, but on the other hand, the basis of the conventional requirements for efficacy, safety and quality to safeguard public health are difficult to apply in the case of traditional medicine. However, when substandard, contaminated and adulterated products are offered for sale, the best interests of the public are not being served.

Currently there are four categories of herbs:

- licensed herbal remedies
- herbal remedies exempt from licensing
- herbal products marketed as food supplements
- herbal products marketed as cosmetics.

Licensed herbal medicines

Full product licence   To receive a product licence, herbal medicines are required to meet safety, quality and efficacy criteria in a similar manner to any other licensed medicines (equivalent to Article 9 of the homeopathic licensing regulations under European directive 92/73/EEC). EU legislation requires herbal products to be authorised for marketing if they are industrially produced and if their presentation or their function, or both, bring them inside its definition of a medicinal product.[31,32]

Well-established and traditional-use medicines   Commission directive 99/83EC in principle gives greater flexibility in the use of bibliographic data for this category of medicines to meet the requirements to demonstrate safety and efficacy.

In September 1999 the European Pharmaceutical Committee set up a working group of member states to investigate the possibility of a directive for 'traditionally used' medicines. The Medicines Control Agency, representing the UK, was asked to act as rapporteur for the group and to develop the first draft of a possible directive, for comment by member states. Subsequently a second draft was drawn up (see below).

Herbal products vary from well-known European herbs to less familiar Asian and south American ones and from botanicals with an excellent safety record to potentially dangerous ones, such as broom and yohimbe. Furthermore, traditional experience with herbs may be a powerful reason for advocating their use, but they may be sold without any of the objective product information needed to counterbalance the often uncritical literature on them. Traditional experience needs to be supplemented with orthodox data from research and postmarketing surveillance. Unfortunately, herbal suppliers and practitioners are not obliged to report suspected adverse reactions. An appeal to pharmacists to report adverse effects of herbal and vitamin products was made in 1994[33] but little effective progress has been made.

However a meeting was held in May 2001 in Bonn to discuss progress in the harmonisation of regulation of herbal medicinal products across the EU, with particular attention being given to the development of a new directive that established a 'traditional use' category.[34] A key difficulty was how to capture the essence of 'tradition' in a regulatory scheme, and whether or not harmonisation on this directive was possible, given the differing views among member states. The scope of the traditional-use directive, now in its second draft, remains controversial. The main requirements are:

- 30 years of traditional use: this takes account of 15 years' non-EU use
- bibliographic data on safety with an expert report
- dossier covering quality issues
- simplified quality dossiers for certain categories, such as herbal teas
- no prescription-only medicines
- special labelling, such as 'efficacy not proven'
- 5-year transitional period once directive in force.

The question of whether it should apply to herbal medicinal products only or to other products has not yet been agreed. It is likely that many Chinese and ayurvedic remedies would not be able to satisfy one of the conditions – that of at least 15 years' use in Europe – and the directive would effectively remove these products from the market. There is a growing need to recognise and respect the culture and traditions of ethnic groups, such as Chinese and ayurvedic remedies, some of which are over 1000 years old.

There are several factors to be considered in awarding a 'traditional use' status:

- the time over which a substance has been used
- the level of exposure among the population
- the coherence of scientific assessments.

For submission based on bibliographic evidence, a full dossier would be required by the regulatory authorities, containing both favourable and unfavourable material.

A speaker at the meeting said that currently the UK measured up poorly with regard to ensuring public access to a wide range of safe, high-quality herbal medicines with appropriate information: licensed products gave too much protection and not enough choice, whereas unlicensed products gave plenty of choice but little protection. The traditional-use directive could apply to products beyond herbals and does not apply to products which are eligible for licensing under directive 65/65/EEC.

Herbal remedies that are exempt from licensing requirements   This exemption applies where herbal remedies meet the conditions set out in Section 12 of the Medicines Act 1968, namely:

- The process to which the plant or plants are subjected consists only of drying, crushing or comminuting.
- The remedy must be sold or supplied under a designation that only

specifies the plant or plants and the process and does not apply any other name to the remedy.

- There must be no specific recommendation on the package label or contained in an insert in the packaging.

For unlicensed herbal remedies there are no specific safeguards on quality and safety. There is also not enough information for the public about unlicensed products. This arrangement gives the public choice, but not enough protection. Herbal remedies form a pot-pourri that ranges from plants that people collect themselves and then take for health reasons to approved medicinal products. Many herbal products available in the UK fall between the far ends of this regulatory range; unlicensed preparations may account for over 80% of herbal sales. These unlicensed products are classified as food supplements to bypass the licence requirements.

Herbal medicines as foods[35]   A typical consumer is unable to appreciate that some medicine-like products have escaped regulatory evaluation by being sold as food supplements. Depending on issues such as claims, presentation and dosage, a single herbal substance can be a food or a medicine. For example, Echinacea may be marketed as a fully licensed product or as a medicine exempt from licensing, garlic as a food or medicine and saw palmetto as a food, a medicine exempt from licensing or potentially as a fully licensed product.

Herbal remedies as cosmetics   Topical preparations, herbal shampoos, bath additives and similar products may be sold as cosmetics. Indications for use may not include medical claims but these are often implied in the advertising terminology.

Other authorities

Australia has developed an integral approach to the herbal market that also covers various non-western herbs. Key elements of the Australian system are the need for more compliance with codes of good manufacturing practice, lists of eligible herbs and certain other substances, and directions on labelling and on allowable indications and claims.

The US Food and Drug Administration (FDA) has relaxed guidelines for the sale of herbal supplements.[36] Its decision allows manufacturers of vitamins, herbs and dietary supplements to market their products for conditions such as morning sickness, hot flushes and memory loss in ageing without first proving that they are safe or effective. The decision marks the latest in a series of legal and regulatory victories for the dietary supplement business, which has been growing since Congress passed a law in 1994 that severely restricted the FDA's authority to regulate it. The new law, part of the Dietary Supplement Health and Education Act, allows manufacturers of supplements to sell products without the FDA's rigorous safety and efficacy review, which is required of drugs, as long as they make claims related only to body structure or function and not to disease. The new rule was first proposed in April 1998. At the time, the agency said that natural states like ageing, pregnancy, menopause and adolescence could be associated with abnormal conditions, such as morning sickness or the premenstrual syndrome, that are diseases. Products aimed at these conditions would have required FDA approval. However, after reviewing thousands of public comments from industry representatives, consumers and others, the agency became convinced that such conditions were not diseases, so claims about them did not qualify as claims about disease. Under the new rule, uncommon or serious conditions associated with these life stages will still be treated as diseases. For example, a company may market a dietary supplement for teenagers who have acne but not for acne so severe that the symptoms include cysts. This move angered and surprised consumer advocates, who claimed that the authorities had caved in to the manufacturers' lobby.

UK

At the time of writing the UK Medicines Control Agency is designing a licensing system for herbal remedies. When implemented the scheme will constitute a significant step forward towards the safer use of industrially produced herbal products. Concerns over the use of herbs by traditional healers in ethnic communities are likely to remain, especially as quantities of raw materials sufficient for treating small numbers of patients are obtained through suitcase smuggling.

It has to be acknowledged that the push for better licensing controls has not been universally supported. It is felt by some that there is a threat to the existence of many products, which may be withdrawn by producers if the cost of complying with new legislation makes the product too expensive to market.[37]

The practice of medical herbalism

The herbal practitioner

The herbal practitioners' activities are covered by Part III of the Supply of Herbal Remedies Order 1977, which lists remedies that may be used in the surgery during a consultation. There are special exemptions through the terms of the Medicines Act 1968 [Sections 12(1) and 56 (2)]. Conditions that need to be satisfied include the following:

- The practitioner must supply remedies from premises in private practice 'so as to exclude the public'.
- The maximum permitted dose must not be exceeded for a list of certain remedies.
- The practitioner must exercise his or her personal judgement in the physical presence of the patient prior to prescribing treatment.
- For systemic treatment, remedies are subject to a maximum dose restriction – all labelling on these medicines must clearly show the date, correct dosage and instructions for use.
- Proper clinical records must be kept.
- Herbal practitioners often prepare their own tinctures, using ethanol, for which registration with Customs and Excise is required.

Training of herbalists

Prospective members of the UK National Institute for Medical Herbalists, a professional body that accredits courses of training, are expected to follow a programme of academic study (normally 3–5 years' duration) and to complete a minimum of 500 h of clinical training.

Schools and universities offering courses in herbal medicine must apply to the National Institute for Medical Herbalists Accreditation Board and pass through the accreditation procedure to enable their graduates to become practising members of the National Institute for Medical Herbalists. Each course must reach the minimum standards as set out in the Accreditation Board's guidelines. Core subjects studied include anatomy, physiology, pathology, diagnosis, pharmacology, pharmacognosy, botany, materia medica, communication skills and complementary medicine, as well as nutritional and herbal therapeutics. Critical skills and research methodology are also required. Clinical practice is supervised by experienced practitioners.

Applications of herbalism

A wide range of conditions respond to treatment and/or management with herbal medicines. Herbal medicine may be used alone or to complement other orthodox or non-orthodox treatments. Some of the most common conditions are listed below. The list is not meant to be exhaustive but is designed to give some idea of the scope of what may be achieved. For further detailed information the reader is referred to the excellent text by Mills and Bone from which Table 5.3 is adapted.[38]

Herbalism and pharmacy

Most pharmacists are likely to become involved with herbalism through the sale of OTC products that are prepackaged and labelled with indications and instructions. The Royal Pharmaceutical Society of Great

Table 5.3 Applications of herbalism in common conditions

Generalised conditions
- Autoimmune conditions
- Acute inflammation of muscles, joints and connective tissues
- Psoriasis and other skin conditions

Debility
- Chronic fatigue syndrome
- Fatigue and debility after illnesss
- Fatigue linked to depression
- Support during terminal illness

Fevers
- Fevers resulting from infectious causes
- Febrile symptoms of non-infectious origin

Infectious disease
Unlike homeopathy, which is not directly effective on body invaders, herbalism may be used in these circumstances. The following conditions respond:

- Acute gastrointestinal, respiratory and urinary infections
- Topical bacterial infections
- Minor to moderate febrile infections
- Minor to moderate chronic bacterial, fungal and viral infections

Malignant diseases
- Cancers of varying types
- Symptoms resulting from cancer
- Problems with body systems

Table 5.3 continued

Cardiovascular system
- Hypertension
- Angina
- Ongoing symptoms of cardiac disease
- Recuperation from cardiac disease

Gastrointestinal system
- Dyspepsia, gastrointestinal reflux
- Food intolerance and allergies
- Constipation and diarrhoea

Genitourinary system
- Urinary tract infections
- Benign prostate hypertrophy
- Impaired lactation

Menopausal problems
- Premenstrual syndrome

Nervous system
- Anxiety states
- Insomnia
- Nervous exhaustion
- Pain control
- Stress symptoms

Respiratory system
- Upper respiratory tract infections
- Allergic rhinitis
- Bronchitis
- Asthma

Skin diseases
- Acne
- Allergic reactions
- Eczema

Adapted from Mills and Bone.[38]

Britain (RPSGB) has produced a factsheet on herbal products that gives useful information.[39] It notes that pharmacists supplying herbal products have a professional responsibility not to recommend any product where they have any reason to doubt its safety or quality, and only to offer advice on herbal products if they have appropriate knowledge. Whenever possible, only licensed products should be offered for sale.

It is possible to dispense herbal preparations extemporaneously in response to requests for assistance, similar to homeopathic counter prescribing. There is a small, but growing market for dispensing herbal prescriptions. One large UK multiple is installing herbal dispensaries in a selected number of its stores. New Zealand has an excellent example of combining orthodox and herbal practice (Figures 5.3 and 5.4).

When to use herbalism

Herbal medicine is particularly useful in two situations:

- Where a well-established herbal compound is used for a short, self-limiting condition such as a cold or the flu, for which other OTC remedies would normally be appropriate, the course of treatment is not more than a couple of weeks and no serious adverse effects have been reported in the scientific literature. Examples are the use of Echinacea to ward off or reduce the effects of a cold or ginger to prevent motion sickness.

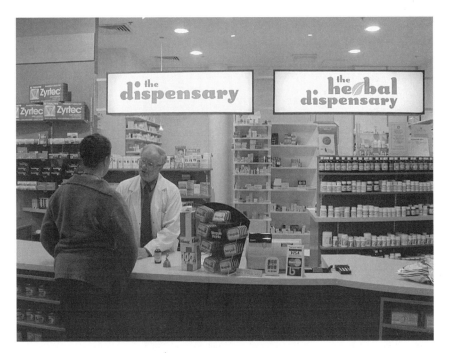

Figure 5.3 Integrating orthodox and herbal pharmacy at the Meridian Pharmacy, Dunedin, New Zealand.

- In the case of a more serious or ongoing illness, where no effective orthodox treatment exists and where there is some evidence from the scientific literature that a particular herbal compound may help. In this kind of situation, it is extremely important that the person is under the close supervision of a physician well versed in the disease in question and who has reviewed the available studies on the herb to be used. An example of this situation is the use of milk thistle extract in the treatment of cirrhosis of the liver.

Because of all of the problems with dosage, testing and the presence of toxins in herbs, there is an understandable temptation to rely on conventional pharmaceuticals in the OTC environment. However, herbs remain one of the few inexpensive sources of treatment for a number of conditions. Ginkgo biloba appears to be one of the only compounds that is claimed to improve memory (as opposed to stimulants, which improve concentration only). It may even slow the progression of Alzheimer's disease. Milk thistle is one of only a handful of compounds that may reverse liver damage.

Herbs remain the primary medicinal agents for most people in the Third World – the majority of the world's population.

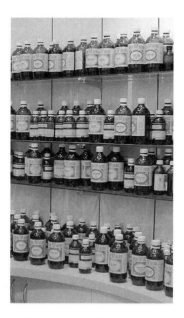

Figure 5.4 Herbal tincture dispensing stock.

Presentation of OTC products

Oral dose forms

Personal experience suggests that the availability of herbal specialities in elegant OTC pharmaceutical presentations as tablets or capsules (Figures 5.5 and 5.6) has provided a quick and easy way of self-treating. An important advantage of this form of dosage is that palatability is greatly improved. However, these tablets do not allow the same flexibility in the dose regime as liquid or crude drug formulations. Furthermore, it has been suggested that the substantial amount of processing required in making tablets and capsules may cause some denaturing of the active

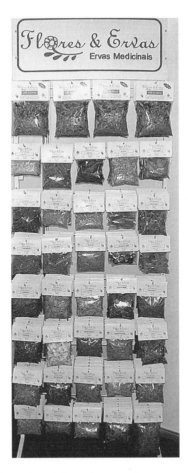

Figure 5.5 Display of powdered drugs for over-the-counter supply (Brazil).

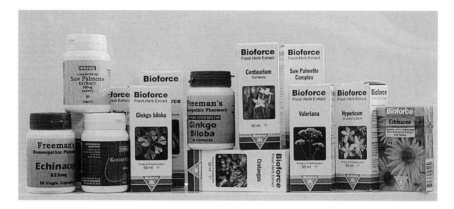

Figure 5.6 Examples of common branded and generic over-the-counter herbal products.

herbal principals. In addition, as such tablets usually contain purified ingredients, the synergistic effect will be lost.

Powdered drugs have a substantial therapeutic advantage in that all the active constituents are included in the dose form rather than just those obtained during the extraction process. Drugs containing tannins are best given as powder because tannins are only slowly dissolved from the herb matrix and are therefore still being released in an active form when the powdered herb reaches the colon.[40] It is important to give instructions to consume water along with or after ingestion of a powder, depending on the nature of the medicine being taken.

Topical products

A wide range of topical OTC products are available, including creams, gels, lotions and ointments. There have been some problems with the adulteration of Chinese herbal ointments (see section on safety issues, below).

Applications for topical formulations   Conditions that may be treated with topical herbal preparations include:

- burns
- infestations
- minor wounds and skin abrasions
- oral inflammatory conditions
- rheumatic conditions
- skin eruptions
- soft-tissue injuries, e.g. muscular sprains and strains.

Examples of the therapeutic classes of topical medicines

Demulcents   These are herbs with a soothing effect on the skin. These are generally mucilages that form the basis of creams and poultices. Aloe vera, marshmallow (*Althaea*) and slippery elm bark (*Ulmus fulva*) are examples.

Anti-inflammatories   Marigold (Calendula) and camomile (*Matricaria chamomilla*) both possess anti-inflammatory properties and are used to treat skin inflammations. Echinacea is another example (Figure 5.7). Knitbone (Symphytum) is also claimed to be effective. In an open uncontrolled study, 105 patients with locomotor system symptoms were treated twice daily with an ointment containing a Symphytum active substance complex.[41] A clear therapeutic effect was noted on chronic and subacute symptoms, which were accompanied mainly by functional disturbances and pain in the musculature. The preparation was effective against muscle pain, swelling and overstrain. Activity was weaker against degenerative conditions, for which the ointment may have an adjuvant role with the aim of improving muscular dysfunction and alleviating pain.

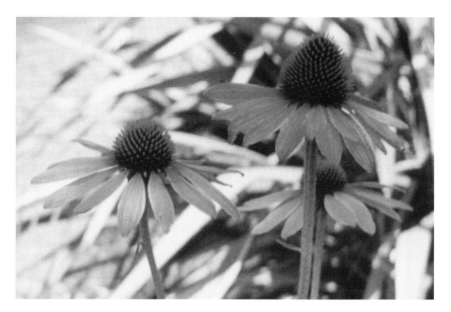

Figure 5.7 *Echinacea purpurea*, often called 'the herbal antibiotic'.

Antiseptics and disinfectants[42]   This section gives an indication of just how many herbal remedies may be available for a given application. Furthermore, most of this chapter has been written with reference to European herbs; in this section some examples of the plethora of traditional herbs from the native Antipodean communities are included.

Antiseptic literally means 'against putrefaction' or 'prevention of sepsis' but the term is usually used to describe agents applied to living tissues in order to destroy or inhibit the growth of infectious microorganisms. Disinfectants kill pathogenic agents and usually involve inanimate surfaces. Some naturally occurring remedies possess antimicrobial effects, and are effective in topical formulations as antiseptics and disinfectants.

Although the bacterial origin of infection was unknown before Pasteur's work in Paris and Lister's work at Glasgow Royal Infirmary, antiseptics and disinfectants have been used empirically since the ancient Egyptians started embalming bodies.

What follows is a review of the most common natural (i.e. nonsynthetic) antiseptics and disinfectants. Many have no apparent scientific explanation for their action, but are nevertheless still in use, relying on the users' cultural traditions for maintaining a belief in efficacy.

Bilberry (*Vaccinium myrtilus*)   Also known as huckleberry, the bilberry is related to the blueberry and cranberry. The fruit contains 7% tannic acid and a blue pigment, and is used, occasionally with the leaves, in an antiseptic mouthwash, together with the roots of the anti-inflammatory herb Tormentilla (*Potentilla* spp.). The latter contains 15–20% tannic acid and a red pigment and is used as an infusion on cuts, wounds, abrasions and sunburn.

Blackcurrant (*Ribes nigrum*)   This aromatic perennial shrub was formerly used in folk medicine as an infusion or gargle to treat sore throats. It is not considered to be of great medical importance now.

Burnet saxifrage (*Pimpinelia saxifraga*)   This herb is native to Europe, but has been introduced and naturalised in New Zealand and the USA. It may be used as a gargle or externally, as a poultice or bath, to treat wounds.

Herb bennet (*Geum urbanum*)   This can be applied to wounds to reduce inflammation and used as a gargle for sore gums and halitosis. It is rarely used now, except in folk medicine.

Hop (*Humulus lupulus*)   Native to northern temperature zones, the hop is best known for its involvement in brewing. A weak antibiotic, it has been used for urinary infections, and also occasionally as an application for skin conditions.

Horsetail (*Equisetum arvense*)   Horsetail or bottlebrush is native to Europe and thrives on moist wasteground. It contains silicic acid and a number of water-soluble silicic compounds, and is used in a poultice to aid wound healing. It is a mild antiseptic and is useful for eczema.

Juniper (*Juniper communis*)   Juniper is applied externally to wounds and, with garlic, rosemary and Echinacea, it is used in poultices. It is also used internally as a urinary antiseptic, especially in cystitis.

Marjoram, wild (*Organum vulgare*)   Native to Europe, although now cultivated elsewhere, this herb grows on hillsides and in dry woodland. It has an aromatic scent. It may be used externally in baths, inhalants or poultices where an antiseptic action is required.

Nettle, stinging (*Urtica dioica*)   A major ingredient of this oil is formic acid, with varying amounts of histamine, chlorophyll, iron, plant enzymes and minerals. In the stinging hairs there is a nettle poison. Nettle is popular as an external application.

Peppermint (*Mentha piperita*)   One of the oldest and best-known European medicinal herbs, peppermint is said to produce a gentle disinfectant effect (preventing fermentation) when there are abnormal decomposition processes in the stomach. Both the herb and its oil may be used externally in baths to treat cuts and skin rashes. The oil contains about 50% menthol.

Sage, common (*Salvia officinalis*)   This has been used as the constituent of a gargle, together with acriflavine and benzocaine. Another effective mixture is to bring equal parts of camomile flowers and sage leaves to the boil with milk, then cover the mixture and leave it to infuse. This can then be used as an antiseptic mouthwash.

Savory, summer (*Satureja hotyrndid*)   This is most commonly used as a culinary herb, but it also possesses medicinal properties and is an effective antiseptic gargle. Winter savory (*Satureja montana*) has similar properties.

Silver birch (*Betula pendula*) This deciduous tree can grow up to 20 m in height, and is common throughout central and northern Europe. The infusion is said to be a diuretic, while the buds and leaves may be added to bathwater to obtain a mild antiseptic action.

Speedwell, common (*Veronica officianlis*)   The speedwell is still listed in the herbal materia medica, but its efficacy is uncertain. It is included in cough mixtures as a weak expectorant with some antiseptic properties.

Tea tree oil (*Melaleuca*)   Tea tree leaves contain about 2% of a pale lemon-coloured volatile oil with a strong nutmeg odour. The oil comprises about 60% terpenes and has germicidal activity. A study has found the oil to be effective in vitro against *Staphylococcus aureus* (see Chapter 7).[43]

Thyme, garden (*Thymus vulgaris*)   Garden thyme is widely used as a culinary herb, being cultivated since the sixteenth century. The German apothecary Neuman first isolated the plant's essential oil in 1725 and this powerfully antiseptic substance is still used in pharmaceutical preparations. The oil contains up to 40% thymol. It has rubefacient properties.

Thyme, wild (*Thymus serpyllum*)   This is used in herb baths and pillows. It is also used as a poultice with onion, myrrh and melilot.

Wormwood (*Artemesia absinthium*)   Also known as absinthe or green ginger, wormwood is one of the most bitter herbs, but despite this has been a major ingredient of aperitifs and herb wines. Vermouth is a French variation of the original German name *Wemut*. It is thought to have antiseptic properties and may be used externally as a liniment.

Wintergreen and **myrrh** are also used with other herbs in poultices and decoctions. Other herbs said to have antiseptic properties include **fennel**, **hyssop** and **nasturtium** species.

Astringents Decoctions of tannin-containing drugs suspended in gum tragacanth are used to treat wounds. Examples are witch hazel (Hamamelis) and tormentil root (*Potentilla*).

Other formulations Other formulations include bath additives, inhalations (e.g. camomile), mucilages (e.g. slippery elm), plasters (e.g. belladonna and cayenne), poultices (e.g. comfrey and marshmallow) and suppositories. Mullein oil (Verbascum) is used as eardrops for deafness associated with earwax; eyebright (Euphrasia) is used for the eyes. Ideally both preparations should be sterile and extreme caution should be exercised in preparing them extemporaneously to minimise the chances of bacterial contamination. Eyebright, in liquid form, is often bought by clients to use as an eye wash. It should always be diluted with freshly boiled and cooled water before use.

Responding to requests for advice

Information to help colleagues respond to requests for advice is provided at the end of this chapter.

Counselling patients

Pharmacists should discourage the use of herbal products by patients when the source, active ingredients and composition are uncertain. Also, the consumption of herbs and herbal preparations by patients on certain medications should be controlled, monitored or avoided when the active ingredient is known to act either antagonistically or synergistically with the prescribed medication. Such safety issues are addressed in detail below.

It is prudent to counsel self-treating clients to observe the following guidelines:

- Try to choose a remedy that is specific for the condition being treated; if in doubt, seek advice from the pharmacist or health shop assistant.
- If you are taking OM seek advice from the pharmacist about the likelihood of interactions.
- Do not take several medicines concurrently unless specifically directed to do so by a qualified medical herbalist.
- Use the lowest dose appropriate for the symptoms being treated; if a little works, a lot more will not necessarily work better and may be dangerous.
- Make sure you understand the dosage instructions.

- If symptoms do not improve significantly within 7 days, seek advice from your family doctor.
- Do not self-treat for lengthy periods without seeking professional help to ensure that appropriate medication is being used.

Pregnant and nursing mothers

An American study has investigated the frequency of use of herbal and alternative medicine by women during pregnancy.[44] Two hundred and fifty pregnant women attending antenatal clinics were prospectively enrolled in a cross-sectional survey about the use of herbal and alternative medical therapies. Two hundred and forty-two women completed surveys (97%). Of the respondents, 9.1% reported use of herbal supplements during the current pregnancy; 7.5% were using these agents at least weekly. The herbs most commonly used during pregnancy were garlic, aloe, camomile, peppermint, ginger, Echinacea, pumpkin seeds and ginseng. There are no comparative statistics for the UK but it is likely that the use is rather less due to the fact that in the USA these products are considered to be food supplements whereas in the UK they are medicines.

Pregnant and lactating women should be as careful about medicinal herbs as they are about conventional medicines.[45] Some compounds in herbs can cross the placenta and may be linked to birth defects or other problems in newborns. Some herbs may be passed to babies via breast milk. The use of black and blue cohosh, feverfew, garlic, ginseng and St John's wort during pregnancy is not recommended. Valerian is not recommended for lactating women (see materia medica section). The remedy Caulophyllum is also contraindicated.[46] In homeopathy this remedy is actually recommended for administration immediately prior to and during childbirth.

Lavender (*Lavendula angustifolia*) is one herbal remedy that is recommended for administration during pregnancy and for postpartum support. Dandelion (*Taraxacum officinales*), nettle (*Urtica dioica*) and red raspberry leaf (*Rubus idaeus*) are also used for this purpose.

An Australian trial that examined the safety and efficacy of raspberry leaf products consumed by a group of 51 mothers during their pregnancy, by comparison with a group of 57 mothers who did not, found that this herb can be consumed by women during their pregnancy to shorten labour with no identified side-effects for the women or their babies.[47] The findings also suggested that women who ingest raspberry leaf might be less likely to receive an artificial rupture of their membranes, or require a caesarean section, forceps or vacuum birth than the women in the control group.

Cranberry juice may provide a useful alternative to OM for the treatment and prophylaxis of urinary tract infection caused by *Escherichia coli* in pregnant women.[48]

The dietary balance of fatty acids is important, and is usually expressed in terms of ratios, comparing omega-6 oils to omega-3 oils.[49] It has been suggested that the most beneficial ratio for human brain function is a 1:1 mixture of the two. The actual ratio for most people in industrialised nations is estimated to be from 20:1 to 30:1 in favour of omega-6 oils. In mother's breast milk the ratio may be as high as 45:1. Infant feeds are estimated to have a ratio of about 10:1. Supplementing with omega-3 oils during pregnancy is often recommended. Flax (and fish) oils are the main sources but could have an adverse effect during pregnancy due to the lignan content.[50]

Pediatric use

Although most medicines have similar actions in persons of all age groups, the required dosage and potential adverse reactions tend to vary. This must be taken into consideration when prescribing for children, particularly infants. Children and infants are much more sensitive than adults to the effects of all medicines and so herbs should be given to these patients with great care. Doses should be carefully calculated. The following formulae may be used to calculate the appropriate amounts of herbs to be administered to children:

Clark's rule:

$$\frac{\text{Weight in lb}}{150} \times \text{adult dose} = \text{child's dose}$$

Young's rule (for children 2 years and older)

$$\frac{\text{Age in years}}{\text{Age in years} + 12} \times \text{adult dose} = \text{child's dose}$$

Body surface area (BSA)

$$\frac{\text{BSA child}}{1.73} \times \text{adult dose} = \text{child's dose}$$

where 1.73 = average adult BSA

There are three main advantages in using herbal medicines for children:[51]

- Many phytomedicines have a relatively good benefit:risk ratio.
- Many herbal medicines for pediatric use fall into the gentle classification, with actions that are perfectly adequate for children.
- The methods of administration (e.g. inhalation, baths, ointments and syrups) commonly used in phytotherapy are particularly acceptable to children; this, together with the cooperation of parents, who are often in favour of this therapy, provides for good concordance.

However, there is also a potential risk to children resulting from unintended access to medication. The accidental ingestion of a diuretic herbal medicine by a 2-year-old, requiring hospital admission and electrolyte monitoring, has prompted one physician to call for the mandatory use of child-resistant closures on containers bought OTC in the UK.[52] The degree of control demanded of prescribable drugs does not extend to those of herbal type. In view of the increasing use of such medicines, there is likely to be an increased risk of accidental ingestion. Childproof containers should be a legal requirement for herbal medicines and parents should be cautioned to store such medicines out of the reach of children.

Liquid preparations are extremely useful for children, although the taste may be rather unpalatable, because the dose can be easily and accurately adjusted down to very small amounts with the aid of an oral syringe.

Caution should be exercised in applying camomile products to the gums of teething children. Valerian should not be given to children under the age of 3 years (see materia medica section).

The elderly

Interaction between medicinal herbs is a major concern, especially for elderly patients, who may well be taking a substantial portfolio of prescription drugs. It may not be possible to obtain satisfactory answers to questions about the names of these drugs, partly because patients may have forgotten the name or because they have been taking the medicines for so long they do not consider them to be worthy of mention.

It may be better to recommend that such patients take homeopathic medicines instead of herbal medicines in view of the lack of toxic effects with the former.

Sports care

In the quest to find energy for that extra hundredth of a second and the medal it may bring, sports persons are constantly seeking products to enhance performance. Word goes from mouth to mouth about some new discovery and it is taken without too much thought for safety or even legality. Ginseng is one such example. Unfortunately, these drugs are often obtained in less developed countries where control is non-existent and adulterants, the names of which do not appear on the label, may be on the International Olympic Committee list of banned substances.

As a general rule, athletes should be instructed not to take herbal remedies unless they can be certain of purity.

Evidence

Many orthodox treatments were originally taken from herbal use, and the majority of conventional drug prescriptions are still said to have a plant-derived component, but recent renewed interest has focused on the traditional use of whole-plant products. Western mainstream research has lagged behind the public shift in usage and this style of evidence is in its early stages of development. For all complementary and alternative medicine (CAM), the Cochrane Collaboration on Complementary Medicine as of March 2000 noted 4700 randomised controlled trials (RCTs) and 204 systematic reviews, of which 1561 trials relating to herbalism met the required criteria.[53]

The investigations that have been carried out on herbal medicines vary widely. St John's wort, for example, has been extensively studied using both in vivo (animal and human) and in vitro studies. Other medicines have been much less studied and rely on folkloric evidence for continued use. For a thorough evaluation of herbal products the following procedures should ideally be performed:

- The active principal should be isolated and investigated.
- An extract from the entire plant from which the active principal was isolated should be investigated.
- A comparison of the herbal preparation with a similar synthetic pharmaceutical product should be carried out in a randomised double-blind trial.

Such a rigorous investigation is well beyond the resources of most manufacturers. For now, most of the evidence base remains traditional knowledge and experience based on centuries of use, centred on clinical effectiveness. The principal sources are:

- bibliographical – compiled from literature; meta-analysis of research studies
- observational studies – audit
- clinical experience – anecdotal
- scientific analysis to identify active ingredients
- RCTs where possible (still limited, partly from resource constraints).

These sources have formed the basis of most current herbal pharmacopoeias, for example the German Commission E monographs[54] have reviewed existing data and traditional knowledge, and then applied the principle of reasonable certainty. These monographs have been criticised in recent months since they are expert opinion rather than reviews. The monographs of the European Scientific Cooperative on Phytotherapy (ESCOP) provide another source of information.

Evidence for applications, where it exists, is quoted in the materia medica and repertory sections at the end of this chapter.

Reasons for negative outcomes

There exist a number of reasons why clients do not observe a positive outcome after taking herbal remedies.

- The most obvious is that an inappropriate treatment has been chosen.
- Clients may have used old herbs (herbs lose potency with age and the herbs on some health food store shelves are literally years old).
- Clients may be using powdered herbs in capsules when really an extract is the only way to get a dose concentrated enough for physiological effect (gingko biloba is an example of a herb best used in concentrate form). Even using fresh herbs, many people do not brew medicinal teas correctly. Such a tea should be quite concentrated and the technique for making it is more elaborate than just dumping a teabag in water and letting it sit for a couple of minutes.
- Clients may also not have used the herb in a manner that delivers the active agent. In many herbs (for example, valerian) the active ingredient is an oil and so not soluble in water. Hence, steeping the herb in water and brewing a tea will not produce much of the active compound. In these cases, extracts in oil or glycerine (or sometimes in alcohol) or directly consuming the powdered herb are the best way to deliver the agent.
- Inappropriate dose regimes may also be responsible for a negative result (see the section on incorrect dosage or instructions below).

Safety

Herbal remedies are complex mixtures of chemicals, many of which have not been subjected to rigorous testing. Unlike homeopathy, material doses are being administered, and given the non-standardisation of many of the medicines, it is quite likely that instances of adverse drug reactions will occur, particularly as the number of people using herbalism is rising at a substantial rate.

In this section the major potential sources of problems are discussed.

Lack of appropriate treatment

Incomplete practitioner education, leading to individuals prescribing outwith their limits of competence, and inappropriate self-treatment have implications for safety issues. Conditions that are not treated correctly because of misdiagnosis or because they were missed altogether may become more acute or lead to the lengthening of incapacitation.

Toxic effects and interactions

Many people who use herbal preparations believe that such preparations are safe in all respects because they are naturally occurring; they think that all the active ingredients fall into the gentle group classification. In fact this is far from the truth and some herbal preparations can be potentially dangerous, even in therapeutic doses. Comfrey (Symphytum) was found to contain pyrrolizidine alkaloids in quantities that could be hepatotoxic[55] and it was withdrawn from sale in its crude form some years ago. Other herbal species (e.g. coltsfoot, Echinacea and Senecio) also contain pyrrolizidines but remain available.

An initial surveillance of case enquiries between 1983 and 1988 and in 1981 by the US National Poisons Unit identified 5563 enquiries related to traditional herbal medicines and food supplements. Following a detailed assessment, a link was found between exposure and reported clinical effects in 49 cases, indicating a need for continuous surveillance of such exposures.[56] The patient's age, genetic constitution, nutritional state, concomitant diseases and concurrent medication may affect the risk and severity of adverse events, as can consumption of large amounts or a wide variety of herbal preparations or long-term use.[57] However, a number of other factors make an assessment of adverse effects associated with herbal products more complex than for pharmaceuticals. A classification has been reported for adverse reactions from herbal products.[58]

Intrinsic effects[59]

Intrinsic effects are adverse effects that result from the herb itself and may be either predictable and dose-dependent, or unpredictable.[60] Yohimbine, an alkaloid found in the bark of the tree *Pausinystalia yohimbe*, has α_2-adrenoceptor antagonistic activity, and is taken for male impotence. It can cause hypertension and anxiety in a predictable dose-related manner. The drug has also been found to have an unpredictable reaction and is known to cause a serious bronchospasm in some patients.[61] Comfrey has already been mentioned above; another example of a drug causing concern is Aristolochia (see below).[62]

Four popular herbal supplements are currently being subjected to safety checks under the US National Toxicology Program.[63] The programme, a coalition of agencies that includes the FDA, the National Institutes of Health and the Centers for Disease Control and Prevention, is testing aloe vera, which is commonly used to soothe burned skin, but is increasingly common as a beverage, with claims that it can fight disease by 'cleansing' the digestive tract. It can cause skin irritation.[64] Researchers have noted some similarities between aloe vera and croton oil, a known carcinogen. The other herbs being investigated are ginseng, kava and milk thistle. More than 30 substances are tested by the programme each year through rodent and in vitro studies. No human subjects are used.

Intrinsic effects also include the effects resulting from misuse, accidental overdose or interactions with orthodox pharmaceuticals. Excessive doses of ginseng, considered to be abuse of the remedy, have been reported to cause agitation, insomnia and raised blood pressure. Similar abuse of liquorice may cause oedema and hypertension. An Australian patient who overdosed on a herbal laxative taken as a weight control remedy suffered neuropathy and coma.[65] The remedy contained podophyllin.

Interactions between medicinal herbs and OM are a major concern for the clinical herbalist.[66] Herbal preparations may be inducers of various drug-metabolising enzymes.[67] This may result in a reduction in the blood levels and therapeutic effect of some medicines metabolised by these enzymes. Because the level of active ingredients may vary from one preparation to another, and patients may switch between preparations, the degree of induction is likely to vary. Concurrent use of herbs may mimic, magnify or oppose the effect of drugs. The following examples serve to illustrate the problem:

- The UK Committee on the Safety of Medicine has recommended that St John's wort should not be used with ciclosporin, digoxin, indinavir, oral contraceptives, theophylline and warfarin. It is thought that St John's wort affects neurotransmitters in the brain and may interact with psychotropic medicines, including selective serotonin reuptake inhibitors.

- Kava (*Piper methysticum*) has gained recent popularity because of its relaxing effects, both as a recreational herb and as a treatment for anxiety.[68] A recent case report suggests caution before using kava along with benzodiazepine drugs. A patient apparently lapsed into a 'semicomatose state' due to an interaction between kava and the drug alprazolam (Xanax).[69] The benzodiazepines generally lose effect within 8–12 h, but secondary metabolites capable of interacting with other substances linger in the blood for 24 h or more afterwards. Interactions between alcohol and the benzodiazepine drugs are well known – alcohol potentiates their effects – but herbal interactions have not been studied or previously recorded.

- Another example is the concurrent use of ginkgo biloba and the so-called blood-thinning agents.[70] This provides a significant risk. The potentisation caused by using a herb with a similar pharmacological effect[71] could provoke a serious bleeding disorder. The risk is probably greatest with concurrent use of heparin, warfarin and coumarin derivatives, but recent anecdotes indicate that interactions may also occur with aspirin. Another report describes a case of spontaneous bleeding into the eye from the iris within a week of the start of daily treatment in a patient who had been taking ginkgo and aspirin.[72]

- Potentiation of oral and topical corticosteroids by liquorice has been reported.[73]

For a comprehensive list of the large number of potential interactions between orthodox drugs and herbal remedies, the reader is referred to the excellent book *Herbal Medicines* by Carol Newall and colleagues.[74] An abbreviated list of interactions is provided in Table 5.4.

It would be appropriate for pharmacists whose advice is sought on potential interactions to check that the medicines concerned do not fall into the same therapeutic group, when potentisation could occur, or into opposite therapeutic groups, when antagonism would be possible.

During the early part of this new century there was much discussion about the availability of St John's wort and the drug was restricted to private prescription in Ireland. There were two main

Table 5.4 Examples of potential interactions between orthodox medicines and herbal remedies

Orthodox drug type	Example of interacting herbal remedy	Potential outcome
Gastrointestinal		
Antacids	Comfrey	Exacerbation of symptoms
Antidiarrhoeals	Senna	Antagonist effect
Laxatives	Senna	Potentiation
Cardiovascular		
Antihypertensives	Garlic, hawthorn	Potentiation
	Blue cohosh, ginger	Antagonist effect
Beta-blockers	Coltsfoot	Antagonist effect
	Alfalfa	Hypertension
Diuretics	Garlic, ginger, St John's wort	Difficulty in controlling diuresis, hypertension
Respiratory		
Antiallergics	St John's wort, valerian	Potentiation of drowsiness associated with antihistamines
Central nervous system		
Analgesics	Dandelion, elder	Increased risk of toxicity with non-steroidal anti-inflammatory drugs
	Liquorice	Decreased plasma concentration of drug
Antidepressants	Comfrey, ginseng	Hypotension with monoamine oxidase inhibitors
	St John's wort	Antagonist effect
Antiepileptics	Borage, evening primrose, sage	May enhance risk of seizure
Anxiolytics, hypnotics	Hops, valerian, St John's wort	Potentiation
Endocrine		
Antidiabetic	Alfalfa, damiana	Potentiation
	Devil's claw, ginseng	Antagonist effect
Hypo- and hyper-thyroidism drugs	Fucus, horseradish, myrrh	Interfere with orthodox therapy
Corticosteroids	Dandelion, elder	Increased potassium loss
	Liquorice	Increased water and sodium retention
Oral contraceptives	Alfalfa, ginseng, St John's wort	Reduction in effectiveness

Adapted from Newall C A, Anderson L A, Philipson J D. *Herbal Medicines: A Guide for Healthcare Professionals*. London: Pharmaceutical Press, 1996: 277–280.

reasons for this action, including possible interactions with a number of common medicines, such as anticoagulant drugs and oral contraceptives, and an assertion that people should not really be self-treating anxiety and depression, albeit of a mild variety. At the time of writing the position remains unsettled but murmurings about a possible restriction in the UK are still circulating.

Herbal drugs may be used recreationally, the best example being cannabis; repeated use may lead to dependence and behavioural changes. Although its use is currently illegal in the UK, several trials are seeking to establish medicinal applications, particularly for the treatment of pain. A recent recreational development involves the use of an obscure hallucinogenic Mexican herb *Salvia divinorum*, which is chewed or smoked. It is supplied in the UK in dried form, ostensibly as incense. Leaves may be 'enhanced' by impregnation with the hallucinogen salvinorin A.

Some culinary herbs also contain potentially toxic constituents. The safe use of these herbs is ensured by limiting the level of constituent allowed in a particular food product to a level not considered to represent a health hazard. The irritant principal present in the volatile oil of parsley, apiole, is said to be both abortifacient and hepatotoxic.[75] Excessive ingestion of ginseng may cause agitation, insomnia and raised blood pressure.

Examples of the adverse effects that may occur with herbal ingredients are summarised in Table 5.5. They include allergic, cardiac, hepatic, hormonal, irritant, purgative and toxic effects.

Extrinsic effects

Other sources of potential danger in the use of herbal medicines are associated with a number of extrinsic effects related to problems in commercial manufacture or extemporaneous compounding.

Failure of good manufacturing practice The failure of good manufacturing practice leads to inaccurate application (or even absence) of standard operating procedures and consequent batch-to-batch variability. This can be a serious problem with herbal preparations as the companies producing these items do not use adequate standards for quality, purity and reliability, uniformity and reproducibility of the herbal product.

Adulteration Herbal products should be free not only from toxic botanical adulterants but also from other contaminants such as substantial residues, pesticides (e.g. organic phosphates), toxic metals[76] (e.g arsenic, cadmium, lead or mercury) and even conventional pharmaceuticals (e.g.

Table 5.5 Examples of adverse drug reactions caused by herbal ingredients

Potential ADR caused by active ingredient	Active ingredient thought to cause ADR (if known)	Examples of herbs that could be implicated
Allergic		
Hypersensitivity	Sesquiterpene lactones	Arnica, feverfew
Phototoxicity	Furanocoumarins	Celery, wild carrot
Immunity problems	Canavanine	Alfalfa
Cardiac	Cardiac glycosides	Squill
Endocrine		
Hypoglycaemic		Alfalfa, ginseng
Hyperthyroid	Iodine	Fucus
Hormonal	Triterpenoids	Liquorice
	Isoflavonoids	Alfalfa
	Saponins	Ginseng
	Antiandrogenic agents	Saw palmetto
Irritant		
Gastrointestinal	Pyrrolizidine alkaloids	Comfrey
Renal	Aescin	Horse chestnut
Toxic		
Hepatotoxic	Pyrrolizidine alkaloids	Comfrey
Mitogenic	Proteins	Mistletoe
Convulsant	Volatile oil constituents	Camphor

Adapted from Newall C A, Anderson L A, Philipson J D. *Herbal Medicines: A Guide for Healthcare Professionals*. London: Pharmaceutical Press, 1996: 8.

corticosteroids or non-steroidal anti-inflammatory drugs).[77] This could lead to potential toxicity in overdose, the signs and symptoms of which are often recognised late.[78] In the USA it was reported that one case of arsenic poisoning resulting from the ingestion of herbal tea has occurred, and in another case small amounts of cocaine were said to have been found in two herbal teas. Topical presentations can also be a source of problems. A study found that eight of the 11 herbal creams being used by patients attending a medical practice (at a cost of up to £35 per week) contained the controlled steroid dexamethasone. Concentrations of the drug varied from 64 to 1500 µg/g,[79] with the highest concentration being prescribed for the face of a 4-month-old baby with eczema. Worryingly, the concentration of dexamethasone in creams prescribed for children was 5.2 times higher than that in those prescribed for adults. The risk of adverse reactions with such potent steroids is increased by their inappropriate use and application to areas of thin skin such as flexures and the face. Furthermore, many of the preparations were supplied in unlabelled containers without clear instructions. The authors called for closer regulation of herbal medicines to ensure adequate labelling and to prevent dispensing of unlicensed products in the guise of herbal treatments. Accidental contaminants may also include allergens, pollen, insect parts, moulds and mould spores.[80] Some plants come from nature with a microbial burden that needs to be reduced during processing.[81]

Misidentification The problem of nomenclature exists in herbalism as well as in homeopathy, with at least four different methods of naming plants: the common English name, the transliterated name from another language (often Chinese or Indian), the latinised pharmaceutical name and the scientific name.[82] It is important that physical and microscopic identification methods are used. This will ensure that the correct species of plant (and later, the correct part of the plant) according to the appropriate herbal pharmacopoeia is used to make the remedy.

Substitution Many herbal medicines do not have both the common and the Latin name of the herb on the label. The suspicion exists that some companies do not give the Latin name because the common name is shared by several different herbs, only one or two of which are medicinal (and therefore usually more expensive). There are several different species of ginseng with different properties and a wide variation in cost. By using only the common name, companies are able to substitute a less effective or even completely non-medicinal herb for the medicinal variety, without making untruthful declarations on the label.

A report of nine cases of nephritis in young women taking a Belgian slimming treatment[84] led to the discovery that *Aristolochia fangchi* containing the nephrotoxic component aristolochic acid had been introduced in place of *Stephania terrandra*. Eighty cases have now been identified, and many have developed terminal renal failure.

Lack of standardisation The amount of pharmacologically active ingredient available in a herbal remedy may vary widely from plant to plant, so accurately regulating dosage can be difficult. For example, glycyrrhizic acid, one of the primary pharmacologic agents in liquorice root, occurs naturally in concentrations ranging on average from 2 to 7%, and in some rare plants it is as high as 27%. A plant with a 7% glycyrrhizic acid concentration is delivering a dose more than twice that of a plant with a 2% concentration. It is therefore important to use a standardised herbal preparation whenever possible. Extracts of many herbs have been analysed for the percentage of active ingredient and adjusted so that every bottle contains the same amount. There are extracts of ginkgo biloba that are standardised to 24% ginkgoglides and in the USA a brand of echinacea has been standardised to 4% echinacosides. Some branded extracts refer to the percentage concentration of the raw herb present, rather than the amount of active principal, still leaving the problem of varying dosages. For example, the leading UK brand of tincture states on the label simply that 'the product has been prepared from *Echinacea purpurea* herb and root' and that '15 drops contains the equivalent of 285 mg of whole fresh plant or 64.5 mg of whole dried plant'. Another British supplier offers far more comprehensive information for its ginkgo biloba. The label states: 'each tablet provides on average ginkgo biloba extract 60 mg (equivalent to 300 mg of ginkgo biloba leaf) which has been standardised to contain 24% ginkgo flavine-glycosides, giving flavone-glycosides 1.4 mg ginkgolides and biloaliides 3.6 mg'. It should be acknowledged that standardisation is not possible in all cases. For many herbal medicines the active ingredients have not been isolated and in other cases no reliable quantitative test exists. Another difficulty may be that the wrong active ingredient is being used to standardise the herb. Hypericin is no longer thought to be the main active consituent of St John's wort, since the concentration of this product may be changed without an apparent change in antidepressant activity.[83]

Incomplete labelling There have been numerous incidents of herbal products, mainly obtained in or from less developed countries, that do not declare all constituents on the label. Thus, a mixture may contain herbs in addition to those declared as adulterants or substitutions. This could lead to adverse reactions or, in the case of a sports person, a positive drug test for a banned substance of which the unfortunate athlete had no knowledge.

Incorrect dosage or instructions In general terms herbal remedies are safe if used according to instructions and within a safe dosage range. There are so many different pharmaceutical forms in which medicines can be taken, some standardised and some not, that calculating the correct dose is difficult – in some cases impossible – for the client. It is important that guidance is given on the label. Dose suggestions given in texts often reflect a consensus opinion amongst herbal practitioners using different methods and philosophies, so there is no definitive answer to the question 'What is the recommended dose for this medicine?' The activity of crude plant material may differ from that of the purified constituents, as some constituents may modify the toxicity of others. Clear instructions are vital.

Monitoring adverse effects

The complexities of processing herbal medicine data in comparison with OM have been highlighted.[85] Areas of concern with respect to the safety of herbal medicines were also highlighted following the recent introduction of a classification system for herbal medicines.

Between 1968 and 1997, 8985 individual case reports received by the World Health Organization Adverse Reactions Monitoring Centre in Uppsala, Sweden, involved herbal medicines. Germany submitted the most reports (1796), followed by France (1479), the USA (1073) and the UK (993). The majority of reports concerned non-critical reactions. In 21 of the 2487 critical cases a fatality was involved. The number of reports for specific remedies was small, although it was possible to determine trends in some cases. For example, echinacea appeared to be responsible for acute hypersensitivity and anaphylaxis. The authors concluded that the adverse effects of herbal products were inadequately documented.[85]

The RPSGB recommends that any suspected adverse reactions in the UK should be reported to the Committee on Safety of Medicines using the yellow card system.

Conclusion

The information available on safety issues, whether from the comparatively small number of scientific investigations or from anecdotal data collected by both medical and non-medically qualified practitioners, forms the basis of advice that can be given to potential patients. Used judiciously, herbal remedies are as safe as OM but, like OM, the potential for non-beneficial outcomes if the medicines are used inappropriately is a real possibility.

The treatment of herbal poisoning[86]

• If contact dermatitis is caused by direct exposure to plants such as poison ivy, it should be treated by cleaning the area and offering symptomatic treatment, which may or may not include antihistamines. If a caustic plant such as rue comes into contact with the oral mucosa, milk may be given and the patient observed to make sure airway closure does not occur.

- Gastrointestinal distress is a common symptom of plant poisoning and may require ongoing fluid replacement.
- Renal toxicity and primary renal failure from plants such as rhubarb leaves and autumn crocus may require urinary alkalinisation to treat haemolysis, and correction of calcium balance to treat oxalate ingestion; rhubarb leaves are a good source of soluble oxalate salts.
- Herbal teas prepared from oleander, foxglove or lily of the valley may cause hyperkalaemia and heart block. Treatment may include use of muscarinic cholinergic blockers such as atropine and phenytoin, cardiac pacing and potassium-removal techniques.
- Ingestion of ergot alkaloids may cause arterial vasospasm; therapy may include close medical observation, nitroprusside or adrenergic blocking agents.
- Atropine-like symptoms produced by plants such as jimsonweed may require simple observation or the judicious use of physostigmine.
- Nicotine, found in both domestic and wild tobaccos, may produce sequential peripheral ganglionic stimulation, then blockade, and may result in seizures, paralysis and death. Treatment includes control of seizures and provision of ventilatory support.
- Ingestion of volatile oils such as pennyroyal or eucalyptus, which are irritants and central nervous system depressants, may cause seizures and aspiration. Medical personnel should observe the patient closely, and be ready to treat aspiration; the risk of aspiration may contraindicate induction of emesis. Non-oily cathartics may be used, since oily cathartics may increase absorption of the toxins.
- Plant resins, such as those found in American ipecac, flowering spurge and common spurge, may cause severe vomiting and catharsis, central nervous system effects and muscle weakness. There are no known antidotes; treatment includes reduction of gastrointestinal effects and maintenance of hydration.
- Plant alkaloids, such as those found in monkshood and Senecio, may produce jaundice and mimic alcoholism, hepatitis or Reye's syndrome. Treatment is supportive and will depend on the degree of hepatic failure. Plants such as pokeberries or poke weed, which contain certain mitogens, may cause severe gastroenteritis, respiratory stress or plasmacytosis. Treatment is symptomatic.

The Royal Pharmaceutical Society herbaria

The Royal Pharmaceutical Society's collection of dried plant specimens, plant extracts and plant parts of medicinal value was established in 1842,[87] to assist detailed investigations into crude drugs and the establishment of standards.[88] Zoological and mineral specimens were added later. Prior to this date drugs, foods and spices had for many years been subject to gross adulteration, simply because there were no standards by which they could be identified or their quality controlled. The herbaria and associated items (collectively referred to as a 'museum' in the literature) was originally housed on the ground floor at the Society's headquarters in 17 Bloomsbury Square, London.

A succession of professors from the School of Pharmacy took charge of the collection on a part-time basis until 1872 when Edward Morrell Holmes was appointed full-time curator at a salary of £150 per annum. Holmes is credited with setting up an active centre of study alongside the herbaria. He remained in charge for 50 years, after which the position became part-time again. One of Holmes' successors was Dr T. Wallis, who took over in 1925, researching, maintaining and extending the collection until Professor Jack Rowson was appointed full-time curator in 1948. Rowson developed the research potential of the museum until his departure in 1957. Dr Wallis then took control again with a technical assistant until 1969 when the collection was transferred to Bradford School of Pharmacy for 13 years,[89] a move that did not meet with universal approval within the profession,[90] but nevertheless prompted the unveiling of a plaque to commemorate the occasion.[91] When the University of Bradford informed the Society that it no longer wished to maintain the collection, the RPSGB Council decided that it should be gifted to the Royal Botanic Gardens, Kew,[92] where the herbaria became largely dispersed within the Economic Botany Collections (EBC) in 1983. The zoological and mineral specimens also went to Kew but have remained as a separate collection within the EBC. This proved to be a more popular arrangement.[93] The collections were subsequently moved to their present site in the Sir Joseph Banks building in 1989.[94]

The EBC was founded by the first official Director of the Gardens, Sir William Hooker. His rationale for establishing the EBC was:

> to render great service, not only to the scientific botanist, but to the merchant, the manufacturer, the physician, the chemist, the druggist, the dyer, the carpenter and the cabinet-maker and artisans of every description, who might here find the raw materials employed in their several professions correctly named.[95]

The 9000 specimens in the Society's herbaria range from south American strychnos, European mandrake root and African rauwolfia to Chinese rhubarb and arrow poisons from Borneo. There is a large and important selection of quinine barks, resins (e.g. frankincense and myrrh), specimens of aloe, cinnamon and opium poppy and a large seed collection. Associated documentation and correspondence concerning collection of the material make fascinating reading.

An indefinite exhibition of particularly interesting items from the EBC (including items clearly labelled as being from the RPSGB collection), entitled 'People and Plants', may be viewed at Kew during normal opening hours.

The complete EBC is not on public view but is available for study by prior arrangement with the curator.

Future directions for herbalism

It seems likely in the foreseeable future that the two streams of plant use will continue side by side. Whole plants will continue to be used as traditional herbal practices are expanded and integrated into orthodox medical practice, and active constituents will be isolated as a basis for the development of modern drugs. For both practices a large pool of plant material is available. This is diminishing fast, however; for example, in Madagascar 90% of forests has been lost in 15 years.

It seems critical to preserve and study the richness of this fauna, as well as the knowledge and experience of traditional healers and healing systems, especially for those peoples of the world who do not have access to, or cannot afford, pharmaceuticals. As western medicine extends to these people, models of integrated local clinics are appearing. Local herbalists are still using medicines from villagers' local forests, but now in cooperation with a doctor. Indeed, when there is a choice people are pluralistic. In Asia OM is used for symptomatic relief of acute conditions and traditional medicine for underlying and chronic problems. The so-called underdeveloped world has given a lead that the industrial world is beginning to follow.

Materia medica

The following is an abbreviated materia medica of common remedies.

Alfalfa (Lucerne)[96]

Source: The leaves and flowering tops of *Medicago sativa*.

Active ingredients: Alkaloids, coumarin derivatives, flavones, isoflavones, proteins and amino acids, sterols, sugars.

Uses: Aperient, bactericidal, cardiotonic, diuretic, emetic, stimulant.

Common applications: Urinary and bowel problems; peptic ulcer. Skin inflammation. Often used to treat arthritis and diabetes, but no firm clinical evidence of effectiveness exists.

Presentation: Infusions for internal and external use. Tablets also available.

Daily dose: 10–15 g.[97]

Adverse drug reactions (ADR): Alfalfa use in humans has been associated with systemic lupus erythematosus – an inflammatory connective tissue disease – other skin reactions, gastrointestinal disturbances and raised serum urate levels. Saponins interfere with the utilisation of vitamin E. Eating large quantities of alfalfa seeds over extended periods can cause reversible blood abnormalities.[98]

Aloe vera

Source: Prepared from the clear jelly-like mucilage obtained from the parenchymal tissue making up the inner portion of the leaves of *Aloe vera* (syn. *A. barbadensis*, *A. vulgaris*).[99]

Active ingredients: Mono- and polysaccharides, lipids, saponins, vitamins and minerals.[100]

Uses: Cathartic. Assists healing of wounds and burns, although evidence of latter confused.[101] Anti-inflammatory.

Common applications: Constituent of topical pharmaceutical and sunburn preparations. Included in various cosmetics, including hair-care products and bath additives.

Presentation: Gel, lotions, ointments and creams.

Daily dose: None documented.[74]

ADR: Often confused with aloes (dried leaf juice), which has a potent laxative action. Ingestion of gel adulterated with leaf juice may cause diarrhoea.

Camomile, German[102]

Source: Flowers of *Matricaria recutita* (or *M. chamomilla*).
Chamaemelum nobile (Roman camomile) is also used, but less widely.

Constituents:[103] A major component responsible for most of the plant's
medicinal qualities is known as alpha bisabolol. Other constituents
include a complex mixture of flavonoids (of which apigenin is an
important element) and coumarins, sesquiterpenoids and spiroethers.

Uses: Antiemetic, antispasmodic, mild sedative, anti-inflammatory and
wound healing.

Common applications: Digestive upset and indigestion, inflammation
of gastrointestinal tract, teething, inflammation of mucous membranes,
mild insomnia and anxiety.

Presentation: Dried flower heads, liquid extract, tincture, tea. Oral
preparations for infant colic and teething. External preparations, oint-
ments/creams (Kamillosan) for cracked nipples, nappy rash. Constituent of cosmetics and haircare products. Essential oil is also used.

Daily dose: 1.5–3.0 g camomile flowers, infusion, liquid extract and
tincture taken orally three times daily.

ADR: Individuals with a known allergy to ragweed, asters, chrysanthe-
mums and other botanical species related to *M. recutita* should be cautious in taking products containing German camomile.[104] Individuals
with existing asthma, urticaria or other allergic conditions should also
use camomile products with caution because of the possibility that their
symptoms will be exacerbated. The application of camomile products
to the gums of teething children is also cautioned against.[104] However,
despite this practice being relatively common, I have never been advised
of any adverse reaction. The reason for the warning is unclear; it may
relate to the potential induction of an allergenic response. Concentrated
tea may have an emetic effect; the infusion should not be allowed in
contact with the eyes.[105]

Cohosh, black[106]

Source: Rhizome and roots of *Cimicifuga racemosa*.

Constituents: Alkaloids, tannins, terpenoids, various acids and volatile
oils.

Uses: Some oestrogenic activity.

Common applications:[107] Stimulation of menstruation, treatment of menopausal symptoms, premenstrual syndrome (a main constituent of Lydia Pinkham's Vegetable Compound).

Presentation: Dried rhizome, liquid extract and tincture.

Daily dose: Dried rhizome 0.3–2 g or by decoction three times daily, 0.3–2 ml liquid extract (BP 1898), 2–4 ml tincture (BPC 1934).

ADR: Black cohosh is contraindicated in pregnancy; an overdose may cause premature birth.[108]

Cohosh, blue[109]

Source: Roots and rhizomes of *Caulophyllum thalictroides*.

Constituents: Alkaloids, saponins with a number of other compounds, including gum, resins and phosphoric acid.

Uses: Antispasmodic, antirheumatic.

Common applications: Amenorrhoea, threatened abortion and conditions associated with uterine atony.

Presentation: Dried rhizome or root and liquid extract.

Daily dose: Rhizome/root 0.3–1 g or by decoction three times daily. Liquid extract (1:1 in 70% alcohol) 0.5–1 ml three times daily.

ADR: Reputed to be abortifacient and should only be taken if required after labour has commenced, not during pregnancy. Self-treatment with this drug is generally considered inappropriate because of the nature of its action.

Echinacea[110]

Source: The rhizome and root of *Echinacea pallida* and *E. augustifolia* (USA) and whole plant of *E. purpurea* (Europe).

Constituents: Polysaccharides, glycoproteins, alkylamides and caffeic acid derivatives. Exact constituents vary with species.

Uses: Thought to be immunostimulant, increasing the body's healing powers. Thought to act indirectly by facilitating increased phagocyte activity rather than by acting on bacterial invaders directly. Stimulates cell-mediated immune system. Anti-inflammatory.

Common applications: Common cold, fevers, upper respiratory tract infections,[111] oral inflammation, minor skin abrasions and wounds.

Presentation: Liquid extract and tincture used to increase immunity in colds and flu. Capsules and external preparations used for boils, burns, inflammatory conditions, wounds.

Daily dose:[112] 6–9 ml of expressed juice (concentration = 2.5:1); tincture 30–60 drops three times daily.

ADR: Nausea. Maximum duration of use 8 weeks.[113] Individuals with allergies to the sunflower family (Asteraceae or Compositae) may experience mild allergic symptoms when ingesting echinacea.[30]

Feverfew[114]

Source: Aerial parts, especially leaves, of *Tanacetum parthenium* (syn. *Chrysanthemum parthenium*).

Constituents: Sesquiterpene lactones (parthenolide), flavonoids, melatonin.

Uses: Treatment and prevention of migraine.[115] Anti-inflammatory,[116] possible antiarthritic.[117] Suggested that it may inhibit prostaglandin production and serotonin.

Common applications: Migraine, arthritis.

Presentation: People may chew fresh leaves. Also available as air-dried or freeze-dried herb and as capsules or tablets containing dried herb. Also liquid extract.

Daily dose:[118] 50 mg–1.2 g of powdered leaf; three cups of infusion daily. 125 mg of dried feverfew leaf preparation standardised to 0.2% parthenolide daily.[119]

ADR: Mouth ulceration or gastric disturbance[120] and inflammation of lips and tongue.[102] May be contraindicated in pregnancy.

Garlic

Source: The fresh bulb of *Allium sativum*, cultivated worldwide.

Constituents: Sulphur-containing compounds (including aalicin, ajoenes and aliiin), enzymes (including alliinase), flavonoids.

Uses: Antihypertensive,[121] antithrombotic,[122] lipid-lowering agent,[123] antimicrobial. Protective effect against cancer.[124]

Common applications: Common cold, hypertension, gastrointestinal ailments, possibly including side-effects of paracetamol (acetamenophen),[125] cholesterol-lowering agent.[126] Garlic was called 'the great panacea' by Galen. The antiseptic action is said to be effective against bacteria acid fungi, and the cloves are used in India and China to treat amoebic dysentery.

Presentation: Available as dried powder, 'odourless' extracts, capsules. Sometimes eaten raw against colds and influenza.

Daily dose:[127] 1–2 fresh garlic cloves (about 4 g) or 8 mg essential oil.

ADR: Garlic should be avoided before undergoing surgical procedures due to possible postsurgical bleeding.[128] Heartburn, flatulence and gastrointestinal upset have been reported, usually at doses equivalent to five or more cloves daily.[129] Contact dermatitis (caused by direct skin contact with raw garlic) is also possible. A possible interaction with warfarin has been reported.[130] Garlic may be contraindicated in pregnancy and breastfeeding.[131] The odour of garlic is noticeable in the milk of lactating women who take the herb. This has been reported to cause colic in nursing children.

Ginger

Source: Usually powdered dried root of *Zingiberis officinalis*; may also be from whole fresh root, when it is known as green ginger.

Constituents: Oleoresins (gingerols and shogaols), essential oil (zigiberene).

Uses: Antiemetic, antinauseant, anti-inflammatory, antimicrobial. Possible gastroprotective and haematological properties.[132] Ginger is one of three most commonly used 'hot' remedies, the others being black pepper and cayenne pepper (*Capsicum*). They are given to stimulate metabolism and often act as a facilitating agent alongside other herbs whose stimulatory activity may be augmented.

Common applications: Loss of appetite, motion sickness,[133] inflammatory conditions.

Presentation: Dried herb, capsules, tea. Liniment for topical use.

Daily dose:[134] 2–4 g. The antiemetic dose is 2 g of freshly powdered drug. May also be used as 10–20 drops of tincture in water with meals.[135]

ADR: Occasional dyspepsia, but no significant risk when consumed at stated dose levels. Large overdose may cause depression and cardiac arrhythmias.[82] May be contraindindicated in pregnancy.[125] Possible risk of increased bleeding following surgery.[136]

Ginkgo biloba[137,138]

Source: Concentrated extract of the leaves of the tree *Ginkgo biloba*; prepared by extraction of dried green leaves with acetone/water solvent.

Constituents:[139] Flavonoids (flavone glycosides), diterpenes (ginkgolides), sesquiterpenes (bilobalides).

Uses: Claimed to be effective in treating ailments associated with ageing and cerebral insufficiency.[140] Increases blood flow.[141] Claimed to enhance cognitive function and memory.[142,143] Antioxidant. Tinnitus.[144] Effects of poor circulation.

Common applications: Tinnitus, vertigo, symptoms of the early stages of Alzheimer's, Raynaud's syndrome, intermittent claudication.

Presentation: Tea, capsules, tablets.

Daily dose:[17] The equivalent of 300 mg dried leaf, 40 mg of extract, standardised to 24% flavone glycosides and 6% terpenoids, three times daily.[132]

ADR: Occasional gastrointestinal disturbances, headache and allergic skin reactions (especially from handling ginkgo fruit). The herb has also been reported to cause spontaneous bleeding and may interact with anticoagulants and antiplatelet agents.[145]

Ginseng[146]

Source: Main and lateral root parts of several species of *Panax*, including *P. ginseng* (Chinese or Asian), *P. japonicus* (Korean), *P. quinquefolium* (American/Canadian) and *Eleutherococcus senticosus* (Siberian). The latter is not a member of the *Panax* genus and is therefore not a true ginseng.

Active ingredients: Contains a complex mixture of at least 13 saponins, known as ginsenosides, and a small amount of volatile oil. Siberian ginseng contains no appreciable amount of saponins but instead contains lignans, coumarins and polysaccharides.

Uses:[147] *Pan* = all, *akos* = cure, thus 'panacea' and *gin* = man, *seng* = essence. The Chinese believe that ginseng represents a crystallisation of the essence of the earth in the form of man. Immunomodulatory activity.

Applications: Promoted as a tonic and stimulant, improving stamina and sexual performance. Believed to improve performance and recovery in athletes.

Common applications: Stress, fatigue, strengthens immune function, increases endurance. General tonic.[148] Anti-ageing.[149] Folkloric use in diabetes.

Presentation: Dried herb, decoction.

Daily dose: 1–2 g root or equivalent. The decoction is taken three to four times daily over 3–4 weeks.

ADR: Mild irritability and excitation, insomnia, diarrhoea. Not recommended during pregnancy.[150] Ginseng is thought to have an additive effect when used concomitantly with monoamine oxidase inhibitors.[151] Clients should be advised against taking ginseng at night as it may cause insomnia.

Hawthorn[152]

Source: Extract from berries, flowers and leaves of several species of *Crataegus*, including *Crataegus oxycanthoides* (*C. laevigata*) and *C. monogyna*.

Constituents:[153] Flavonoids (including quercetin glycosides and flavone-C-glycosides) and oligomeric procyanidins.

Uses: Beneficial effects on coronary blood flow, blood pressure and heart rate;[154] decreases cardiac output. Slow-acting therefore has long-term use.

Common applications:[155,156] Hypotension; treatment of angina. To facilitate maximum effort in sport.

Presentation: Decoction, liquid extract, tea, capsules/tablets.

Daily dose: 5 g drug (in five to six divided doses) or 900 mg extract for minimum 6 weeks' duration.

ADR: None known. Possible interaction with orthodox hypotensive drugs.

Kava[157,158]

Source: The rootstock derived from *Piper methysticum*.

Constituents: Kavalactones, including the pyrones kavain (kawain), dihydrokavain, methysticin, dihydromethysticin and yangonin. The alkaloids cepharadione A (an isoquinoline) and pipmethystine (a pyridone, in the leaf only) and miscellaneous flavonoids and benzyl-ketones.[159]

Uses: Treatment of anxiety[160,161] and as a muscle relaxant. Antimicrobial, antiseptic, mild analgesic, antispasmodic, diuretic, stimulant, tonic.

Common applications: Genitourinary infections, vaginitis, pruritus, geriatric incontinence. Powerful soporific. Used as liquid to cause mood elevation and feeling of relaxation (especially in the Pacific Islands). Treatment of stress-related headaches and muscle spasm; possible alternative to benzodiazepines.[162,163]

Presentation: Powder, liquid extract, lotion.

Daily dose: 2–4 g three times daily of herb, decoction (30 g to 5000 ml) half a cup three times daily, lotion (30 g to 250 ml glycerine) as necessary for itching.

ADR: Excessive consumption can result in disturbances of vision (photophobia, diplopia and oculomotor paralysis), yellowing of the skin, problems with equilibrium, dizziness and ultimately stupor.[157] A possible interaction between kava and alprazolam has been noted.[164]

Milk thistle (St Mary's thistle)

Source: Extract from fruit (seeds) of *Silybum marianus* (syn. *Carduus marianus*).

Constituents: Flavanolignans (especially silymarin and its derivative silybin), fixed oil, flavonoids and sterols.

Uses: Free radical scavenger; hepatoprotective activity.[165–167] Said to facilitate lactation in nursing mothers.

Common applications: Loss of appetite. Liver and gallbladder complaints,[168,169] dyspepsia. Occasional reports of use in psoriasis.[170]

Presentation: Capsules, liquid extract and tincture. Injection claimed to be most effective, tea the least effective.[171]

Daily dose: (i) 12–15 g drug or 200–300 mg of silymarin calculated as silybin;[172] (ii) 200 mg of standardised extract (70% silymarin) three times daily;[153] (iii) 20 drops of tincture three times daily.

ADR: Occasional diarrhoea.

St John's wort[173]

Source: Extract from the fresh or dried leaves and the golden yellow flowering tops of *Hypericum perforatum*.

Constituents: Anthracene derivatives (including hypericin and pseudo-hypericin), flavonoids, phenolics (including hyperforin), procyanidins and volatile oil.

Uses: Affinity for nervous tissue; antidepressant. Also used as anxiolytic, sedative and antiviral.

Common applications: Mild antidepressant. In a meta-analysis of 23 randomised trials, including a total of 1757 outpatients with mild or moderate depressive disorders, hypericum was found to be significantly superior to placebo.[174] St John's wort is said to be as effective as imipramine.[175,176] Menopausal symptoms of psychological origin.[177] Blood and crush injuries orally and topically. Topical application also for neuralgias and myalgias.

Presentation: Capsules, tablets, liquid extract, infusion, tincture, topical oil or cream/ointment.

Daily dose: 2–4 g of dried drug as an infusion three times daily[178] or equivalent of 1.0–2.7 mg of total hypericin.

ADR: Stated to be 'minor', but headache, nausea, dizziness, dry mouth and photosensitivity have been reported.[179] Slight in vitro uterotonic activity has been reported[171] as well as the above, so probably wise to avoid use during pregnancy. St John's wort may represent a potential and possibly overlooked cause for drug interactions in transplant recipients.[180]

The following drugs should not be used in combination with St John's wort or preparations containing derivatives of hypericum:[63,181] monoamine oxidase inhibitors (phenelzine, tranylcypromine and isocarboxazid), selective serotonin reuptake inhibitors (fluoxetine), dibenzazepine derivatives (amitriptyline, protriptyline, nortriptyline, desipramine, amoxapine, imipramine, doxepine, perphenazine, carbamazepine, cyclobenzapine, clomipramine, maprotiline and trimipramine) and sympathomimetics [amphetamines, ephedrine (found in many cold and hayfever remedies), methyldopa, dopamine, levodopa and trytophan].

In view of the current interest in this herb the clinically important interactions of St John's wort are summarised in Table 5.6.

Saw palmetto[182]

Source: Powdered partially dried and fresh ripe fruit of the North American tree *Sabal serrulata* (syn. *Serenoa repens*). Seeds are nutty with vanilla aroma; characteristic 'soapy' taste.

Constituents: Rich in fatty acids and phytosterols (notably beta-sitosterol). Also contains flavonoids and polysaccharides.

Table 5.6 Examples of clinically important interactions of St John's wort

Orthodox drug	Effect of interaction
Anticonvulsants	Reduced blood levels; possible risk of seizures
Ciclosporin	Reduced blood levels with risk of transplant rejection
Digoxin	Reduced blood levels and loss of control of heart rhythm or heart failure
HIV protease inhibitors	Reduced blood levels with possible loss of HIV suppression
Oral contraceptives	Reduced blood levels with risk of conception and breakthrough bleeding
SSRIs	Increased serotonergic effects with increased incidence of adverse reactions
Theophylline	Reduced blood levels and loss of control of asthma or chronic airflow limitation
Triptans	Increased serotonergic effects with increased incidence of adverse reactions
Warfarin	Reduced anticoagulant effect and resultant need for increased dose

HIV, human immunodeficiency virus; SSRIs, selective serotonin reuptake inhibitors.
From *Committee on Safety of Medicines Fact Sheet for Healthcare Professionals*. London: Medicines Control Agency, 2000, with permission.

Uses: Has a phyto-oestrogenic effect.

Common applications: Claimed treatment for benign prostatic hypertrophy.[183,184] Also promoted as a urinary tonic, as a diuretic, for cystitis and irritable bladder, and as a male reproductive tonic.

Presentation: Liquid extract, capsules/tablets.

Daily dose: 2–4 g of dried herb or equivalent.

ADR: Occasional gastric problems have been reported.[185] Because of its antiandrogen and oestrogenic activity, saw palmetto may interact with orthodox hormonal therapy, including hormone replacement therapy and oral contraceptives.[186]

Valerian[187]

Source: Dried root and rhizome of *Valeriana officianalis* dried at temperatures below 40°C.

Constituents: Valepotriates, volatile oil, sesquiterpenes, pyridine alkaloids and caffeic acid derivatives.

Uses:[188] Sedative, hypnotic and for treating exhaustion and excitability.

Common applications: Used for insomnia.[189] Valerian is reputed to have muscle-relaxing properties and is used alone or in combination with other herbs in the management of musculoskeletal conditions.[190]

Presentation: Available in a number of official and OTC preparations, teabags and mixtures. Extracts, powders and tinctures. Unpleasant nauseous odour.

Daily dose:[191] 3–9 g of drug in divided doses; 2–6 ml liquid extract.

ADR: Occasionally headaches, excitability and insomnia.[192] Valerian may potentiate the effects of central nervous system-depressant drugs, including alcohol. The herb should be used with caution in children under 3 years of age and in pregnant or lactating women.[147]

Repertory

This list is not designed to be exhaustive; it is merely an indication of remedies that can be used to treat various commonly occurring, mainly acute, conditions.

Anxiety, depression, stress

Anxiety: St John's wort (hypericum), Asian ginseng

Depression: Ginkgo biloba

Insomnia: Hops (*Humulus lupulus*), scullcap (*Scutellaria baicalensis*)

Sedatives: Lemon balm (*Melissa officinalis*), valerian (*Valeriana officinalis*)

Stress: Kava (*Piper methysticum*)

Coughs

Coltsfoot, ephedra (*Ephedra* spp.), horehound (*Marrubium vulgare*), liquorice, mullein (*Verbascum*), thyme (*Thymus vulgaris*), wild cherry bark (*Prunus serotina*)

Ear and eye conditions

Ear infections: Echinacea (*E. purpurea*)

Ear wax: Mullein (*Verbascum*)

Eye problems: Eyebright (*Euphrasia*)

Gastrointestinal conditions

Colic: Camomile (*Matricaria chamonilla*)

Constipation: Aloe (*Aloe barbadensis*), senna, rhubarb, cascara (*Cascara sagrada*), dandelion (*Taraxacum officinalis*)

Diarrhoea: Barberry (*Berberis vulgaris*), bilberry (*Vaccinium myrtillus*)

Haemorrhoids: Horse chestnut (*Aesculus hippocastanumn*)

Morning sickness: Ginger, horehound

Motion sickness: Ginger

Nausea and vomiting: Ginger

Heartburn and indigestion: Devil's claw (*Harpagophytum procumbens*), gentian (*Gentiana lutea*), liquorice (*Glycyrrhiza* spp.), peppermint

Influenza and colds, sore throat

Elderflower, garlic golden seal (*Hydrastis*), nettle, rose, usnea (*Usnea barbata*)

Menstrual problems

Menopause: Alfalfa (*Medicago sativa*), black cohosh (*Cimicifuga racemosa*), sage (*Salvia officinalis*)

Painful menstruation: Black cohosh (*Cimicifuga racemosa*), blue cohosh (*Caulophyllum thalictroides*), cramp bark (*Viburnum opulus*)

Premenstrual syndrome: Chaste berry (*Vitex agnus castus*)

Motion sickness

Ginger (*Zingiber officinale*)

Rheumatics

Devil's claw (*Harpagophytum procumbens*), turmeric (*Curcuma longa*), yucca (*Yucca* spp.)

Skin conditions

Abrasions, superficial: Marigold (*Calendula officinalis*)

Acne: Burdock (*Arctium lappa*), tea tree (*Melaleuca alternifolia*)

Athlete's foot: Myrrh (*Commiphora molmol*), tea tree (*Melaleuca alternifolia*)

Eczema: Borage (*Borago officinalis*), sarsasparilla (*Smilax* spp.)

Psoriasis: Cayenne (*Capsicum* spp.)

Wound healing: Comfrey (*Symphytum*)

Urinary

Urinary tract infections: Cranberry (*Vaccinium macrocarpen*), uva ursi (*Arctostaphylos uva-ursi*)

More information

National Institute of Medical Herbalists (NIMH)
56 Longbrook Street,
Exeter
Devon EX4 6AH
Tel: 01392 426022
www.btinternet.com/~nimh/

British Herbal Medicine Association (BHMA)
Sun House, Church Street
Stroud
Gloucestershire
Tel: 01453 751389

The Scottish School of Herbal Medicine (validated by the University of Wales)
Unit 22, Six Harmony Row
Glasgow
G51 3BA
Tel: 0141 401 8889
www.herbalmedicine.org.uk

European Scientific Cooperative on Phythotherapy (ESCOP)
Uitwaardenstraat 13
NL-8081 HJ Elburg
The Netherlands

References

1. Kayne S. Plants, medicines and environmental awareness. *Health Homoeopathy* 1993; 5: 12–14.
2. World Health Organization. *Traditional Medicine*. WHO fact sheet N134. Geneva: World Health Organization, 1996.
3. Huxtable R J. The pharmacology of extinction. *J Ethnopharmacol* 1992; 27: 1–11.
4. Holloway H. Sustaining the Amazon. *Sci Am* 1993; 269: 77–84.
5. Orr D. India accuses US of stealing ancient cures. *London Times* 1999; July 31.
6. WWF International Report. *Booming Medicinal Plant Trade Lacks Controls*. Godalming, Surrey: WWF, 1993.
7. Anon. Ozone hole cuts plant growth. *Independent* 1993; 11 June.
8. Dueck Th A, Elderson J. Influence of ammonia and sulphur dioxide on the growth and competitive ability of *Arnica montana* and *Viola canina*. *New Phytol* 1992; 122: 507–514.

9. Bellamy D. Something in the air. *BBC Wildlife* 1993; 11: 31–34.
10. Sitwell N. *The Shell Guide to Britain's Threatened Wildlife*. London: Collins, 1993.
11. Anon. Threatened wild flowers saved by EC's arable farm policy. *Independent* 1993; 19 July.
12. Fellows L. What can higher plants offer the industry? *Pharm J* 1993; 250: 658.
13. Farnsworth N R. The role of ethnopharmacology in drug development. Cited in: Kayne S. Plants, medicines and environmental awareness. *Health Homoeopathy* 1993; 5: 12–14.
14. Norfolk D. *The Therapeutic Garden*. London: Bantam Press, 1999.
15. Balentine D A, Albano M C, Nair M G. Role of medicinal plants, herbs and spices in protecting human life. *Nutr Rev* 1999; 57: S41–S45.
16. Bartram T. *Encyclopedia of Herbal Medicine*. Christchurch, Dorset: Grace, 1995: 224.
17. Directive EC 65/65. Brussels: EU Secretariat, 1995.
18. Ratsch C. *Plants of Love*. Berkeley, CA: Ten Speed Press, 1997.
19. Kapoor L D. *Opium Poppy*. New York: Food Products Press, 1997: xiii.
20. Hutchens A R. *Indian Herbology of North America*. Boston, MA: Shambhala, 1991: xxix.
21. Mills S, Bone K. *Principles and Practices of Phytotherapy*. London: Churchill Livingstone, 1999: 80–86.
22. Wren R C. *Potter's New Cyclopaedia of Botanical Drugs and Preparations*. Saffron Walden: C W Daniel, 1988.
23. Weiss R F. *Herbal Medicine*. Beaconsfield: Beaconsfield Publishers, 1988.
24. BHMA Scientific Committee. *British Herbal Pharmacopoeia*, vol. 1. Bournemouth: BHMA, 1996.
25. Evans W C. *Trease and Evans Pharmacognosy*, 14th edn. London: W B Saunders, 1996.
26. Mills S, Bone K. *Principles and Practices of Phytotherapy*. London: Churchill Livingstone, 1999: 23–79.
27. Schilcher H. *Phytotherapy in Paediatrics*, 2nd edn. Stuttgart: Medpharm, 1992: 16–18.
28. Munzel K, Huber K. Extraction procedures in the preparation of chamomile fluid extract. *Pharma Acta Helv* 1961; 36: 194–204.
29. Meier B. The extraction strength of ethanol/water mixtures commonly used for the processing of herbal drugs. *Planta Med* 1991; 57 (suppl. 2): A26.
30. De Smet A G M. Should herbal medicine-like products be licensed as medicines? *BMJ* 1995; 310: 1023–1024.
31. Sale of pharmaceutical plants. *Official J Eur Commun C* 1994; November 14: 317/17.
32. Thompson R. *The Single Market for Pharmaceuticals*. London: Butterworths, 1994: 17–45, 141–151.
33. Perharic L, Shaw D, Murray V. An appeal to pharmacists to report adverse effects of herbal and vitamin products. *Pharm J* 1994; 252: 479.
34. Barnes J. Developments in the regulation of herbal medicinal products – report of the 6th International European Scientific Co-operative on Phytotherapy Symposium, Bonn May 2001. *Pharm J* 2001; 264: 794.
35. Mason P. The regulation of herbal products in Europe – from diversity to harmonisation. *Pharm J* 2000; 264: 856–857.

36. Gottlieb S. News extra. *BMJ* 2000; 320: 208.
37. Judge E. 'Natural' is not necessarily 'safe'. *London Times* 1999; June 26.
38. Mills S, Bone K. *Principles and Practices of Phytotherapy*. London: Churchill Livingstone, 1999: 132–255.
39. RPSGB. *Herbal Medicines Fact Sheet*. London: RPSGB, 2000.
40. Mills S, Bone K. *Principles and Practices of Phytotherapy*. London: Churchill Livingstone, 1999: 121.
41. Kucera M, Kalal J, Polesna Z. Effects of symphytum ointment on muscular symptoms and functional locomotor disturbances. *Adv Ther* 2000; 17: 204–210.
42. Kayne S, Hayes P. Natural antiseptics and disinfectants. *NZ Pharm* 1996; 16: 23–26.
43. Carson C F, Cookson B D, Farrelly H D, Riley T V. Susceptibility of methicillin-resistant *Staphylococcus aureus* to the essential oil of *Melaleuca alternifolia*. *J Antimicrob Chemother* 1995; 35: 421–424.
44. Gibson P S, Powrie R, Star J. Herbal and alternative medicine use during pregnancy: a cross-sectional survey. *Obstet Gynecol* 2001; 97 (suppl. 1): S44–S45.
45. Brinker F. *Herb Contraindications and Drug Interactions*, 2nd edn. Sandy, Oregon: Electric Medical Publications, 1998: 173–185.
46. Mills S, Bone K. *Principles and Practices of Phytotherapy*. London: Churchill Livingstone, 1999: 99.
47. Parsons M, Simpson M, Ponton T. Raspberry leaf and its effect on labour: safety and efficacy. *J Aust Coll Midwives* 1999; 12: 20–25.
48. Kontiokari T, Sundoqvist K, Nuutinen M *et al.* Randomised trial of cranberry–lingonberry juice and *Lactobacillus* GG drink for the prevention of urinary tract infections in women. *BMJ* 2001; 322: 1571–1574.
49. Kayne S B. Getting to know the good guys. *Chemist Druggist* 2001; 255: 22–23.
50. Rapport L, Lockwood B. Flaxseed and flaxseed oil. *Pharm J* 2001; 266: 287–289.
51. Schilcher H. *Phytotherapy in Paediatrics*. Stuttgart: Medpharm Scientific Publishers, 1997: 15–16.
52. Houlder A-M. Herbal medicines – should they be in child resistant containers? *BMJ* 1995; 310: 1473.
53. *Cochrane Collab Complement Med Field Newslett* 2000; 6: 2.
54. Blumenthal M, Busse W, Goldberg A *et al. The Complete German Commission E Monographs: Therapeutic Guide to Herbal Medicine*. Austin, TX: American Botanical Council, 1998: 685.
55. Betz J H, Eppey R M, Taylor W C, Andrzejewski D. Determination of pyrrolizidine alkaloids in commercial comfrey products (*Symphytum* sp.). *J Pharm Sci* 1994; 83: 649–653.
56. Perharic L, Shaw D, Murray V. Toxic effects of herbal medicines and food supplements. *Lancet* 1993; 342: 180–181.
57. De Smet P. Health risks of herbal remedies. *Drug Safety* 1995; 13: 81–93.
58. Drew A K, Myers S P. Safety issues in herbal medicine: implications for the health professions. *Med J Aust* 1997; 166: 538–541.
59. Newall C A, Anderson L, Phillipson J D. *Herbal Medicines*. London: Pharmaceutical Press, 1996: 7–9.

60. Winterhoff H. Toxicological aspects of phytomedicine. *Eur Phytotelegram* 1994; 6: 17–20.
61. De Smet P A G M, Smeets O S N M. Potential risk of health foood products containing yohimbe extract. *BMJ* 1994; 309: 958.
62. Breckenridge A. Letter from CSM. Renal failure associated with aristolochia in some Chinese herbal medicines. *CEM/CMO/99/8*. London: CSM, 1999: 27 July.
63. Gottlieb S. News. *BMJ* 1999; 319: 336.
64. Goldfrank L, Lewin N, Flomenbaum N, Howland M A. The pernicious panacea – herbal medicine. *Hosp Phys* 1982; 18: 64–67.
65. Dobb G J, Edis R H. Coma and neuropathy after ingestion of herbal laxative containing podophyllin. *Med J Aust* 1984; 140: 496–498.
66. Brinker F. *Herb Contraindications and Drug Interactions*, 2nd edn. Sandy, Oregon: Electric Medical Publications, 1998.
67. Breckenridge A. Message from chairman CSM, concerning important interactions between St John's wort (*Hypericum perforatum*) preparations and prescription medicines. London: Committee on Safety of Medicines/Medicines Control Agency, 2000.
68. Bergner P. Herb–drug interaction. *Med Herbalism* 1997; 9: 1.
69. Almeida J C, Grimsley E W. Coma from the health food store: interaction between kava and alprazolam. *Ann Intern Med* 1996; 125: 940–941.
70. Kleijnen J, Knipschild P. Ginkgo biloba. *Lancet* 1992; 340: 1136–1139.
71. Rowin J, Lewis S L. Spontaneous bilateral subdural hematomas associated with chronic Ginkgo biloba ingestion. *Neurology* 1996; 46: 1775–1776.
72. Rosenblatt M, Mindel J. Spontaneous hyphema associated with ingestion of Ginkgo biloba extract. *N Engl J Med* 1997; 336: 1108.
73. Fugh-Berman A. Herb–drug interactions. *Lancet* 2000; 355: 134–138.
74. Newall C A, Anderson L, Phillipson J D. *Herbal Medicines*. London: Pharmaceutical Press, 1996: 277–280.
75. Tisserand R, Balacs T. *Essential Oil Safety*. Edinburgh: Churchill Livingstone, 1995.
76. Ko R J. Adulterants in Asian patent medicines. *N Engl J Med* 1998; 339: 847.
77. De Smet P A G M. The safety of herbal products. In: Jonas W B, Levi J S, eds. *Essentials of Complementary Alternative Medicine*. Baltimore: Lippincott, Williams & Wilkins, 1999: 108.
78. Perchant L, Shaw D, Murray V. Toxic effects of herbal medicines and food supplements. *Lancet* 1993; 342: 180–181.
79. Keane F M, Munn S E, du Vivier A W P *et al*. Analysis of Chinese herbal creams prescribed for dermatological conditions. *BMJ* 1999; 318: 563–564.
80. Cooper C R. Herbal remedies. *Hosp Forum* 1982; 17: 1387–1392.
81. Mills S, Bone K. *Principles and Practices of Phytotherapy*. London: Churchill Livingstone, 1999: 109.
82. But P. Need the correct identification of herbs in herbal poisoning. *Lancet* 1993; 341: 637.
83. Lenoir S, Degenring F, Saller R. A double blind randomized trial to investigate three different concentrations of a standardized fresh plant extract obtained from the shoot tips of *Hypericum perforatum* L. *Phytomedicine* 1999; 6: 141–146.

84. Vanhaelen J-L, Depierreux M, Tielemans C *et al*. Rapidly progressing interstitial renal fibrosis in young women; association with slimming regimen including Chinese herbs. *Lancet* 1993; 341: 387–391.
85. Farah M H, Edwards R, Lindquist M *et al*. International monitoring of adverse health effects associated with herbal medicines. *Pharmacoepidemiol Drug Safety* 2000; 9: 105–112.
86. Kunkel D B, Spoerke D G. Evaluating exposures to plants. *Emerg Med Clin North Am* 1984; 2: 133–144.
87. Anon. History of the collection. *Pharm J* 1989; 243: 545.
88. Shellard E J. Materia medica museum and herbaria. *Pharm J* 1972; 208: 244–246.
89. Anon. Herbarium moves to Bradford. *Pharm J* 1969; 203: 117.
90. Editorial. Future of the Society's herbaria. *Pharm J* 1967; 202: 275.
91. Anon. Unveiling plaque marking transfer of Society's herbaria to Bradford. *Pharm J* 1970; 204: 154.
92. Anon. Monthly meeting of Council – report. *Pharm J* 1982; 229: 545.
93. Trease G E. Reminiscences of the Society's herbaria. *Pharm J* 1982; 229: 655.
94. Anon. The Society's drug collection 'back to life' at Kew. *Pharm J* 1989; 243: 544–545.
95. Royal Botanic Gardens Kew website. www.rbgkew.org.uk/collections/ecbot.html.
96. Berry M. Alfalfa. *Pharm J* 1995; 255: 353–354.
97. *PDR for Herbal Medicines*. Montvale, NJ: Medical Economics Company, 1999: 962.
98. Malinow M R, Bardana J R, Goodnight S H Jr. Pancytopenia during ingestion of alfalfa seed. *Lancet* 1981; i: 615.
99. Tyler V E. *Tyler's Honest Herbal*. New York: Haworth Herbal Press, 1998: 27.
100. Newall C, Anderson L, David Phillipson J. *Herbal Medicines: A Guide for Health Care Professionals*. London: Pharmaceutical Press, 1996: 25–26.
101. Marshall J M. Aloe vera gel. What is the evidence? *Pharm J* 1990; 244: 360–362.
102. Berry M. The chamomiles. *Pharm J* 1995; 254: 191–193.
103. Craker L E, Simon J E (eds) *Herbs, Spices and Medicinal Plants*, vol. 1. Arizona: Onyx Press, 1986: 235–280.
104. Newall C, Anderson L, David Phillipson J. *Herbal Medicines: A Guide for Health Care Professionals*. London: Pharmaceutical Press, 1996: 296.
105. McGuffin M, Hobbs C, Upton R, Goldberg A. *Botanical Safety Handbook*. Boca Raton: CRC Press, 1997: 74.
106. Newall C, Anderson L, David Phillipson J. *Herbal Medicines: A Guide for Health Care Professionals*. London: Pharmaceutical Press, 1996: 80–81.
107. Tyler V E. *Tyler's Honest Herbal*. New York: Haworth Herbal Press, 1998: 51–52.
108. Phillipson J D, Anderson L A. Counterprescribing of herbal remedies – part two. *Pharm J* 1984; 2333: 272–274.
109. Newall C, Anderson L, David Phillipson J. *Herbal Medicines: A Guide for Health Care Professionals*. London: Pharmaceutical Press, 1996: 82–83.
110. Hobbs C. Echinacea – a literature review. *Herbalgram* 1993; 30: 33–49.

111. Lindenmuth G E, Lindenmuth E B. The efficacy of Echinacea compound herbal tea preparation on the severity and duration of upper respiratory and flu symptoms: a randomized double-blind placebo-controlled study. *J Altern Complement Med* 2000; 6: 327–334.

112. *PDR for Herbal Medicines*. Montvale, NJ: Medical Economics Company, 1999: 819.

113. McGuffin M, Hobbs C, Upton R, Goldberg A. *Botanical Safety Handbook*. Boca Raton: CRC Press, 1997: 44.

114. Berry M. Feverfew. *Pharm J* 1994; 253: 806–808.

115. Vogler B K, Pittler M H, Ernst E. Feverfew as a preventative treatment for migraine: a systematic review. *Cephalalgia* 1998; 18: 704–708.

116. Berry M. Feverfew. *Pharm J* 1994; 253: 806–807.

117. Pattrick M, Hepinstall S, Doherty M. Feverfew in rheumatoid arthritis: a double blind, placebo controlled study. *Ann Rheum Dis* 1989; 48: 547–549.

118. *PDR for Herbal Medicines*. Montvale, NJ: Medical Economics Company, 1999: 1172.

119. Awang D. Feverfew fever – a headache for the consumer. *Herbalgram* 1993; 29: 66.

120. McGuffin M, Hobbs C, Upton R, Goldberg A. *Botanical Safety Handbook*. Boca Raton: CRC Press, 1997: 113.

121. Silagy C A, Neil H A W. A meta-analysis of the effect of garlic on blood pressure. *J Hypertens* 1994; 12: 463–468.

122. Kiesewetter H, Jung F, Jung E M *et al*. Effect of garlic on platelet aggregation in patients with increased risk of juvenile ischaemic attack. *Eur J Clin Pharmacol* 1993; 45: 333–336.

123. Silagy C A, Neil H A W. Garlic as a lipid lowering agent – a meta-analysis. *J R Coll Phys Lond* 1994; 28: 39–45.

124. Ernst E. Cardiovascular effects of garlic (*Allium stivum*): a review. *Pharmatherapeutica* 1987; 5: 83–89.

125. Miller L G, Murray W J (eds). *Herbal Medicinals. A Clinical Guide*. Bingha, NY: Pharmaceutical Products Press, 1998: 40.

126. Warshafsky S, Kamer R S, Sivak S L. Effect of garlic on total serum cholesterol. *Ann Intern Med* 1993; 119: 599–605.

127. *PDR for Herbal Medicines*. Montvale, NJ: Medical Economics Company, 1999: 627.

128. Petry J J. Garlic and postoperative bleeding. *Plast Reconstruct Surg* 1995; 96: 483–484.

129. Tyler V E. *Herbs of Choice. The Therapeutic Use of Phytomedicinals*. Binghamton, NY: Pharmaceutical Products Press, 1994: 209.

130. Sunter W. Warfarin and garlic. *Pharm J* 1991; 246: 72.

131. McGuffin M, Hobbs C, Upton R, Goldberg A. *Botanical Safety Handbook*. Boca Raton: CRC Press, 1997: 6–7.

132. Boon H, Smith M. *The Botanical Pharmacy*. Kingston: Quarry Press, 1999: 155–163.

133. Tyler V E. *Tyler's Honest Herbal*. New York: Haworth Herbal Press, 1998: 181–182.

134. *PDR for Herbal Medicines*. Montvale, NJ: Medical Economics Company, 1999: 1230.

135. Weiss R F. *Herbal Medicine*. Beaconsfield: Beaconsfield Publishers, 1988: 48.
136. Backon J. Ginger as an antiemetic: possible side effects due to its thromboxane synthetase activity. *Anaesthesia* 1991; 46: 669–671.
137. Kleijnen J, Knipschild P. Ginkgo biloba. *Lancet* 1992; 340: 1136–1139.
138. Houghton P. Gingko. *Pharm J* 1994; 253: 122–123.
139. Pang Z. Ginkgo biloba: history, current staus and future prospects. *J Altern Complement Med* 1996; 2: 359–363.
140. Vorberg G. *Ginkgo biloba* extract (GBE): a long term study of cerebral insufficiency in geriatric patients. *Clin Trials J* 1985; 22: 149–157.
141. Jung F, Mrowietz C, Kiesewetter H, Wenzel E. Effect of *Ginkgo biloba* on fluidity of blood and peripheral microcirculation in volunteers. *Arzneimittelforschung* 1990; 40: 589–593.
142. Ernst E, Pittler M H. Ginkgo biloba for dementia: a systematic review of double blind placebo controlled trials. *Clin Drug Invest* 1999; 17: 301–308.
143. Kennedy D O, Scholey A B, Wesnes K A. The dose-dependent cognitive effect of acute administration of *Ginkgo biloba* to healthy young volunteers. *Psychopharmacol* 2000; 151: 416–423.
144. Ernst E, Stevinson C. Ginkgo biloba for tinnitus: a review. *Clin Otolaryngeal* 1999; 24: 164–167.
145. Fessenden J M, Wittenborn W, Clarke L. Gingko biloba: a case report of herbal medicine and bleeding postoperatively from a laparoscopic cholecystectomy. *Am Surg* 2001; 67: 33–35.
146. Raman A. Ginseng. *Pharm J* 1995; 254: 150–152.
147. Vogler B K, Pittler M H, Ernst E. The efficacy of ginseng. A systematic review of randomized clinical trials. *Eur J Clin Pharmacol* 1999; 55: 567–575.
148. Schulz V, Hänsel R, Tyler V E. *Rational Phytotherapy: A Physicians' Guide to Herbal Medicine*. Berlin: Springer, 1998: 270–272.
149. Xiao P G, Xing S T, Wang L W. Immunological aspects of Chinese medicinal plants as antiageing drugs. *J Ethnopharmacol* 1993; 38: 167–175.
150. McGuffin M, Hobbs C, Upton R, Goldberg A. *Botanical Safety Handbook*. Boca Raton: CRC Press, 1997: 81.
151. Stockley I. *Drug Interactions. A Sourcebook of Adverse Interactions, Their Mechanisms, Clinical Importance, and Management*, 3rd edn. Cambridge, UK: Blackwell Scientific Press, 1994.
152. Weiss R F. *Herbal Medicine*. Beaconsfield: Beaconsfield Publishers, 1988: 162–169.
153. Mills S, Bone K. *Principles and Practices of Phytotherapy*. London: Churchill Livingstone, 1999: 439–447.
154. Rodale J I. *The Hawthorn Berry for the Heart*. Womaus, PA: Rodale Books, 1971.
155. Newall C A, Anderson L, Phillipson J D. *Herbal Medicines*. London: Pharmaceutical Press, 1996: 157–158.
156. Tyler V E. *Tyler's Honest Herbal*. New York: Haworth Herbal Press, 1998: 206.
157. Bartram T. *Encyclopedia of Herbal Medicine*. Christchurch: Grace Publishers, 1885: 259.
158. Singh Y D, Blumenthal M. Kava: an overview. *HerbalGram* 1997; 39: 34–55.

159. Boon H, Smith M. *The Botanical Pharmacy*. Kingston: Quarry Press, 1999: 133.
160. Woelk H. The treatment of patients with anxiety. A double blind study: kava extract WS1490 vs. benzodiazepine. *Z Allgem Med* 1993; 69: 271–277.
161. Lehmann E, Kinzler E, Friedemann J. Efficacy of a special kava extract (*Piper methysticum*) in patients with states of anxiety, tension, and excitedness of non-mental origin – a double-blind, placebo-controlled study of four weeks' treatment. *Phytomedicine* 1996; 3: 113–119.
162. Tyler V E. *Tyler's Honest Herbal*. New York: Haworth Herbal Press, 1998: 230.
163. Bone K. Kava – a safe herbal treatment for anxiety. *Br J Phytother* 1993; 3: 147–153.
164. Almeida J, Grimsley E. Coma from the health food store: interaction between kava and alprazolam. *Ann Intern Med* 1996; 125: 940–941.
165. Hobbs C. *Milk Thistle: The Liver Herb*, 2nd edn. Santa Cruz, CA: Botanica Press, 1992: 14–24.
166. Plomteux G, Albert A, Heusghem C. Hepatoprotector action of silymarin, in human acute viral hepatitis. *Int Res Commun Syst* 1977; 5: 259.
167. Blumenthal M, Brusse W R, Goldberg A *et al*. *The Complete German Commission E Monographs*. Austin, Texas: American Botanical Council, 1998: 685.
168. Flora K, Hahn M, Rosen H, Benner K. Milk thistle (*Silybum marianum*) for the therapy of liver disease. *Am J Gastroenterol* 1998; 93: 139–143.
169. Weiss R F. *Herbal Medicine*. Beaconsfield: Beaconsfield Publishers, 1988: 83.
170. Boon H, Smith M. *The Botanical Pharmacy*. Kingston: Quarry Press, 1999: 250–254.
171. Tyler V E. *Tyler's Honest Herbal*. New York: Haworth Herbal Press, 1998: 254.
172. *PDR for Herbal Medicines*. Montvale, NJ: Medical Economics Company, 1999: 1139.
173. Mills S, Bone K. *Principles and Practice of Phytotherapy*. Edinburgh: Churchill Livingstone, 2000: 542–552.
174. Linde K, Ramirez G, Mulrow C *et al*. St John's wort for depression – an overview and meta-analysis of randomised clinical trials. *BMJ* 1996; 313: 253–258.
175. Vorbach E U, Arnoldt K H, Hubner W-D. Efficacy and tolerability of St John's wort extract LI 160 versus imipramine in patients with severe depressive episodes according to ICD-10. *Pharmacopsychiatry* 1997; 30 (suppl. 2): 81–85.
176. Woelk H. Comparison of St John's wort and imipramine for treating depression: randomized controlled trial. *BMJ* 2000; 321: 536–539.
177. Grube B, Walper A, Wheatley M D. St John's wort extract: efficacy for menopausal symptoms of psychological origin. *Adv Ther* 1999; 16: 177–186.
178. Newall C A, Anderson L, Phillipson J D. *Herbal Medicines*. London: Pharmaceutical Press, 1996: 250–251.
179. Ernst E, Rand J I, Barnes J, Stevinson C. Adverse effects profile of the herbal antidepressant St John's wort (*Hypericum perforatum*). *Eur J Clin Pharmacol* 1998; 54: 589–594.
180. Barone G W, Gurley B J, Ketel B L, Abul-Ezz S R. Herbal supplements: a potential for drug interactions in transplant recipients. *Transplantation* 2001; 71: 239–241.

181. Boon H, Smith M. *The Botanical Pharmacy*. Kingston: Quarry Press, 1999: 283–290.
182. Mills S, Bone K. *Principles and Practice of Phytotherapy*. Edinburgh: Churchill Livingstone, 2000: 523–533.
183. Champault G, Patel J C, Bonnard A M. A double-blind trial of an extract of the plant *Serenoa repens* in benign prostatic hyperplasia. *Br J Clin Pharmacol* 1984; 19: 461–462.
184. Braeckman J. The extract of *Seronoa repens* in the treatment of benign pro-static hyperplasia: a multicentre open study. *Curr Ther Res* 1994; 55: 776–785.
185. McGuffin M, Hobbs C, Upton R, Goldberg A. *Botanical Safety Handbook*. Boca Raton: CRC Press, 1997: 107.
186. Newall C A, Anderson L, Phillipson J D. *Herbal Medicines*. London: Pharma-ceutical Press, 1996: 238.
187. Houghton P. Valerian. *Pharm J* 1994; 253: 95–96.
188. Hobbs C. Valerian – a literature review. *Herbalgram* 1989; 21: 19–35.
189. Stevinson C, Ernst E. Valerian for insomnia: a systematic review of random-ized clinical trials. *Sleep Med* 2000; 1: 91–99.
190. Boon H, Smith M. *The Botanical Pharmacy*. Kingston: Quarry Press, 1999: 308–313.
191. Mills S, Bone K. *Principles and Practice of Phytotherapy*. Edinburgh: Churchill Livingstone, 2000: 542–581.
192. McGuffin M, Hobbs C, Upton R, Goldberg A. *Botanical Safety Handbook*. Boca Raton: CRC Press, 1997: 120.

6

Aromatherapy

Aromatherapy is currently growing in popularity and may well overtake the other complementary therapies in the near future. Medicinal and cosmetic uses are sometimes difficult to separate and there is often confusion in consumer's minds as to the different qualities of oils available for purchase.

Definition

The word 'aromatherapy' entered the English language in the early 1980s to describe the use of fragrant essential oils to affect or alter a person's mood or behaviour.[1]

History

The practice of using oils to treat illnesses is reputed to be at least 6000 years old and to have followed the westward course of civilisation beginning in the oriental cultures of China, India, Persia and Egypt. The earliest Hindu scriptures mention several hundred perfumes and aromatic products, classifying their use for both liturgical and therapeutic applications.[2]

The Egyptians are known to have used plant products for many reasons, including medicine, massage therapy, preservation and mummification. Aromatic oils were made by soaking plant materials in base oils or fats. There is some evidence that later Egyptians experimented with crude methods of distillation.[1] The Greeks used aromatics and essential oils in warfare to stimulate aggression and heal battle wounds. Dioscorides, a first-century Greek surgeon in Nero's Roman army, included a chapter on oils in his medical encyclopedia, which remained a standard medical text for more than 1000 years.

Modern aromatherapy owes its emergence to numerous European pharmacists and apothecaries, chiefly in France and Germany, whose improved methods of distillation and investigations on the nature and value of essential oils during the seventeenth and early eighteenth centuries contributed much to its wider acceptance. However, although by the end of the eighteenth century almost every herbalist and many physicians used essential oils to varying degrees, the practice received a major setback with the advent of chemistry. Using newly discovered techniques, alchemists began to extract what they believed to be active principals rather than using the plant and later even synthesised simple chemical drugs. The enthusiasm for naturally occurring treatments within the medically oriented professions receded until there was a revival in the 1920s.

The term *aromathérapie* is attributed to the French chemist René-Maurice Gattefossé, who published a book on the subject in 1937 and is generally considered to be the founder of modern aromatherapy.[3] The first English translation of the book was published in 1993.[4] Gattefossé is said to have become interested in the study of essential oils in 1910 following a laboratory explosion in which he burnt his hand severely while working in his family perfumery. He is said to have plunged his hand into a conveniently placed bath of lavender oil. The hand not only healed within a few hours, but did so without scarring. This experience led him to investigate many essential oils and record the chemical constituents of each. During the First World War he used essential oils successfully to treat burns and prevent gangrene. With the advent of powerful modern drugs and in common with other complementary disciplines, aromatherapy fell into decline during the middle years of the twentieth century. In the 1960s a French doctor, Jean Valnet, who as an army surgeon had treated wounded soldiers with aromatherapy, followed up the work of Gattefossé. Together with one of his students, Margaret Maury, a biochemist, Valnet developed a method of applying the oils using massage. Maury introduced aromatherapy to the UK in the 1950s. Since then aromatherapy has enjoyed a considerable resurgence, with about 5000 trained aromatherapists now practising in the UK. It is now the fastest-growing complementary discipline in this country.

Theory

The basis for the action of aromatherapy is similar to modern pharmacology, with active principals entering the biochemical pathways, albeit in much smaller doses. Aromatherapy is thought to work at psychological, physiological and cellular levels.

Two mechanisms of action have been identified: olfactory stimulation and dermal action.

Olfactory stimulation

Aromatherapists believe that olfactory stimulation plays an important role in their treatment, the sense of smell being the most immediate of our senses. Olfactory stimulants enter the nose, reaching the olfactory bulb. From here nerve impulses move on to the limbic system of the brain, where the areas of the amygdala and the hippocampus are associated with emotional and learning processes respectively. Learning processes are thought to be responsible for the memories evoked by various different odours (see below).

Dermal action

Medical aromatherapy may involve direct physiological action on the body, with active compounds being absorbed into the blood stream through the skin. Absorption may be enhanced by warming the skin or by massage (see below).

Production of aromatherapy oils

Essential oils – composition and production

Essential oils are fragrant and highly volatile aromatic compounds generated by plants through photosynthesis.[5] They are used in:

- foods, as flavourings (e.g. orange or lemon oil)
- toiletries (e.g. cosmetics, perfumes and toothpaste)
- orthodox medicines [e.g. clove oil for toothache, peppermint oil for indigestion and eucalyptus as an inhalation, and are the constituents of many over-the-counter (OTC) patented products]
- complementary medicine.

The first three applications are the most important commercially, with only about 4% of production being directed towards complementary use.

The terms 'essential oils' and 'essences' are often used interchangeably to cover all the oils used by aromatherapists. Strictly speaking, the former term should only be applied to those oils derived from a plant after distillation (see below).

Extraction

The starting materials for true essential oils are 'essences'. These are produced in highly specialised secretory cells that may be in the leaf, bark or other parts of the plant.[6] They may be stored within the same cell in which they are made or they may pass into a storage cell or duct. These cells are often just below the surface of the leaf and the essence may be released if the leaf is crushed, giving off a characteristic aroma. In other plants, storage ducts are in minute hairs on the leaf. These plants are highly aromatic and release their fragrance when simply brushed against. The proportion of essence in the plant varies with species and this accounts in part for the varying prices of essential oils. The particular plant used, and the part of that plant used, can have a significant effect on the final product.[7]

The best-quality essential oils are obtained from essences derived from a whole plant or plant parts (Table 6.1) by vapour or steam distillation. Ideally, a copper or stainless steel still that separates the plant material and steam is used. The separate chamber ensures that hot water will not break down or dilute the essential oils. The application of heat during the distillation process initiates certain chemical changes. The oil is slowly liberated from the plant material.

Other methods involving the passage of steam through the plant material, extraction with volatile solvents and cold pressing (mainly for citrus oils) are also available. Some plants may produce several oils as different sections of the plant are processed, e.g. from the leaves, flowers and fruit.

Table 6.1 Source of extracted essential oils

Part used for oil	Example
Bark	Cinnamon
Blossom	Orange (neroli)
Bulbs	Garlic
Dried flower buds	Clove
Flowers	Jasmine, lavender, rose
Fruits	Lemon, mandarin
Grass	Lemongrass
Leaves	Eucalyptus, geranium, peppermint
Root tuber	Ginger
Seeds	Fennel
Wood	Sandalwood

Varying amounts of essential oil can be extracted from a particular plant. Over 100 kg of rose petals are required to obtain about 50 ml of essential oil, while lavender and lemon plants yield far greater quantities.

Some widely used products (e.g. citrus fruits and bergamot) are really essences, which are obtained by expression. This involves a simple crushing pressure, and these products are not really essential oils. The active principal of the citrus fruit is found in the outer coloured layer of the rind and the pulp, and the white pith must be removed before extraction can proceeed. The peel is then squeezed and the resulting juice left to stand until the aromatic oil can be separated off.

Other oils (jasmine, neroli and rose) are obtained by enfleurage or solvent extraction without any distillation. These are neither essential oils nor essences and are classified as 'absolutes'.

All these variations are usually included in the aromatherapist's armamentarium under the general heading 'essential oils'.

Composition

Essential oils are highly complex chemicals containing perhaps as many as 100 or more constituents, many of which may be present in concentrations as low as 1%. Examples of typical chemical constituents in essential oils and their therapeutic properties are indicated in Table 6.2. Aromatherapists believe that the many constituents of essential oils combine synergistically, making the final therapeutic effect better than could be predicted from the sum of individual chemical group activities.

Table 6.2 Constituents of essential oils

Constituents	Therapeutic properties
Acids	Anti-inflammatory, hypothermic
Alcohols	Astringent
Aldehydes	Anti-inflammatory, astringent, bactericidal, hypothermic
Coumarins	Sedative, calming action
Dienes	Anticoagulant, antispasmodic
Esters	Antispasmodic, sedative
Ethers	Sedative, antispasmodic
Ketones	Anticoagulant, sedative, mucinolytic
Oxides	Mucinolytic, decongestant, expectorant
Phenols	Anthelmintic, bactericidal, fungicidal
Sesquiterpenes	Antiallergic properties
Terpenes	Bactericidal, fungicidal, tonic

This synergy works both to enhance outcomes directly and to reduce the possibility of side-effects by some constituents cancelling out the potentially damaging effects of others. This is known as 'quenching'.

An oil usually contains between three and five chemical groups. Because of the synergistic effects it is not possible to determine the therapeutic properties by simply listing the properties associated with each constituent. The influence of one chemical group on another results in specific therapeutic properties. For example, studies on mice have shown lavender oil to be a more effective sedative than its two major constituents in isolation. One of the chemical groups is usually present in greater quantity than the others and the oil is often named for this group, although it does not necessarily show the expected therapeutic characteristics.

Knowledge of environmental effects on essential oil content and the composition of aromatic crops is essential to determine the level of success that can be obtained in therapeutic use. Significant differences among essential oil contents can be observed between plants grown under field conditions and those grown in greenhouses.[8]

Chemotypes

Oils derived from the same source but with different characteristics are known as 'chemotypes'. There may be more than one chemotype for a given essential oil. For example:

- Most thyme oils on the market are rich in thymol, a compound with irritant properties; other chemotypes of thyme oil exist, which may contain little or no thymol, markedly changing its therapeutic potential.
- There are three commercial types of camomile oil – German (*Matricaria recutica*), Roman or English (*Chamamaelium nobile*) and Moroccan (*Ormenis multicaulis*), all differing in genus and composition.
- Eucalyptus oil can be extracted from 120 different species and at least three entirely different commercial oils are available.

Care should be taken to read the labels of such products to ascertain whether the ingredients are as expected. The selling price of an oil may reflect its composition.

The chemical constituents of an essential oil represent a mixture of many organic compounds that have related, but distinct, types of chemical structure, giving the oil its odour, therapeutic properties and, in some cases its toxicity.[9] These constituents can vary with a number of different factors:

- The characteristics of the soil and climate in which the plants have been grown can affect the composition of the oil. In drought or other extreme climatic circumstances, or if there are nutritional deficiencies in the soil, the plant's essential oils help to facilitate survival. The amount of essential oil in a plant is inversely proportional to the amount of water present. As the plant dries out it produces essential oils to compensate for the loss of water. Thus, the aroma from dried flowers is often more intense than that from fresh leafy material. Furthermore, the aroma from specimens of certain cultivated species may differ from that of similar wild species.[10] The wild variety of *Rosmarinus officinalis* (rosemary), which grows in various parts of Europe, contains an ester and ketone as its main active ingredients. The same variety cultivated in a greenhouse contains an oxide as the main chemical group. Geographical location may also affect the nature of the essential oil. The Mediterranean version of rosemary has a ketone as the main constituent and smells quite different to the wild or greenhouse varieties. The effect of various combinations of day and night temperatures and day lengths have been studied using dill plants in environmentally controlled chambers.[11] The concentration of essential oil was found to be highest during high-temperature periods; exposure to light was also important.
- Different stages of a plant's development may affect the oil's characteristics. For example, when *Verbena officinalis* is in bloom it gives off a pleasant perfume. However, soon after blooming this is replaced by a bitter odour. Hence plants destined for oil extraction must be harvested at specific times of the year.
- In many cases the time of day and environmental conditions at the time of harvesting are also important in determining the chemical and therapeutic nature of the essential oil. The period of time that elapses between collection of raw plant material and distillation must be as short as possible because chemical changes are initiated immediately after cutting. Significant differences in the essential oil content have been observed in camomile during protracted storage of harvested plants. After 31 months' storage at 16°C approximately 50% of the initial oil content was maintained.[12]
- Differences in production techniques and manufacturing equipment will result in differences in the quality and composition of the resultant oil.[4]
- Degradation from incorrect storage conditions can occur. The main degrading factor is atmospheric oxygen, which causes the oxidation of active principals, especially terpenes, and this process is

enhanced by heat and light. Chemical change can result in the appearance of toxic chemicals. Terpene degradation in certain oils leads to compounds that can act as skin sensitisers being formed.

Despite its name, an essential oil may or may not necessarily be oily in consistency. For example, the cedar tree produces a non-oily substance known as thujone that is very poisonous and should not be used in aromatherapy.[13] Tansy oil is a safe chemotype; it contains little or no thujone but unfortunately is not commercially available. Other oils may not represent a naturally occurring state, but are changed for commercial reasons. White camphor oil is only a fraction of true camphor oil, while cornmint oil almost always has its menthol content halved.

Quality of oils

Apart from the intrinsic nature of the oil and the possibility that its chemotypes may be confused, oils are liable to adulteration and contamination, possibilities that are said to be widespread.[14] Possible adulterants include other essential oils, chemotypes and synthetic chemicals. Contaminants may include herbicides and pesticides. It is possible to detect these foreign materials using gas chromatography, mass spectroscopy, high-performance liquid chromatography, and nuclear magnetic resonance: for consumers, it is important that aromatherapy products are purchased from a reputable source.

'Oils' may be fabricated by combining the same components as are found in the naturally occurring oil. There are probably no particular dangers associated with using these fabricated oils other than the possibility of allergic skin reactions. Examples of commonly fabricated oils include melissa and verbena. Other oils may be totally synthetic, for example wintergreen oil is almost always made from the chemical methyl salicylate.

Some oils are marketed as both essences and essential oils. The significant price difference between the two variants can be confusing to consumers who do not appreciate the fact that the former have not been subject to distillation.

Storage

It is recommended that essential oils should be used within 1 year of opening the container. Because of the potential increase in the rate of degradation as a result of heat and light, oils should be packed in amber bottles and kept in a cool place, preferably a refrigerator. Under these circumstances the lifespan of the oil may be doubled. Some oils become viscous if stored in a refrigerator, making them rather difficult to pour if they are not allowed to reach room temperature before use.

Incorrect storage may lead to the production of impurities that can cause dermatological problems.

Aromatherapy in practice

The term 'aromatherapy' is commonly applied both to treating ill health (i.e. therapy) and cosmetic use, which relies on 'fragrancing'. Making a distinction between the two is not always possible: the use of aromatherapy in epilepsy, for example, is clearly designed to be therapeutic,[15] but where largely psychological factors might be involved a clear distinction is not easy.

Four basic types of use may be identified:[16]

- cosmetic – aromas are of a pleasurable type (bath essences, soaps)
- holistic aromatherapy for general stress
- environmental fragrancing – evocative scents of wartime Britain have been used to treat depression and memory loss in old people. According to a report in the *London Times* psychiatrists believe that certain odours, from damp washing to the fires of the Blitz, bring unique breakthroughs for the elderly, whose nostalgic memories of youth have otherwise been lost. A highly characteristic odour pervaded the stations of the Glasgow Underground prior to the system's modernisation. The City's Transport Museum has tried to recreate this environment in one of its displays
- medicinal or clinical aromatherapy – used in the treatment of various conditions and where outcomes are measurable.

Aromatherapy practitioners claim to be able to help a range of conditions, including eczema, digestive problems, muscular aches and pains, premenstrual syndrome, asthma, insomnia and headaches. Because aromatherapy encourages relaxation, it is thought that patients suffering from stress-related conditions can also benefit.[17] Another aspect of aromatherapy is an enhanced feel-good factor, which may improve self-esteem, following a massage or a bath with essential oils. The current interpretation of the word 'perfume' illustrates the divergent course taken by modern fragrancing away from traditional aromatics.[18] As recently as the nineteenth century, 'to perfume' still meant 'to disinfect', i.e. to fumigate by using scent or, more literally, through smoke (i.e. per fume). When our ancestors scented themselves and their possessions or took a nosegay or scented handkerchief it was with a dual mood-enhancing and germicidal objective. Only in the past century or so has the purpose of fragrancing been divided between the aesthetic objectives of the modern perfume industry and the therapeutic objectives of aromatherapy. Aromas have also been used as a marketing tool. For example, supermarkets are known to release aromas of newly baked bread or percolating coffee to enhance sales. According to the Director of the Smell and Taste Treatment and Research Foundation of Chicago, 'Smell and taste are an enormous part of our everyday lives and *much* more than just a biological response'.[19]

Aromatherapy in France and Germany, in direct contrast to that in the UK and the USA, involves medically qualified doctors using essential oils as conventional internal medicines.

As a way of including both medical and non-medical practice, the term 'olfactory remediation' has been suggested to describe the umbrella beneath which aromatherapy may coexist with a more scientific practice that also employs essential oils.[20] In this model aromatherapy is considered to be a largely experience-oriented discipline with a reliance on healing rather than scientific principles. It is usually practised by non-health professionals, who aim to treat a wide range of physical, mental and emotional symptoms, as well as being prescribed for general well-being.

The second area of olfactory remediation is not called aromatherapy formally, although its results may affect its practice. In this area olfactory stimulation is used therapeutically in a more specific manner to alleviate particular medical conditions only where appropriate. Studies on clinical outcomes have been published. Health professionals, especially nurses, are often involved in this variant. Although it is conceivable that pharmacists may be involved in both methods of using essential oils it is olfactory stimulation to which this chapter refers.

Route of administration

Essential oils may be administered by one or more of the following routes:

- topically
- internally by mouth
- externally by inhalation
- rectally or vaginally.

Topically

Essential oils are included in several patented OTC products, including Vicks rub and Tiger Balm, where the ointment base serves as a carrier for both transdermal absorption and inhalation.

Normally the oils are used in liquid form, although various gel and cream formulations exist. As the oils are highly concentrated they should not generally be applied to the skin undiluted, except under supervision. The use of aromatherapy oils contained in a vegetable carrier oil by skin massage is the most frequent route of administration. Aromatherapists dilute essential oils (0.5 ml/10 ml) with carrier oils, such as sweet almond, walnut, wheatgerm and hazelnut, which contain active vitamins and fatty acids. Other possible carrier oils are rapeseed, sunflower and soya bean.[21] Lavender oil enters the circulation within 5–10 min, with maximal blood concentrations being achieved after approximately 20 min.

The rate of essential oil absorption through the skin varies with a number of factors:

- **Temperature.** A modest rise in the temperature of the skin is likely to cause enhanced blood flow and therefore lead to increased absorption of the essential oil. Many years ago the absorption of methyl salicylate was investigated and found to be enhanced by a rise in skin temperature consistent with taking a bath.[22] If the temperature is too high, the volatile oils will evaporate, reducing the amount of essential oil available for absorption.

- **Water.** The presence of water influences the rate of absorption; it is thus beneficial to have a shower or bath prior to applying essential oils.

- **Skin occlusion.** Covering the skin with a non-permeable dressing causes a change in the local environment: both temperature and hydration increase. As stated above, this will facilitate a more rapid absorption of essential oil. An American study with perfumes showed that almost 20 times as much fragrance was absorbed through the skin when it was covered than when it was left uncovered.[23] The application of a greasy ointment will have a partial occlusive effect in that it retards evaporation of water away from the skin. However, this also retards the passage of the essential oil and ointment bases are useful only for local effects.

- **Presence of detergent.** Detergents and soaps increase skin permeability, thus a good wash before aromatherapy is likely to be beneficial. The fat-solubility of oil-based liniments and other oily topical applications (e.g. oily creams) helps the penetration of essential oils.

Part of the aromatherapy treatment is the act of massage itself (Chapter 13) and this is extremely useful in the relief of stress and tension. Ready-blended oils, comprising several essential oils mixed in a carrier, are available for specific purposes, e.g. rheumatics or insomnia. Massage also provides the means for establishing a positive patient–practitioner healing relationship.[24] Aromatherapy massage is a mixture of Swedish (soft-tissue massage), shiatsu (massage at acupuncture points) and neuromuscular massage. Gentle rubbing movements may be used in some cases. Essential oils can also be added to bath water. Here the cosmetic and medical applications become entwined. Clients often find it helpful to relax in a pleasantly scented bath for 20–30 min and this can also be used to relieve muscular strains and sprains. About 6–8 drops of oil are suggested. The oil is normally eliminated from the body within about 90 min.

Compresses may also be used for skin conditions.

Internally by mouth

Some essential oils are used as orthodox medicines and are given orally. The oral use of peppermint oil[25] and some components of essential oils, such as pinene, limonene, camphene and borneol, is documented.[26,27] Various oils of the Umbelliferae family, e.g. caraway, dill and fennel, are used in remedies for indigestion, flatulence and dyspepsia in adults and infants.

In general the oral administration of essential oils is not recommended, except under medical supervision, for it may carry a risk of an adverse reaction occurring. Significant levels of active ingredients in the blood stream are achieved. Oral administration is not routinely used in the UK, although some practitioners do recommend the use of a weak aqueous solution as a mouthwash. Rinsing the mouth four times a day with 15 ml of a 5% solution of tea tree oil has been shown to be effective in treating oral thrush.[28] Gargles and mouthwashes made from essential oils should not be swallowed.

Externally by inhalation

Many conditions respond extremely well to essential oil inhalation. There are several commercially available inhalation products that include essential oils in their formulation (Karvol, Vicks) as well as the standard inhalation of camphor and menthol BP. The oils can be inhaled using the old-fashioned bowl of hot water and towel over the head method or simply from 1–2 drops on a handkerchief or tissue. A few drops on the pillow may help a restless client sleep, but direct contact with the skin should be avoided. A variety of steam inhalers and fan-assisted apparatus are available. Used as a room fragrance, essential oils create a pleasant atmosphere, enhancing the mood and even creating a suitable ambiance for meditation (Figure 6.1).

Other routes of administration

Rectal (suppositories) or vaginal administration (pessaries or douches) using appropriate presentations are found to be useful for localised symptoms. Being lined with mucous membranes, the rectum and vagina are both sensitive to irritation.

Metabolism[29]

Essential oil components are metabolised differently according to the route of administration.

After external application most essential oil components are likely to pass through the skin and enter the blood stream.[30]

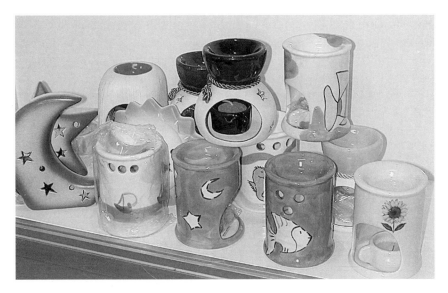

Figure 6.1 Aromatherapy burners; a small candle facilitates vaporisation.

Inhaled components pass to the lungs or olfactory system. The olfactory nerves lie in the upper part of the nose and are directly connected to the brain. From the main body of each olfactory cell several fine cilia extend into the layer of mucus in the nose. The tips of these filaments have receptors that can detect the presence of any aromatic particles. Essential oils and other aromatic substances are extremely volatile and are taken into the nose as vapour, dissolving in the mucosal layer. The olfactory nerves can only detect the odour when it is in this form. Information about the odour passes to the body of the cell from the cilia and from here longer nerve fibres transmit the information through the limbic system to the part of the brain associated with emotion, motivation and thought.

Orally administered essential oils are absorbed through the large and small intestine, and subsequently enter the circulation.[31] Most essential oils are fat-soluble but as they pass to the liver enzymic action will change them to more water-soluble structures, facilitating urinary excretion. Fat-soluble substances usually pass readily into the central nervous system and the liver, more slowly into muscle and finally into adipose tissue, where a store of essential oil components may be built up slowly because of low blood flow. Once lodged in fat, most substances are inactive.

Essential oils are often electrically charged at body pH and can adhere easily to electrically charged molecules such as proteins. Ketones, esters, aldehydes and carboxylic acids, all of which are found in essential oils, tend to bind to plasma albumin, a soluble protein that is present in the blood in very high concentrations. Although it is not known whether this mechanism, which is found in drug metabolism, applies to essential oils, these two facts make it a likely hypothesis.

The metabolic pathways of essential oils are summarised in Figure 6.2.

Choice of oil

As with methods applicable to other complementary therapies, the choice of a particular oil will depend on the individual patient. Patients with similar symptoms may be prescribed different oils or mixtures of oils. Aromatherapy oils may be classified into groups according to their effects, two of which are stimulants and sedatives.

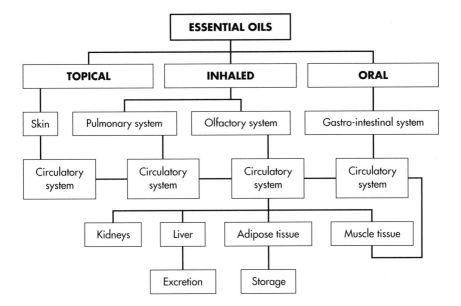

Figure 6.2 Absorption pathways of essential oils.

Stimulants

These oils are useful in the short term, in a crisis or when exceptional effort is required, or in convalescence in small amounts to help restore some vitality. They include basil, black pepper, eucalyptus, peppermint and rosemary; rosemary is the most widely used. There is some debate as to whether stimulant oils should be used during pregnancy. Such decisions should be left in the hands of a qualified aromatherapist.

Sedatives

A number of essential oils are considered to be primarily calming or sedative. These include bergamot, camomile, lavender, marjoram, melissa and sandalwood. The most effective ways of using these oils are in massage and in baths, especially before going to bed.

Some oils have been shown to have both sedative and stimulant properties depending on the way in which they are used. These include geranium, neroli (orange flower) and rosewood.

Blends of oils for treating a variety of conditions are available. Most textbooks will give an indication of oils that can be mixed in a suitable carrier.

Conditions treated

Examples of common applications of aromatherapy in the pharmacy environment, together with appropriate routes of administration, are summarised in Table 6.3.

Evidence

Robust evidence for the benefits of aromatherapy is scarce. The quality of published trials is generally low and the range of conditions treated diverse. There are few trials of aromatherapy on human subjects, most studies having used animal or tissue culture models.[32] The randomised controlled trial (RCT) literature on aromatherapy has been evaluated in order to define whether or not any clinical indication is backed up by evidence.[33] Studies on the local effects of oils and those involving healthy volunteers were excluded. Six RCTs were located, one each for the common

Table 6.3 Examples of essential oils and their uses

Condition to treat	Essential oil	Route of administration
Arthritis	Camomile, juniper, rosemary	Massage, bath additive
Athlete's foot	Lavender, tea tree	Footbath
Blisters	Lavender	Topical application
Burns	Lavender, camomile, eucalyptus, tea tree	Topical application, bath
Chilblains	Juniper, lavender, marjoram, rosemary	Topical application
Colds	Eucalyptus, orange, tea tree	Inhalation, massage/rub throat and chest
Coughs	Eucalyptus, lavender	Inhalation, massage/rub throat and chest
Influenza	Eucalyptus, juniper, lavender, tea tree	Inhalation, massage/rub throat and chest
Insect bites	Camomile, lavender, tea tree	Topical application, bath, compress
Irritable bowel syndrome	Camomile	Massage abdomen, bath
Migraine	Lavender, marjoram, rosemary	Inhalation, massage head and neck
Muscle injuries	Eucalyptus, marjoram, rosemary, tangerine	Massage/rub affected area
Nausea	Lavender, mint	Inhalation
Sore throat	Lavender, sandalwood, tea tree	Massage/rub throat and upper chest

cold, prophylaxis of bronchitis, smoking withdrawal symptoms, perineal discomfort after childbirth, anxiety and alopecia. With one exception these were all positive. A further six trials were found concerning the use of aromatherapy for anxiety and well-being in a variety of patient types in the hospital environment. Positive results were recorded in five of these studies, suggesting that aromatherapy may have an anxiolytic effect but that the evidence for other applications was not 'compelling'.

A randomised trial assessing the effectiveness of aromatherapy in reducing preoperative anxiety in women undergoing abortions has been carried out. Aromatherapy appeared to be no more effective than having patients sniff other pleasant odours in reducing preprocedure anxiety.[34]

An investigation into the use of aromatherapy in the management of acute postoperative pain concluded that further research was necessary before a firm conclusion could be reached.[35]

The use of aromatherapy during childbirth is becoming an increasingly popular care option with mothers and midwives. An evaluation of a midwifery aromatherapy service for mothers in labour has been reported.[36] This study, of 8058 mothers in childbirth, is the largest research initiative so far undertaken in the use of aromatherapy within a healthcare setting. The study took place over a period of 8 years and a total of 10 essential oils were used plus a carrier oil, administered to the participants via skin absorption and inhalation. The study found little direct evidence that the practice of aromatherapy reduced the need for pain relief during labour or the incidence of operative delivery. However, a key finding of this study suggests that two essential oils, clary sage and camomile, are effective in alleviating pain. The evidence from this study suggests that aromatherapy can be effective in reducing maternal anxiety, fear and/or pain during labour. The use of aromatherapy appeared to facilitate a further reduction in the use of systemic opioids in the study centre, from 6% in 1990 to 0.4% in 1997 (per woman).

Aromatherapy and massage have gained wide popularity amongst nurses in clinical practice. An RCT has shown that a statistically significant psychological benefit was derived from giving foot massage to patients following cardiac surgery.[37] Evidence from an audit into the effects of aromatherapy massage in palliative and terminal care suggested that most patients derived some benefit.[38] The effect of massage with 1% Roman camomile in carrier oil has been investigated in patients receiving palliative care.[39] The control group was given massage alone. Anxiety scores improved in both groups but the aromatherapy group showed significant improvement in physical symptoms and quality of life. Other workers have not found significant improvements when using aromatherapy and massage over massage alone.[40]

Another study investigated the effects of aromatherapy and massage on disturbed behaviour in severe dementia.[41] Only four patients completed the evaluation. The opinion of the staff involved was that all four patients benefited from the treatment, but in fact only one of the participants showed an improvement of statistical significance. A number of other studies have demonstrated positive effects from massage.[42]

Aromatherapy has been used by some patients suffering from epilepsy as a means of controlling their seizures. Certain oils, notably rosemary, can cause an increase in seizure frequency, so the appropriate oil must be carefully selected.

Statistically significant differences have been noted between groups of patients suffering from a common cold who inhaled a mixture of camphor (35%), menthol (56%) and eucalyptus (9%) compared with those using a hot-water vapour control. Only 24 adults were involved in the trial.[43]

Essential oils as antiseptics

Many essential oils and their constituents have antimicrobial properties.[44] Indeed, essential oils have been used externally to eradicate fungal or bacterial infections for hundreds of years.[45] At the time of the Black Death, apothecaries would wrap scarves soaked in essential oils such as camphor around their necks and over their mouths when visiting sick patients.

In the years just prior to the First World War and following an article in *Nature*, Even, a French pharmacist, impregnated gauze with the essential oils bergamot, geranium, lavender and rosemary.[46] These volatile oils were selected because in his opinion they had the greatest antiseptic value while being the least irritating. The fragranced dressing was used to cover suppurating wounds. During the Great War Australian soldiers used tea tree oil (see below).

Several other essential oils are said to have antimicrobial qualities, including cinnamon, salvia (sage), sandalwood and thymus (thyme).

Essential oils of eucalyptus, lavender and thyme in the proportion 2:2:4 provide an effective disinfectant, and tissues impregnated with the mixture are recommended for wiping toilet seats, baths and basins in areas of uncertain pedigree! A disinfectant suitable for tropical countries has oregano added, the essential oil of which contains up to 15% thymol.

Although lavender oil is often assumed to be 'very antiseptic',[47] studies carried out on a range of commercial lavender oils have shown a wide variation in antibacterial effect.[48] Nevertheless, a few drops of lavender, lemongrass and thyme are reported as being effective in disinfecting mattresses. A wide variation in activity in other essential oils has also been reported.[49]

Peppermint is one of the oldest and best-known European medicinal herbs, and is reputed to produce a gentle disinfectant effect (preventing fermentation) when there are abnormal decomposition processes in the stomach. Both the herb and its oil may be used externally in baths to treat cuts and skin rashes. The oil contains about 50% menthol.

One of the most widely used antiseptic oils in recent years has been tea tree oil.[50] The oil is obtained from the leaves of *Melaleuca* spp., historically used by Australian aboriginals and New Zealand Maoris to treat skin abrasions and infections. The name was invented by Captain Cook, whose crew used the leaves to make tea and to flavour beer. Tea tree oil was distributed to Australian soldiers during the First World War as a disinfectant, leading to a high demand for its products locally. In recent years the oil has become widely available in Europe. It contains terpinoids and is effective against fungus and bacteria, including *Pneumococcus*, *Staphylococcus*,[51] *Streptococcus* and those resistant to some orthodox antibiotics.[52] A 3-month single-blind study has shown topical application of 5% tea tree oil gel in patients suffering from acne is at least as beneficial as 3% benzyl peroxide, with fewer side-effects.[53] A double-blind study found that a 10% tea tree oil cream was as effective as clotrimazole in the treatment of athlete's foot.[54] It has been pointed out that topical application of a gel or lotion in this fashion does not really constitute true aromatherapy.[55]

The aromatogram[56]

The aromatogram is a laboratory test that allows aromatherapists to analyse in vitro the antibacterial activity of essential oils and to select more accurately those considered to be the most effective in destroying a particular microbial infection. The test is conducted much like the conventional culture test for antibiotic activity.

Safety

One of the concerns with aromatherapy is its marketable strengths, which suggests that the consumer does not have to be an expert aromatherapist to use the oils.[57] Indeed, the availability of essential oils in the high street and advice columns in magazines and newspapers could be interpreted as evidence of total safety.

It is important to view the possibility of side-effects in context, for they are only likely to occur with prolonged use of high concentrations and in people with acute hepatic or renal problems. However, clearly some of the chemical groups present in essential oils are potentially toxic and clients should be instructed that essential oils should be used judiciously and according to instructions.

Most of the data on toxicity relate to the ingestion of essential oils. Oral administration is extremely rare in the UK, so the reports available refer to poisoning from accidental or intentional ingestion of large amounts of essential oils, including citronella[58,59] and eucalyptus. Death is usual after consuming about 30 ml of the latter, following severe cardiovascular, respiratory and central nervous effects.[60] There are many recorded cases of poisoning by essential oils in young children.

Camphor and sassafras are claimed to be carcinogenic and their use is generally contraindicated in aromatherapy. Camphorated oil is not an essential oil and so cases of poisoning due to ingestion of this are not included here.

In general, toxicity is dose-dependent: the more of an oil that is used, the higher the potential toxicity.

Potential toxic effects

Potential side-effects include dermal toxicity, skin sensitisation (allergy), phototoxicity and dependence.[61]

Dermal toxicity   Skin irritation is a relatively common reaction to the application of several essential oils, although this risk may be reduced by dilution. Some oils may cause a dermatological reaction after prolonged use. Severely irritant essential oils include horseradish and mustard; moderately or strongly irritant oils include cinnamon, clove, oregano, parsley, rue and wintergreen. Tea tree oil has also been cited as causing dermatitis.[62]

Skin sensitisation (allergy)   Allergies to camomile have been reported,[63] with two cases of nipple dermatis after the application of an OTC product containing the essential oil.[64] The most notorious oils for causing allergies are costus (formerly used widely in perfumes) and verbena. Cinnamon, garlic and laurel leaf oil can also cause sensitisation reactions to varying degrees. Skin rashes and itching have been reported following the application of tea tree oil.[65] Table 6.4 shows a number of commonly used essential oils for which sensitising constituents have been identified.[66] Aromatherapists themselves may be subject to sensitisation, particularly if they are handling significant quantities of oils on a daily basis.[67]

Phototoxicity[68]   Certain essential oils (e.g. verbena, bergamot and the citrus oils, including grapefruit, lemon, lime and orange) may cause increased photosensitivity in some individuals if the skin is exposed to direct sunlight shortly after application (see section on aromatherapy during pregnancy, below). Substances known to be phototoxic include many with antiseptic properties that are added to toiletries and suntan preparations. Phototoxic components (psoralens or furanocoumarins) are present in a limited number of essential oils and in small amounts, normally less than 2%, but nevertheless they are still capable of causing a reaction, even if the essential oil is diluted substantially. One report concerns a woman who was treated for minor burns after 20 min spent on a sunbed immediately after taking a sauna where there were a few drops of lemon oil on the burner.

It has been found that the bergapten component of bergamot oil produces abnormally dark pigmentation and reddening of the surrounding skin after exposure to an ultraviolet lamp. This condition is known as berloque dermatitis or bergapten dermatitis. The darkened patches of skin can remain for several years. To ensure that the risk of photosensitivity is reduced to a minimum, maximum-use levels have been set for some common essential oils. These are summarised in Table 6.5.

Table 6.4 Main sensitising constituent of some common essential oils

Essential oil	Main sensitising constituent
Bergamot	Coumarins
Camphor	Terpene
Dill	Carvone
Eucalyptus	Creole and phellandrene
Fennel	Phellandrene
Lemon	Limonene
Lemongrass	Citral
Pine oil	Borneol
Rose oil	Citronelle
Spearmint	Limonene

Table 6.5 Maximum dose levels to ensure risk of photosensitivity is minimised[67]

Verbena	0.05%
Bergamot	0.4%
Lime	0.7% (expressed)
Rue	0.78%
Orange	1.4% (expressed)
Lemon	2.0% (expressed)
Grapefruit	4.0% (expressed)

Dependence   It is possible that the repeated application of rubs and ointments containing large amounts of essential oils (e.g. Vicks or Tiger Balm) may lead to some dependence, with the product being used long after it needs to be. Pharmacists should be alert to this possibility.

Interactions with orthodox medicines[69]

There may be interactions between orthodox medicines and essential oils. Possible problems include enhanced transdermal penetration, potentiation effect of warfarin, monoamine oxidase inhibition and the induction of cytochrome P_{450}, an important detoxifying enzyme that is induced by alcohol and certain drugs, including carbamazepine, diphenhydramine, nicotine, nitrazepam, phenobarbital, phenytoin and progestogens. Any essential oil taken orally that also induces this enzyme may potentiate the toxic effect of a drug.

Common drugs that are incompatible with topically applied oils include aspirin (clove and garlic), paracetamol (basil, camphor, cinnamon, clove), pethidine (parsley) and warfarin (cinnamon, clove, garlic, wintergreen).

Interaction with homeopathic medicines

Traditionally it is said that homeopathic remedies are inactivated by aromatic oils, thus the two should not be used concurrently. There is no firm evidence to substantiate this perception, but it is usual to instruct patients to leave 1–2 h between brushing the teeth with a peppermint toothpaste and taking a homeopathic medicine.

Aromatherapy during pregnancy

Authorities are divided as to the advisability of using aromatherapy oils during pregnancy as there are no reliable data on potential teratogenic, abortifacient and emmenagogic risks. However, it is probable that the components of essential oils can cross the placental barrier and a number are contraindicated or should be used with caution during pregnancy (see below).[70]

One of the most versatile essential oils, lavender, is classified by some aromatherapists as emmenagogic (i.e. it may cause uterine bleeding and/or a miscarriage) and is restricted to the later stages of pregnancy or not used at all. Other authorities promote its use throughout pregnancy. Other essential oils said to be emmenagogic are calendula, jasmine, juniper, marjoram, melissa, nutmeg, peppermint and thyme. There is no evidence that, even if these oils are potentially emmenagogic in the small amounts used during aromatherapy, they would necessarily be abortifacients.

Aromatherapists sometimes recommend that new mothers add 6–8 drops of lavender oil to bathwater following childbirth, but a study found no evidence that such a practice was effective in reducing perineal discomfort.[71]

There are accounts in the literature of women attempting to bring on menstruation[72] or induce abortions with pennyroyal, an essential oil that is in any case contraindicated in aromatherapy because of hepatotoxicity.[73] Extra care should be taken with topical use of essential oils during pregnancy. For aromatherapy massage over large areas of skin a maximum concentration of 2% essential oil is recommended. The phototoxic risk mentioned above is particularly important in pregnant women, who already have raised melanocytic hormone levels and are therefore more likely to burn in strong sunlight. These oils should only be used by qualified practitioners for short periods and mothers advised to keep out of the sun for between 2 and 12 h after therapy, depending on the concentration of oil used.

An example of a special topical formulation for nursing mothers is in use at the Maternity Unit at the Southern General Hospital in Glasgow. It comprises a mixture of three oils – cypress, geranium and lavender – in the proprietary gel known as KY and is applied three times a day to the vaginal area.

A summary of oils that may be used in pregnancy and those that should be avoided is given below:

- Oils that are generally considered safe to use during pregnancy: camomile, ginger, lavender, rose, sandalwood.
- Oils that may be used externally during pregnancy: anise, mace, nutmeg, rosemary, spike lavender.

- Oils that should be avoided during pregnancy: oils rich in apinol, e.g. parsley leaf and seed, and oils rich in sabinyl acetate, e.g. sage and savin.

Aromatherapy in the pharmacy

OTC supply

A list of common aromatherapy oils and their main indications is provided at the end of this chapter.

Reducing the risks of adverse reactions

Containers and labelling

Inadequate labelling and lack of appropriate guidance on how the product should be used at the point of sale are two major inadequacies that could be rectified relatively easily. Containers that restrict the delivery of contents to drops, facilitating more accurate dilution, are essential.

Counselling

Clients intending to self-treat should be advised to take the following precautions:[74]

- Never eat or drink essential oils except under medical supervision.
- Never use concentrated essential oils directly on the skin; always dilute with a suitable carrier oil (e.g. almond oil) – a typical dilution for massage is 15 drops of essential oil to 50 ml of a carrier oil.
- Be aware that some oils (e.g. bergamot, lemon and orange) can react with sunlight and burn the skin.
- Clients in an 'at-risk category' (infants, the elderly, pregnant women, or those who have kidney or liver problems, etc.) should seek professional advice before attempting to treat ongoing conditions.
- Do not use homeopathic and aromatherapy remedies concurrently.

Table 6.6 Characteristics and uses of a selection of common oils

Oil	Characteristics	Examples of indications
Bergamot	Uplifting	Anxiety, appetite loss, skin problems
Camomile	Comforting	Muscle/joints, skin, soothing, calming
Clary sage	Relaxing	Sedative, stress/tension
Clove	Stimulating	Antiseptic, toothache
Eucalyptus	Energising	Antiseptic, respiratory, antiviral
Geranium	Uplifting	Anxiety, skin problems
Ginger	Warming	Colds/flu, stomach problems
Lavender	Relaxing	Muscle/joints, skin problems, soothing
Lemon	Refreshing	Antiseptic, cols/flu/sore throat, tonic, skin
Patchouli	Soothing/sensual	Anxiety, skin problems
Peppermint	Stimulating	Anxiety, cooling, feet, insect repellant
Rosemary	Reviving	Circulation, mental processes, lethargy
Sandalwood	Balancing	Urinary, throat, skin problems
Tea tree	Revitalising	Antibacterial, fungal (thrush)
Ylang ylang	Relaxing, sensual	Respiration regulation, shock, trauma

Common oils and their uses

Table 6.6 gives a summary of the most common oils together with examples of their indications.

More information

Aromatherapy Organisations Council
PO Box 19834
London
SE25 6WF
Tel/fax: 020 8251 7912

Association of Medical Aromatherapists
Abergare, Rhu Point
Helensburgh
Dumbartonshire
G84 8NF
Tel: 0141 332 4924

International Federation of Aromatherapists
Stamford House
2–4 Chiswick High Road

London
W4 1TH
Tel: 020 8742 2605
www.int-fed-aromatherapy.co.uk

References

1. *Unabridged Electronic Dictionary* (CD-Rom). New York: Random House, 1994.
2. Damian P, Damian K. *Aromatherapy. Scent and Psyche*. Rochester, Vermont: Healing Arts Press, 1995: 3.
3. Gattefossé R-M. *Aromathérapie: Les Huiles Essentielles Hormones Végétales*. Paris: Girardot, 1937.
4. Gattefossé R-M. *Gattefossé's Aromatherapy*. Tisserand R (ed.) Saffron Walden: C W Daniel, 1993.
5. Kayne S B. The sweet smell of health. *Chemist Druggist* 1998; 21 March: i–v.
6. Davis P. *Aromatherapy – An A–Z*. Saffron Walden: C W Daniel, 1995: 110–115.
7. Buckle J. Aromatherapy. Does it matter which lavender essential oil is used? *Nurs Times* 1993; 89: 32–35.
8. Morales M R, Simon J E, Charles D J. Comparison of essential oil content and composition between field and greenhouse grown genotypes of methyl cinnamate basil. *J Herbs Spices Medicinal Plants* 1990; 1: 25–35.
9. Tisserand R, Balacs T. *Essential Oil Safety*. Edinburgh: Churchill Livingstone, 1996: 8.
10. Serrentino J. *How Natural Remedies Work*. Washington: Hartley and Marks, 1991.
11. Halva S, Craker L E, Simon J E, Charles D J. Growth and essential oil in dill, *Anethum graveolens* in response to temperature and photoperiod. *J Herbs Spices Medicinal Plants* 1993; 1: 47–56.
12. Letchmo W. Effect of storage temperatures and duration on the essential oil and flavenoids of chamomile. *J Herbs Spices Medicinal Plants* 1993; 1: 13–26.
13. Davis P. *Aromatherapy: An A–Z*. Saffron Walden: C W Daniel, 1995.
14. Barnes J. Aromatherapy. *Pharm J* 1998; 260: 862–867.
15. Betts T, Fox C, Rooth K, MacCallum R. An olfactory countermeasure treatment for epileptic seizures using a conditioned arousal response to specific aromatherapy oils. *Epilepsia* 1995; 36 (suppl. 3): S130.
16. Buckle J. Aromatherapy. In: Novey D W (ed.) *Clinician's Complete Reference to Complementary and Alternative Medicine*. St Louis, MO: Mosby, 2000: 653.
17. Anon. Aromatherapy. *Health Which?* 1999; June: 30–31.
18. Damian P, Damian K. *Aromatherapy. Scent and Psyche*. Rochester, VT: Healing Arts Press, 1995: 23–24.
19. Smell and Taste Foundation website. http://www.smellandtaste.org.
20. Martin G N. Olfactory remediation: current evidence and possible applications. *Soc Sci Med* 1996; 43: 63–69.
21. Sadler J. *Aromatherapy*. London: Parragon, 1984.

22. Brown E W, Scott W O. Absorption of methyl salicylate by human skin. *J Pharmacol Exp Ther* 1934; 50: 32–50.

23. Bronaugh R L. In vivo percutaneous absorption of fragrance ingredients in rhesus monkeys and humans. *Food Chem Toxicol* 1990; 28: 369–373.

24. Tisserand R. *The Art of Aromatherapy*. Saffron Walden: C W Daniel, 1990.

25. *British National Formulary*, vol. 41. London: British Medical Association/Royal Pharmaceutical Society of Great Britain, 2001.

26. Somerville K W, Ellis W R, Whitten B H *et al*. Stones in the common bile duct: experience with medical dissolution therapy. *Postgrad Med J* 1985; 61: 313–316.

27. Engelstein E, Kahan E, Servadio C. Rowarinex for the treatment of ureterolithiasis. *J Urol* 1992; 98: 98–100.

28. Jandourek A, Vaishampayan J K, Vazquez J A. Efficacy of melaleuca oral solution for the treatment of fluconazole refractory oral candidiasis in AIDS patients. *AIDS* 1998; 12: 1032–1037.

29. Tisserand R, Balacs T. *Essential Oil Safety*. Edinburgh: Churchill Livingstone, 1996: 35–44.

30. Jager W, Buchbauer G, Jirovetz L, Fritzer M. Percutaneous absorption of lavender oil from a massage oil. *J Soc Cosmet Chem* 1992; 43: 49–54.

31. Kovar K A, Gropper B, Friess D, Ammon H P T. Blood levels of 1.8–cineole and locomotor activity of mice after inhalation and oral administration of rosemary oil. *Planta Med* 1987; 53: 315–318.

32. Lis-Balchin M. Essential oils and aromatherapy; their modern role in healing. *J R Soc Health* 1997; 11: 324–329.

33. Cooke B, Ernst E. Aromatherapy: a systematic review. *Br J Gen Pract* 2000; 50: 493–496.

34. Wiebe E. A randomized trial of aromatherapy to reduce anxiety before abortion. *Effect Clin Pract* 2000; 3: 166–169.

35. Ching M. Contemporary therapy: aromatherapy in the management of acute pain? *Contemp Nurse* 1999; 8: 146–151.

36. Burns E, Blamey C, Ersser S J *et al*. The use of aromatherapy in intrapartum midwifery practice: an observational study. *Complement Ther Nurs Midwifery* 2000; 6: 33–34.

37. Stevenson C. The psychological effects of aromatherapy massage following cardiac surgery. *Complement Ther Med* 1994; 2: 27–35.

38. Evans B. An audit into the effects of aromatherapy massage and the cancer patient in palliative and terminal care. *Complement Ther Med* 1995; 3: 229–241.

39. Wilkinson S. Aromatherapy and massage in palliative care. *Int J Palliat Nurs* 1995; 1: 21–33.

40. Corner J, Cawley N, Hildebrand S. An evaluation of the use of massage and essential oils on the wellbeing of cancer patients. *Int J Palliat Nurs* 1995; 1: 67–73.

41. Brooker D J, Snape M, Johnson E *et al*. Single-case evaluation of the effects of aromatherapy and massage on disturbed behaviour in severe dementia. *Br J Clin Psychol* 1997; 36: 287–296.

42. Stevensen C. Aromatherapy. In: Micozzi M S (ed.) *Fundamentals of Complementary and Alternative Medicine*. Edinburgh: Churchill Livingstone, 1996: 137–148.

43. Cohen B M, Dressler W E. Acute aromatics inhalation modifies the airways. Effects of the common cold. *Respiration* 1982; 43: 285–293.

44. Knobloek K, Pauli A, Iberl B *et al.* Antibacterial and antifungal properties of essential oil components. *J Essent Oil Res* 1989; 1: 119–128.

45. Valnet J. *The Practice of Aromatherapy.* Saffron Walden: C W Daniel, 1982.

46. Gattefossé R-M. *Gattefossé's Aromatherapy.* Tisserand R (ed.) Saffron Walden: C W Daniel, 1993: 107.

47. Cornwell S, Dale A. Lavender oil and perineal repair. *Modern Midwife* 1995; 5: 31–35.

48. Lis-Balchin M. *Aroma Science: The Chemistry and Bioactivity of Essential Oils.* Surrey: Asherwood Publishing, 1995.

49. Lis-Balchin M, Hart S L, Deans S G, Eaglesham E. Comparison of the pharmacological and antimicrobial action of commercial plant essential oils. *J Herbs Spices Medicinal Plants* 1994; 4: 69–86.

50. Schuyler W, Lininger D C, Gaby A R *et al. The Natural Pharmacy.* Rocklin, CA: Prima Publishing, 1999: 463–464.

51. Raman A, Weir U, Bloomfield S F. Antimicrobial effects of tea-tree oil and its major components on *Staphylococcus aureus*, *Staph. epidermidis* and *Propionibacterium acnes*. *Appl Microbiol* 1995; 21: 242–245.

52. Carson C E, Cookson B D, Farrelly H D, Riley T. Susceptibility of methicillin-resistant *Staphylococcus aureus* to the essential oil of *Melaleuca alterifolia*. *J Antimicrob Chemother* 1995; 35: 421–424.

53. Bassett I B, Pannowitz D L, Barnetson R S. A comparative study of tea tree oil versus benzoylperoxide in the treatment of acne. *Med J Aust* 1990; 153: 455–458.

54. Buck D S, Nidorf D M, Addino J G. Comparison of two topical preparations for the treatment of onychomycosis: *Melaleuca alternifolia* (tea tree oil) and clotrimazole. *J Fam Pract* 1994; 38: 601–605.

55. Barnes J. Aromatherapy. *Pharm J* 1998; 260: 862–867.

56. Damian P, Damian K. *Aromatherapy. Scent and Psyche.* Rochester, Vt: Healing Arts Press, 1995: 45–48.

57. Mackereth P. Aromatherapy – nice but not 'essential'. *Complement Ther Nurs Midwifery* 1995; 1: 4–7.

58. Temple W A, Smith N N A, Beasley M. Management of oil of citronella poisoning. *J Toxicol Clin Toxicol* 1991; 29: 257–262.

59. Mant A K. A case of poisoning by oil of citronella. In: Tisserand R, Balacs T (eds) *Essential Oil Safety.* Edinburgh: Churchill Livingstone, 1996: 51.

60. Gurr F W, Scroggie J G. Eucalyptus oil poisoning treated by dialysis and mannitol infusion with an appendix on the analysis of biological fluids for alcohol and eucalyptol. *Aust Ann Med* 1965; 14: 238–249.

61. Tiran D. Aromatherapy in midwifery: benefits and risks. *Complement Ther Nurs Midwifery* 1996; 2: 888–892.

62. DeGroot A C, Weyland J W. Systemic contact dermatitis from tea tree oil. *Contact Dermatitis* 1992; 27: 279–280.

63. Van Ketel W G. Allergy to *Matricaria chamomilla*. *Contact Dermatitis* 1982; 24: 139–140.

64. McGeorge B C, Steele M C. Allergic contact dermatitis of the nipple from Roman camomile. *Contact Dermatitis* 1991; 24: 139–140.

65. Knight T E, Hansen B M. Melaleuca oil (tea tree oil) dermatitis. *Med J Aust* 1994; 30: 423–427.

66. Packham C. Re: Essential oils and aromatherapy: their role in healing – letter to the editor. *J R Soc Health* 1997; 117: 400.

67. Selvaag E, Holm J-O, Thune P. Allergic contact dermatitis in an aromatherapist with multiple sensitisations to essential oils. *Contact Dermatitis* 1995; 33: 334–335.

68. Tisserand R, Balacs T. *Essential Oil Safety*. Edinburgh: Churchill Livingstone, 1996: 83–85.

69. Tisserand R, Balacs T. *Essential Oil Safety*. Edinburgh: Churchill Livingstone, 1996: 41–43.

70. Tiran D. Aromatherapy in midwifery: benefits and risks. *Complement Ther Nurs Midwifery* 1996; 2: 86–92.

71. Dale A, Cornwell S. The role of lavender oil in relieving perineal discomfort following childbirth: a blind randomised clinical trial. *J Adv Nurs* 1994; 19: 89–96.

72. Tisserand R, Balacs T. *Essential Oil Safety*. Edinburgh: Churchill Livingstone, 1996: 93–94.

73. Balacs T. Safety in pregnancy. *Int J Aromather* 1992; 4: 12–15.

74. Anon. Aromatherapy. *Health Which?* 1999; June: 30–31.

7

Flower remedy therapy

In years there has been considerable discussion about the status of flower remedies as to whether they fit in with the homeopathic or herbal systems of classification. They really do not fit in either, having a unique method of preparation and use. They were in fact included in the last two editions of the *British Homeopathic Pharmacopoeia*,[1] much to the disappointment of many homeopaths, as none of the remedies has been subject to provings nor are they used according to the concept of 'like to treat like'. They are used exclusively for mental symptoms and there is a spiritual element in the associated philosophy.

Currently the remedies fall outwith either group's licensing system. Although still known as 'remedies' in Europe, they are called 'essences' in the USA and other countries, causing some confusion with certain aromatherapy products that bear a similar description. It has been stated that homeopathy and flower remedy therapy are clearly different therapies, but some common ground exists and they may have a complementary role, which is perhaps insufficiently recognised.[2]

Definition

Flower remedy therapy is a form of therapy that treats predominantly mental and emotional manifestations of disease, relying on the administration of remedies derived from the flowering parts of plants.

History

There are many variants of flower remedies, but the original and best known are the Bach flower remedies, made at Mount Vernon in Oxfordshire, UK. They were popularised by the physician Edward Bach, who was born in Birmingham, UK, in 1886. It is claimed that Dr Bach was intuitively drawn towards certain wild flowers while walking in the countryside and that he was able to associate them with particular emotions. He believed that these were not just chance occurrences, but indications that he had been led divinely towards a new method of healing. Initially he found 12 remedies, usually referred to as the original healers. These are:

- Agrimony (*Agrimonia eupatoria*), for those not wishing to over-burden others with their problems
- Centaury (*Centaurium umbellatum*), for those who are averse to saying 'no' and are always anxious to please
- Cerato (*Ceratostigma willmottiana*), for those who doubt their ability to make decisions
- Chicory (*Cichorium intybus*), for those who are overprotective of others
- Clematis (*Clematis vitalba*), for lack of interest in present circumstances
- Gentian (*Gentiana amarella*), for those who hesitate in making decisions
- Impatiens (*Impatiens glandulifera*), for those who are quick-thinking but impatient
- Mimulus (*Mimulus gluttatus*), for the timid and shy
- Rock rose (*Helianthemum nummularium*), for those suffering from terror
- Scleranthus (*Scleranthus annuus*), for the indecisive
- Vervain (*Verbena officinalis*), for those with fanatical opinions
- Water violet (*Hottonia palustris*), for those who prefer to be alone.

In 1934 Dr Bach established a healing centre in a small house at Mount Vernon where many of the plants used in his remedies could be grown or were available as wild specimens in the immediate vicinity. He subsequently completed his collection with a further 26 remedies, and considered the final total of 38 to be sufficient to treat the most common negative moods that afflict the human race. The remedies are: aspen, beech, cherry plum, chestnut bud, crab apple, elm, gorse, heather, holly, honeysuckle, hornbeam, larch, mustard, oak, olive, pine, red chestnut, rock water, star of Bethlehem, sweet chestnut, vine, walnut, white chestnut, wild oat, wild rose and willow.

All Bach's remedies can be found growing naturally in the British Isles, with the exception of cerato, olive and vine.

Development of other flower remedies[3,4]

For many years after Edward Bach died no new flower remedies were created. Then in 1982, over 200 essences were produced from the native plants of California according to the methods of Bach, to the opposition of some practitioners who maintain that Bach finished the system when he died. The main themes of the Californian essences are sexuality, social integration, work, life and growth.

Pharmacists in the UK are occasionally asked for Australian bush essences. Created in the early 1980s, these essences have a strong focus on the issues of healing relationships and sexuality, aiming to bring out and cultivate people's positive qualities. This group contains remedies derived from a wide range of Australian plants and trees, including banksia, bottlebrush, jacaranda, paw paw and waratah.

The Alaskan essences, first produced commercially in the summer of 1983 from the native plants of that state, are mainly focused on mental and spiritual ideas, considered to be abstract by many.

There is also a group of 45 flower essences that were developed over a period of 20 years in Yorkshire.

There is currently great interest in essences from the flowers of tropical, subtropical and equatorial regions, for example the Himalayan tree and flower essences, the Amazon orchid essences and the Hawaiian essences. The Christchurch flower essences were assembled in New Zealand and comprise spring, summer and blended essences. Like all the other essences, they do not treat the disease directly, but help to stabilise emotional and psychological stress.

The Bach Centre believed that it had a patent on the manufacturing process for its remedies but this was successfully challenged in court during the 1990s and other companies have now begun to use the Bach method.

Theory

Dr Bach's explanation for the healing power of his medicinal herbs was quite simple: he believed they were divinely enriched. The remedies are not used directly for physical symptoms, but for the state of mind, the rationale being that the state of mind may hinder recovery and also may be the primary cause of certain diseases. This emphasises the idea that all true healing must come from a spiritual level.

Preparation of Bach remedies

There are two methods of preparation:

- The sun method is used to prepare mother tinctures from flowers that bloom during late spring and summer, when the sun is at its strongest. The procedure is carried out where the plants or trees have been gathered, commencing around 9.00 a.m. on a calm settled day. Fifty parts of pure spring water are added to a glass container until the level reaches just below the brim. One part of flower heads is floated on the surface of the water. The container is then left in the sunshine for 3 h, after which the flowers are removed and the remaining solution strained into a glass bottle. It is mixed with an equal quantity of grape brandy, vigorously shaken and stored in a cool dark place.

- The boiling method is used to prepare mother tinctures from flowers and twigs of trees, bushes and plants that bloom early in the year, before there is much sunshine. The material is gathered as before, and one part is added to 10 parts of water in a glass vessel. The resulting mixture is boiled for half an hour and allowed to cool before being diluted with grape brandy and vigorously shaken.

In both cases the resulting mother tinctures are diluted to the equivalent of the fifth decimal homeopathic dilution using 22% ethanol. There is doubt as to whether the dilution process is actually homeopathic, although the manufacturers claim this to be so.

Bach flower therapy in practice

The 38 Bach remedies can be split into six groups according to their principal use:

- fear (aspen, cherry plum, mimulus, red chestnut, rock rose)
- uncertainty (cerato, gentian, gorse, hornbeam, scleranthus, wild oat)
- insufficient interest in present circumstances (chestnut, clematis, heather, honeysuckle, impatiens, mustard, olive, water violet, white chestnut, wild rose)
- oversensitivity to influences and ideas (agrimony, centaury, holly, walnut)
- despondency or despair (crab apple, elm, larch, oak, pine, star of Bethlehem, sweet chestnut, willow)
- overcare for the welfare of others (beech, chicory, vervain, vine, rock water).

For full details on the subtleties of how the remedies are used within each group the reader is referred to more specialised literature from the manufacturers. However, as a guide the most useful remedy from each group is listed in Table 7.1.

One of the difficulties of using Bach remedies is that during the resolution of disease mental symptoms are likely to change, requiring the administration of different treatments. In order to deal with this there is

Table 7.1 Examples of useful Bach flower remedies

Emotion	Bach flower remedy indicated
Confidence, lack of	Larch
Energy, lack of	Olive
Envy	Holly
Indecision or uncertainty	Scleranthus
Overenthusiasm	Vervain
Terror	Rock rose

an extremely useful combination of five Bach flower remedies, known as five-flower remedy or rescue remedy. It was so named for its stabilising and calming effect on the emotions during a crisis. The remedy comprises cherry plum (for the fear of not being able to cope mentally), clematis (for unconsciousness or the 'detached' sensations that often accompany trauma), impatiens (for impatience and agitation), rock rose (for terror) and star of Bethlehem (for the aftereffects of shock). This remedy is often used in place of Arnica, where the mental symptoms resulting from a traumatic episode or overwork are more evident than the physical.

The practice of blending flower remedies appears to be growing. One recently launched range includes nine combination remedies with names such as 'male essence', 'bowel essence' and 'night essence'.

Bach rescue cream is a skin salve that is claimed to help a wide range of skin conditions. The cream contains the same five remedies as the rescue remedy drops plus crab apple (for a sense of uncleanliness). It is broadly used for conditions similar to those for which Arnica might be applicable. However, it is difficult to understand how topical use in this way fits in with the concept of treating mental symptoms.

Administration

Frequency of administration depends to a large extent on each individual patient. If the mood is transient then only one dose might be appropriate, while if the condition persists repeated dosing could be appropriate.

Patients should be instructed to add 2–4 drops of the Bach flower remedy to a cold drink of their choice (fruit juice or still mineral water are both acceptable) and the mixture sipped every 3–5 min for acute problems until the feelings have subsided.

The remedy should be held in the mouth for a moment before swallowing. If no suitable beverage is available, 4 drops of the remedy may be placed under the tongue. For longer use a dose should be taken four times daily.

Bach remedies, particularly rescue remedy, are added to animals' drinking water by owners at similar dose levels during stressful times, e.g. firework displays, travelling or showing.

Flower remedies in the pharmacy

Flower remedies are usually sold in individual bottles or sets (Figure 7.1). The manufacturers provide charts that can be consulted to help with choosing the correct remedy. Rescue remedy is the easiest to counter prescribe because it has clear indications. Colleagues in the southern part of the UK may receive requests from visitors from continental Europe, particularly Germany, where the remedies are expensive and generally in short supply.

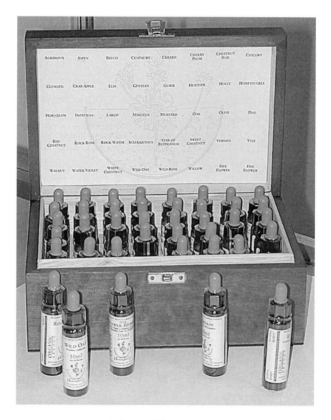

Figure 7.1 An example of a full set of flower essences (Brazil).

Evidence

Numerous anecdotal reports exist in the literature supporting the view that rescue remedy is of substantial benefit in stressful situations for both human and veterinary patients.[5] However, a randomised double-blind clinical trial of 100 university students who had previously suffered from examination nerves, in which participants took one to four doses daily of rescue remedy or identical placebo, revealed no benefit from taking the remedy.[6] However, it should be stressed that this is only one piece of evidence; users do testify to the effectiveness of the product.

More information

The Dr Edward Bach Centre
Mount Vernon
Bakers Lane
Sotwell
Oxon
OX10 0PZ
Tel: 01491 834678
www.bachcentre.com

References

1. *British Homeopathic Pharmacopoeia*, vol. 1. Ilkeston, Derbyshire: BAHM.
2. van Haselen R A. The relationship between homeopathy and the Dr Bach system of flower remedies: a critical appraisal. *Br Homeopath J* 1999; 88: 121–127.
3. Harvey C G, Cochrane A. *The Encyclopaedia of Flower Remedies*. London: Thorson's, 1995.
4. Mansfield P. *Flower Remedies*. London: Optima, 1995.
5. Vlamis G. *Rescue Remedy. The Healing Power of Bach Flower Rescue Remedy*. London: Thorson's, 1994.
6. Armstrong N C, Ernst E. A randomised double blind placebo controlled clinical trial of a Bach flower remedy. *Perfusion* 1999; 12: 440–446.

Part Three

Ethnic traditional therapies

8

Integrating traditional and western medicine

Foolish the doctor who despises the knowledge acquired by the ancients.

Hippocrates

Almost 20 years ago the World Health Organization estimated that 'In many countries, 80% or more of the population living in rural areas are cared for by traditional practitioners and birth attendants'.[1] It has since revised its view, adopting a rather safer position, now stating: 'most of the population of most developing countries regularly use traditional medicine'.[2] Whereas most people use traditional medicine in developing countries, only a minority have regular access to reliable modern medical services.[3]

When many people from less developed countries emigrate they continue to seek medical advice from traditional practitioners working in their own communities, even in countries where all citizens have free access to good-quality western medicine.[4] They have difficulties adjusting to a new lifestyle, let alone to a new system of medicine. It is not surprising that they turn to their own healers, who emigrated before them and practise their trade much the same as they did in their home countries. Although the main reasons for this are probably cultural and linguistic, the role of mistrust and fear should also be acknowledged.

The ethnic medical systems embrace philosophies very different to that of the west. They are derived from a sensitive awareness of the laws of nature and the order of the universe. Practised according to traditional methods, their aim is to maintain health as well as to restore it. The ideas are complex and require much study to grasp their significance and the nuances of practice.

It is appropriate to look at the ways in which traditional (ethnic) medicine and western medicine exist side by side in the countries from which immigrant practitioners can be expected, for it gives us an understanding of how they may approach their profession in the UK and other host communities.

Key policy issues in integration have been outlined by Commonwealth health ministers.[5] Ministers established the Commonwealth Working Group on Traditional and Complementary Health Systems to promote and integrate traditional health systems and complementary medicine into national healthcare.

Medical pluralism – the use of multiple forms of healthcare – is widespread in Asia. Consumers practise integrated healthcare irrespective of whether integration is officially present. In Taiwan, 60% of the public use multiple healing systems, including modern western medicine, Chinese medicine and religious healing. A survey in two village health clinics in China's Zheijang province showed that children with upper respiratory tract infections were being prescribed an average of four separate drugs, always in a combination of western and Chinese medicine.[5] The challenge of integrated healthcare is to generate evidence on which illnesses are best treated through which approach. The Zheijang study found that simultaneous use of both types of treatment was so commonplace that their individual contributions were difficult to assess.

Asia has seen much progress in incorporating its traditional health systems into national policy. Most of this began 30–40 years ago and has accelerated in the past 10 years. In some countries, such as China, the development has been a response to mobilising all healthcare resources to meet national objectives for primary healthcare. In other countries, such as India and South Korea, change has come through politicisation of the traditional health sector and a resultant change in national policy.

Two basic policy models have been followed: an integrated approach, where modern and traditional medicine are integrated through medical education and practice (e.g. China), and a parallel approach, where modern and traditional medicine are separate within the national health system (e.g. India).

Unfortunately, at the present time it is generally recognised that regulation of traditional systems of medicine, the products used in traditional systems and the practitioners of these systems is very weak in most countries.[6] This leads to misuse of the medicines by unqualified practitioners and loss of credibility of the system. In traditional medicine, practitioners and manufacturers (particularly the small ones) usually oppose any steps to strengthen regulation by the health administration. Their fears are that regulation such as applies to allopathic medicine is not suitable for traditional medicine. The World Health Organization has initiated an effort in this direction and may be the appropriate body to help countries not only to develop a regulatory system but to take steps to meet the obligations under the Trade-related Intellectual Property Rights Agreement when this becomes applicable in the developing countries around 2005. It means that traditional healers (hakkims) who come to the UK may practise within a culture that is oblivious to the highly regulated status of western medicine. Health professionals should be vigilant to ensure that any risks to patients are minimised.

All the foregoing may seem to indicate that integrating traditional and western medicine is at best difficult and at worst impossible. Most of the remarks in this chapter have been directed to Chinese and Asian medicine, these two systems being the two traditional disciplines that pharmacists are most likely to meet in the UK. It should be noted that traditional medicines in other cultures also flourish and many are integrated into local healthcare. In their own countries Australian Aboriginals,[7] New Zealand Maoris,[8] North American Indians,[9,10] Africans,[11,12] Pacific Islanders[13] and the peoples of Latin America[14] continue to make important contributions to their national cultures.

Each culture has its own range of remedies, although some elements are common to all. One notable success to cross the cultural divide is tea tree oil, known as melaleuca in Australian bush medicine and manuka in New Zealand. It has become a popular and effective remedy in Europe (Chapter 5).

Traditional healers may be called shamans. They practise a method of healing that is supplemented by rituals and explanatory systems appropriate to their particular culture and environment. The healing often includes meditation, prayer, chanting and traditional music (e.g. Celtic drumming), together with the administration of herbal, and occasionally orthodox, remedies.

Safety

The following safety matters are a source of concern in ethnic medicine: training, uncontrolled products and concurrent therapy.

Training

Practitioners' training varies widely, raising concerns for the quality of the treatment being offered. Little is being done currently to regulate the delivery of traditional healthcare.

Uncontrolled products

Large amounts of traditional medicines are imported into the UK, legally and illegally, and use of such medicines is frequently not admitted when serious illness forces patients to consult western medical practitioners. These medicines carry with them a risk of adverse reactions; the risk needs to be quantified and as far as possible minimised.

An issue under discussion by European regulatory authorities is whether the proposed Herbal Medicines directive (Chapter 5) should extend to traditional medicines containing non-herbal ingredients, such as those used in Chinese and ayurvedic medicine.

The UK Medicines Control Agency (MCA) has established an ethnic medicines forum to encourage and assist the UK ethnic medicines sector to achieve improvements to safety and quality standards in relation to unlicensed ethnic medicines in advance of any improvements to the statutory regime that might emerge from current policy initiatives. Representatives of ayurvedic and traditional Chinese medicine suppliers, manufacturers and practitioners in the UK form part of this forum, as well as the MCA and other bodies in the herbal medicines sector with experience of operating self-regulatory arrangements.

One issue identified by the forum is the lack of understanding of existing law by some of those operating in the ethnic medicines sector. The document *Traditional Ethnic Medicines: Public Health and Compliance with Medicines Law*, published on the MCA website, highlights problem areas.[15] It aims to help consumers make an informed choice and seeks to assist businesses and practitioners to understand certain aspects of medicines law.

Concurrent therapy

Patients with chronic or recurrent conditions are particularly vulnerable as they tend to lose confidence in conventional medicine and resort to self-medication without informing their general practitioner.

What needs to be done to ensure the safety of traditional medicine?

There can be no doubt that safety issues are of extreme concern as the use of traditional therapies increases in a largely uncontrolled manner. Travel by tourists and business people to long-haul destinations has brought increasing numbers of people into contact with other cultures.

Immigration brings different cultures to enrich our own. Whether you consider traditional medicine to have a part to play in modern medicine is for you alone to decide. The fact is, it has arrived without seeking your permission! Healthcare is an emotive subject. The holistic and spiritual qualities associated with oriental medicine appeal to the public, leading to the HYGSE ('Have you got something else?') syndrome.

The risks of participating in traditional Chinese medicine or ayurveda are certainly outweighed by the many benefits that are reported. Adverse reactions are relatively rare, although when they do happen they can be very severe. Perhaps the best solution is to control the practice, improve training and license the medicines. However, there are problems in establishing these ideals.

Practitioners of traditional medicine certainly need to be more aware of the problems of toxicity. In particular, they must learn that infrequent adverse drug reactions will not be recognised without a formal system of reporting. They must participate in such a scheme, and consideration should be given by the MCA to making such reporting compulsory, as it is in Germany. This is an important deficiency and until a formal mandatory system of reporting adverse reactions for traditional medicine becomes available, all healthcare professionals should be aware of the potential difficulties, advise the public of the dangers when-ever necessary, and record and report any problems promptly in main-stream literature.

All practitioners of orthodox and traditional medicine need to be aware of the occurrence and dangers of dual treatment.

Patients need to appreciate that they must disclose exactly what they are taking; such information should be recorded carefully because, as stated above, there is a risk that patients will receive simultaneous western and traditional treatments, particularly when self-treating. This may require a sympathetic non-judgemental approach to questioning. Purchasers of traditional medicines should be advised accordingly.

All practitioners who offer traditional medicines need thorough training and continuing education.[2] Great attention has been paid to the quality of training and further education in orthodox western medicine, and it is time to police more carefully the practice of traditional medi-cine in the UK. For European herbal medicine this should be easy. The training establishments are situated in the UK, which makes guarantee-ing standards and limiting the right to practise to those who are thoroughly trained relatively straightforward. It is much more difficult in the case of traditional Chinese and Indian medicine, as full training cannot currently be obtained in the UK. Verifying the quality of the training given in China and India by identifying appropriate qualifications and recognising them seems prudent. Practitioners who are not qualified should be barred from practice in the UK, and policing this would clearly require a powerful registration body. Ultimately, the creation of academic establishments in the UK, where such training could be given under appropriate regulation, should be considered.

This puts pharmacists firmly into the frame as the healthcare professional whom the public sees most. The opportunities to provide assistance and counselling should not be lost. The significant proportion of pharmacists of Asian origin within the profession should be of great benefit in helping to break down barriers of suspicion between new immigrants and established medical practice.

Traditional ethnic medicine and pharmacy

It is recognised that most community pharmacists will not relish the thought of taking a proactive interest in the highly complicated world of traditional medicine unless they share the origins of their clientele. However, given our extended healthcare role within the multicultural society in which most of us live, the possibilities of coming into contact with traditional Chinese medicine and ayurvedic medicine is possible for a number of reasons:

- concern over interactions between traditional remedies and orthodox medicines
- concern over using traditional remedies during pregnancy
- concern over intrinsic toxicity of traditional remedies and cosmetics, and the safety of some procedures
- the necessity of considering and understanding a patient's total healthcare status when designing pharmaceutical care plans.

The practice of traditional medicine involves concepts with which we in the west are generally unfamiliar. It may be that with more understanding of the therapies involved, some can be incorporated into our own procedures. For example, our focus on treating illness could be shifted more towards maintaining health, a process that has already started. We may be able to understand better the needs of our immigrant communities and perhaps use approaches with which they feel more comfortable.

References

1. Bannerman R H. *Traditional Medicine and Healthcare Coverage*. Geneva: World Health Organization, 1983.
2. *Traditional Medicine*. WHO Fact Sheet N134. Geneva: World Health Organization, 1996.
3. Bodeker G. Lessons on integration from the developing world's experience. *BMJ* 2001; 322: 164–167.
4. Atherton D J. Towards the safer use of traditional remedies. *BMJ* 1994; 308: 673–674.
5. Bodeker G. Traditional (i.e. indigenous) and complementary medicine in the Commonwealth: new partnerships planned with the formal health sector. *J Altern Complement Med* 1999; 5: 97–101.
6. Chaudhury R R. Commentary: challenges in using traditional systems of medicine. *BMJ* 2001; 322: 167.
7. Low T. *Bush Medicine*. North Ryde, NSW: Collins/Angus & Robertson, 1990.
8. Riley M. *Maori Healing and Herbal*. Paparraumu: Viking Sevensen NZ, 1994.
9. Cohen K. Native American medicine. In: Jonas W B, Levin J (eds) *Essentials of Complementary and Alternative Medicine*. Baltimore: Lippincott/Williams & Wilkins, 1999: 233–251.
10. Nauman E. Native American medicine. In: Novery D (ed.) *Clinician's Complete Reference to Complementary Alternative Medicine*. St Louis, MO: Mosby, 2000: 293–308.
11. Sofowora A. Plants in African traditional medicine – a review. In: Evans W C (ed.) *Trease and Evans' Pharmacognosy*, 14th edn. London: W B Saunders, 1996: 511–520.
12. van Wyk B-E, van Oudtshoorn B, Gericke N. *Medicinal Plants of South Africa*. Pretoria: Briza Publications, 1997.
13. Weiner M A. *Secrets of Fijian Medicine*. Berkeley: Quantum Books, 1983.
14. Feldman J. Traditional medicine in Latin America. In: Novery D (ed.) *Clinician's Complete Reference to Complementary Alternative Medicine*. St Louis, MO: Mosby, 2000: 284–292.
15. www.mca.gov.uk.

9

Traditional Chinese medicine

This chapter looks at the basic concepts governing the practice of traditional Chinese medicine (TCM) and then discusses two of the most widely practised disciplines, acupuncture and Chinese herbal medicine (CHM), in some detail.

Pharmacists and other health professionals, particularly those who practise in areas with substantial Chinese immigrant populations, will find it useful to have some background knowledge of this topic. However, the reader should appreciate that this chapter is only designed to be a brief introduction to what is a very wide-ranging and complex subject and it will certainly not equip you to set up as a TCM practitioner!

A number of salient concepts are identified, but for a more indepth explanation you are referred to any of the excellent texts on TCM that may be found on most good booksellers' shelves. You may even be motivated to apply for admission to the new degree course in TCM being offered by the School of Health, Biological and Environmental Sciences at Middlesex University.

Definition

TCM is a generic term used to describe a number of medical practices that originated in China but have now spread throughout the world. It includes not only acupuncture, moxibustion and CHM but also a number of other disciplines including dietary therapy, mind and body exercise (including t'ai chi) and meditation.

History

The earliest Chinese medical treatise known is attributed to the highly esteemed Yellow Emperor (Huangdi) who, according to legendary history, ascended to the throne of China around 2698 BC.[1] It is not known whether the Emperor actually wrote the text, variously entitled *The Yellow Emperor's Classic of Internal Medicine* (the *Nei Ching*) or *The Yellow Emperor's Manual of Corporeal Medicine* (*Huangdi Neijing Suwen*) depending on the literature source consulted. In it he discusses medicine, health, lifestyle, nutrition and contemporary religious beliefs.[2] It is likely that the book was developed by others over the centuries until a definitive version appeared in the first century BC, but it is, none the less, usually ascribed to him. The theories of medicine expounded in the *Nei Ching* remain to this day the most authoritative guide to TCM.

Another significant influence on the development of Chinese medicine was produced in the first or second century AD. Entitled *The Classic of Difficult Issues*, it discusses the origins of the nature of illness, describes an innovative approach to diagnosis and outlines a system of therapeutic needling.

The origins of what might be called modern TCM can be traced back to Zhang Ji, who practised in the Qing Chang mountains close to Chengdu, Szechuan province, in the early years of the third century AD, although it was known to exist in various forms for more than 1000 years before this date.[3] Ji was described as the sage of medicine and probably used traditional methods of healing that were originally linked to Indian practices but were subsequently modified according to Chinese Taoist spiritual philosophy. Another of the famous masters of Chinese medicine active in the third century AD was Hua Tuo, a surgeon and practitioner of a range of therapies.

In the western world TCM, especially acupuncture and CHM, experienced its main expansion during the nineteenth and twentieth centuries as populations moved with developing means of transport. It diffused from immigrant families into host communities and was promoted by subsequent media exposure. The UK's 100-year involvement in Hong Kong led to immigration from the colony and returning merchants, both spawning an interest in all things oriental.

In 1849 the Gold Rush in California brought a large influx of Chinese people to the western USA. They brought their traditional medicine with them and it proved to be popular among the prospectors and their families, particularly as western medicine was largely unavailable in these remote areas. The steady expansion of interest in TCM in the past 30 years in the USA has been attributed to media interest during President Nixon's visit to the People's Republic of China in the early 1970s (see the section on acupuncture, below).

Theory

The Chinese approach to understanding the human body is unique. It is based on a highly sophisticated set of practices designed to cure illness and to maintain health and well-being.[4] Ji was reputed to have said: 'The superior physician helps before the early budding of disease'.[5] These practices also represent an energetic intervention designed to re-establish harmony and equilibrium for each patient according to the holistic principle.

Whenever the practitioner uses acupuncture or herbal medicine, prescribes a set of exercises or proposes a new diet, his or her activities are all considered to be mutually interdependent and necessary to restore (or maintain) health. Acupuncture and CHM are dealt with as separate therapies in this chapter but they would seldom be prescribed in isolation by Chinese practitioners.

TCM is as much a proactive process as a reactive one. That is to say, the principles of TCM may be applied to daily life to stimulate better health without the presence of an illness to initiate it.

There follows a brief outline of the various concepts that are fundamental to an understanding of how Chinese medicine is used. Although they are presented in discrete sections, they are all interlinked, like a jigsaw puzzle. In isolation each piece has little significance.

Yin and yang

According to Emperor Fu His, who lived in the Yellow River area of China approximately 8000 years ago, the world and all life within it comprises pairs of opposites, each giving meaning to the other. They may be viewed as complementary aspects of the whole. Fu His formulated two symbols to represent this idea: a broken line and an unbroken line. These symbols depicted the two major forces in the universe – creation and reception – and how their interaction formed life. This duality was named yin–yang and represents the foundation of Chinese medicine. Thus, the meaning of night is linked to the meaning of day, the ebb of a tide to the flow, and hot with cold. Perhaps the most appropriate link might be that of health and disease, often thought of as being direct opposites. A different view might be that these are both facets of life, each necessary for the other, indeed each giving rise to the other.[6] Thus disease may be thought of as a manifestation of health.

The relationship between the two elements is dynamic; nature constantly moves between the two. An analogy might be provided by considering a cup of coffee that starts as yang; as it cools the yang changes to yin passing through an equilibrium that is just right for drinking. At any stage the application of heat will cause a flow back into yang. This element of change involving energy flows (see below) is seen as a fundamental quality of life.

Yin and yang are now reflected in the well-known entwined symbol, depicted in Figure 9.1.

Thus:

- Yang is a positive state associated with heat, light and vigour: its symbol signifies the sunny side of a mountain.
- Yin is a negative state associated with cold, dark, stillness and passiveness: its symbol signifies the dark side of a mountain.

An example of the yin–yang principle in therapeutics may be provided by considering a patient suffering from a fever, i.e. an excess of yang. Only when the opposites are in equal balance is life in harmony. Too much or too little of either element results in disharmony. Treatment would therefore be seen as the ability to promote the conversion of excess yang into yin, allowing restoration of the equilibrium between the two and a consequent resolution of the fever. A child suffering from colic or diarrhoea would have too much yang; a teenager who could not get up in the morning, too much yin.

As the organs of the body were discovered they were deemed to be yin or yang. Yang organs are vital and solid, including the heart, spleen, lungs, kidneys and liver. Yin organs are hollow and functional,[7] and include the stomach, intestines and bladder. Each organ also has a yin and yang element within it, and it is the overall imbalance that leads to disease.

Rather like the constitutional patient in homeopathy, many ailments may be described as being yin or yang. Thus a yin-deficient patient may be hot and feverish, restless and stressed-out. A yang-deficient patient will feel cold and be pale and lethargic.

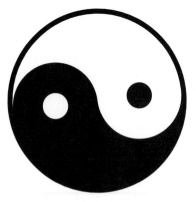

Figure 9.1 The symbol usually employed to depict the idea of yin and yang.

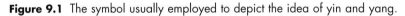

The five elements (wu xing)

According to Chinese philosophy, the body organs are related to one of the five elements: wood, fire, earth, metal and water. These are said to represent the circle of life. Wood is burnt by fire, its ashes fall to support the soil, earth creates metal (ore) that becomes molten with fire (resembling water) and, finally, water nourishes the trees that give us the wood.

The five elements (also known as the five phases) are applied to practice of TCM in a number of different cycles:

- In the sheng (or mother-and-son) cycle organs are considered to be in a familial relationship supporting each other. For example, the kidney might be the 'mother' and the liver her 'son'. Treating the 'mother' organ might provide a route to improving the health of a deficient 'son' organ. This is more of a supporting role: the heart is considered to support the spleen, while the spleen supports the lungs, etc.
- The ke cycle implies a degree of control, as when water 'controls' fire. When an organ is weak it is unable to exert the control necessary to assist other organs. Thus, if the lungs are weak the liver may become too strong, leading to headaches or hypertension.
- The cosmological sequence considers water to be the most important element. As water corresponds to the kidney it reflects the importance that Chinese prescribers place on this organ. It is viewed as the centre of all yin and yang energy in the body and its health is therefore vital.

The five substances

In TCM five substances encompass both tangible and intangible elements within the body. The first three, qi, jing and shen, include qualities such as energy and spirit, and are known as the three treasures. They are believed to be the essential components of an individual's life. The other elements, blood and body fluids, are rather easier for the scientifically trained health professional to understand, although these too have essential intangible properties.

Qi (chee)

Qi is usually translated as simply 'energy' but there is no one English word that conveys its true meaning. It is considered to be a vital or life force similar to that mentioned in Chapter 4 during the discussion on how homeopathy might work.

Qi is responsible for the following day-to-day body functions:[8,9]

- movement, both conscious (voluntary) and unconscious (involuntary)
- transforming food and drink into blood, body fluids and energy
- containment – holding organs, blood vessels and body tissues in their proper places
- protection, from external environmental factors including heat, cold and dampness
- maintenance of body heat.

A number of qi disharmonies may be identified:

- A deficiency in qi (qi xu) will lead to debilitation, protracted recovery from illness, chronic colds, lethargy and other signs of weakness.
- Sinking qi (qi xian) is when qi can no longer perform its holding function and this is reflected in an organ prolapse.
- Stagnation of qi (qi zhu) is caused by an irregular energy flow or blockage – this may be the result of physical injury or emotional stress and its symptoms include indigestion and irritability or swelling and inflammation following a knock.
- Rebellious qi (qi ni) is when qi flow is in the wrong direction, i.e it rebels, for example in the stomach qi is considered to flow downwards; a reverse flow might cause nausea and vomiting.

An excess of qi is not considered to be detrimental.

Jing

The concept of jing, like qi, is difficult to convey in a single English word. It is translated as 'essence' and underpins all aspects of organic life. If jing is plentiful life itself is good, full of harmony and vitality. If jing is lacking then qi will be weak, life will be dull and the person will be susceptible to contracting disease. Jing differs from qi in that the former is responsible for the developmental changes associated with growth throughout the life, while the latter is associated with day-to-day bodily functions. Jing governs fertility, sexuality and growth, and is believed to have 7- or 8-year cycles, during which development and ageing take place.

Jing is responsible for the following:

- governing growth, reproduction and development
- production of bone marrow
- promotion of kidney qi
- determining the basic constitutional strength.

Deficiency of jing is the only disharmony and is said to be more prevalent in men than in women. The following symptoms may be identified:

- developmental disorders, including physical, mental and learning problems – as jing deteriorates with age, so symptoms of baldness, deafness, brittle bones and senility may result
- kidney-related disorders
- poor memory and concentration
- constitutional weakness
- low libido.

Shen

Shen is both mind and spirit. It is based in the heart and governs spiritual, mental and emotional health. It has been described as responsible for 'the sparkle in one's eyes'. Disharmony can range from mild confusion and insomnia to substantial psychiatric disturbances accompanied by irrational behaviour.

Blood

In TCM blood is much more than simply a physical transport system, as in western medicine. It is closely linked to qi and is considered to have the following important functions:

- It nourishes the body by carrying nutrients to all tissues and structures and in so doing it helps to fulfil the nutritive functions of qi.
- It has a moistening and lubricating action.
- It aids clear and stable thought processes.

There are three imbalances:

- Deficiency (xue xu) shows in pale face, dry skin, light-headedness and emaciation.
- Stagnation (xue yu) produces stabbing pains and purple lips and tongue.
- Excessive heat in the blood can cause skin conditions and fever.

Body fluids (jin ye)

Body fluids include external light and watery fluids, such as saliva and tears (known as jin), and the dense thicker fluids that circulate inside the body, e.g gastric juices and joint fluids (known as ye). The function of all the body fluids is to nourish and lubricate the body. They are essential for the maintenance of healthy qi.

Deficient body fluids result in dryness of the eyes, lips and hair, a dry cough and excessive thirst. Excess body fluids can lead to problems known as dampness and phlegm in TCM, characterised by productive coughs, weeping skin rashes and vaginal discharge.

The five substances are summarised in Table 9.1.

The organs (zang fu)

The organs detailed below have a special status in TCM, being the creators and storers of the five substances. They are considered to be closely related to specific emotions and virtues, and if their essential requirements are not fulfilled, ill health will result. They are known as the solid organs and are associated with yin.

The heart governs the circulatory system, but is also the centre of shen. It is positively associated with compassion, love and affection, and negatively with overexcitement. Symptoms of ill health include insomnia and hyperactivity.

The lungs relate to qi and require confidence to function effectively. They are positively associated with conscientiousness and negatively with sadness. Symptoms of ill health include irregular breathing, coughs and susceptibility to colds.

Table 9.1 Summary of the five substances

Basic substance	Main responsibility	Possible symptoms of disharmony (deficiency or excess)
Qi	Day-to-day functions	Debilitation, chronic colds, gastrointestinal problems
Jing	Development	Learning difficulties, kidney problems, ageing, weak constitution
Shen	Consciousness	Anxiety, insomnia, psychiatric problems
Blood	Nourishes, moistens	Paleness, stabbing pains, fever
Body fluids	Moistens, nourishes	Dryness of skin, dry cough; weeping rashes, productive cough (phlegm)

The liver (gan) ensures that qi flows smoothly. Benevolence and a state of agitation are associated with its positive and negative virtues respectively. Symptoms of ill health are irregular periods and bad temper.

The spleen creates qi. Its health depends on a good diet and an unstressful lifestyle. It is positively associated with empathy and negatively with obsession. Symptoms of ill health include poor appetite and diarrhoea.

The kidneys store jing and are associated with long-term growth. Their positive emotion is courage; their negative emotion is fear. Symptoms of ill health include lethargy, diarrhoea, infertility and oedema.

The hollow organs, associated with yang, are the gallbladder, large and small intestines, bladder, stomach and san jaio, also known as the 'triple burner' or 'triple heater'. San jaio has no equivalent anatomical structure in western medicine, although it roughly corresponds to the thoracic and abdominal regions, including all the organs within. It coordinates transformation and transportation of fluids in the body. San jaio also helps move qi and maintain the ambient temperature in the body, a function from which its English name derives.

The meridians or channels

The word 'meridian' as used in TCM entered the English language through a French translation of the Chinese term jing-luo. *Jing* means 'to go through' and *luo* means 'something that connects'. Meridians are the channels that carry qi and blood throughout the body. They form an invisible network close to the surface of the body, which links together all the fundamental textures and organs. Kaptchuk mentions 14 meridians in his book;[10] other writers refer to different numbers ranging from 11 to 20. Because the meridians unify all parts of the body and energy can pass along the channels, they are essential for the maintenance of harmonious balance. Set along the meridians are a number of points used by acupuncturists (see below).

The meridians are named for the organs or functions to which they are attached. Fulder, in his excellent book, explains the function of the meridians thus:[11]

> The meridian of the colon runs from a point on the nail of the index finger along the arm and over the shoulder and neck to the nose from whence it follows a deep pathway down to the colon. Because the meridian system connects the exterior of the body by pathways to the viscera, external factors can penetrate and produce symptoms such as abdominal pain, migraine, etc. Conversely, diseases of the internal organs will produce superficial symptoms that

may appear along the lines of the meridians. Thus, kidney disease can induce back pain, while disease of the gall bladder can bring pain to the shoulder, these being areas through which the respective meridians pass.

Practice of TCM

Diagnosis

A diagnosis is achieved using four traditional methods (si zhen):[12]

* listening carefully to the sound and quality of the patient's voice, (auscultation) and evaluating any breath or body odours (olfaction)
* asking questions to ascertain the features of the illness (inquiry)
* observing the patient's general demeanour, emotional state and shen, and assessing the quality and texture of the skin and the shape, colour and coating of the tongue (inspection)
* palpation of the pulses and body.

Following a full history, the blood pressure and pulses will be read. Chinese medicine recognises up to 28 pulses, which are palpable on the right and left wrists. The right-hand pulses represent conditions of the lung, spleen and kidney, while the left-hand pulses represent conditions of the heart, liver and kidney. The pulse is assessed in seven criteria: depth, fluency, rhythm, size/shape, speed, strength and tension. The experienced practitioner can deduce much information on the patient's past and present health status from reading the pulses and palpating the body.

The aim is to determine which organ or organs might be out of balance by considering all the many elements outlined above, and to take appropriate action to rectify the problem according to the various principles outlined above. It appears to be a daunting task to the western healthcare professional, who is more used to making a decision on appropriate medication based on symptoms determined within a 3–5-min consultation.

A modern diagnosis technique is now also used to enhance the old traditional diagnosis method. With new techniques developed through modern Chinese medicine, pressure reactions convert variances in the patient's pulse into electromagnetic waves. These waves are analysed by a computer and registered as a signal on the screen. This represents the marriage of modern scientific precision with the art of TCM.

Treatment

Treatment is by a range of different therapies; each will be dealt with to varying degrees under the appropriate section headings below.

Evidence

There are a number of difficulties in assembling the evidence of effectiveness for TCM. Much research has been carried out in China but is considered inadmissible because of problems associated with:

- poor translation of studies
- the quality and design of the research not being up to western standards
- the use of unvalidated methods
- methodological difficulties of establishing control groups and sham procedures for the placebo arm of trials (e.g. it is impossible to 'blind' an acupuncturist)
- variations in what is understood by different terms.

It is vital that correct plant species are used when researching traditional herbal medicine and that tests are carried out on material prepared ethnically.[13] The choice of test system might also be difficult because, particularly with Chinese or Indian medicine where the aim may be to correct imbalances in health, there is no outcome to measure in the same way that western medicine allows. For the same reason animal models are unlikely to provide applicable results. Practitioners frequently use mixtures of ingredients and testing standardised individual elements may not be appropriate.

Another significant factor with ethnic medicine is the charisma and seniority of the practitioner, which introduce a significant element of placebo response that cannot be quantified.

Modern Chinese medicine

Since the 1950s, the Chinese government and the government of the Republic of China on Taiwan have put great efforts into promoting the modernisation of Chinese medicine. This has been in response to national planning needs to provide comprehensive healthcare services. Previously, TCM had been viewed as part of an imperial legacy, to be replaced by a secular healthcare system. Integration was guided by health officials trained in modern medicine; harmonisation with modern medicine was the goal. This was accomplished by a science-based approach to the education of TCM and an emphasis on research. As a result, there are now professionals trained in both TCM and modern western medicine, who conduct research on the development of Chinese medicine. Western science methodologies have been employed to analyse the effectiveness of herbs and treatment on various subjects. Many of the differences between TCM and western scientific practices are now being studied for their synergistic potential.

Joint research projects have been undertaken in the USA, involving research institutes such as Stanford University, the College of Physicians and Surgeons of Columbia University and the National Cancer Institute to evaluate the effectiveness of Chinese medicine and improve the classification and selection/prescription of formulas. However, this process of integration has resulted in the loss of important aspects of traditional theory and practice. Fewer acupuncture points are taught than in the classical system, and aspects of the theory of TCM have been de-emphasised.

Hospitals practising TCM still treat 200 million outpatients and almost 3 million inpatients annually. Overall, 95% of general hospitals in China have traditional medicine departments, which treat about 20% of outpatients daily.[14]

Acupuncture (zhen)

Acupuncture is a technique involving the insertion of fine needles into the skin at selected points over the body. Practitioners of acupuncture generally follow one of two broad approaches to the discipline, using either TCM with all its many ramifications for maintaining health, or the simpler symptom-oriented western acupuncture. This section gives an outline of both.

History

The theory that surrounds the practice of traditional acupuncture probably dates back as much as 4000–5000 years, although there are no reliable references in Chinese literature prior to the first century BC. Ancient works were generally written on bamboo strips and silk, and have not survived. The earliest physician reputed to be proficient in acupuncture techniques was Bian Que in around 500 BC.

The oldest known text to include a reference to acupuncture is attributed to *The Yellow Emperor's Classic of Internal Medicine* (the *Nei*

Ching), which developed over the centuries until a definitive version appeared in the first century BC. The names and reputed functions of all the acupuncture points were established by about 259 AD when *The Classic of Acupuncture (Zhen Jiu Jia Jing)* was published. Acupuncture continued to flourish in China, especially throughout the Ming period (1368–1644). Subsequently, it went into gradual decline until 1822, when it was finally banned by Emperor Dao Guang, who disapproved of its practices. In the early part of the twentieth century acupuncture became part of the ongoing debate as to whether Chinese culture should be overtaken by western influences or maintain its own traditions. With the arrival of western medicine, acupuncture was increasingly relegated to rural and remote backwaters.

In the 1950s the discipline was reintroduced by the communist authorities, who saw TCM as a solution to the problem of providing healthcare to an ever-growing population. Acupuncture developed once again as people were quickly trained and pressed into service. Today it is practised alongside western medicine.

News of the success of acupuncture was brought to the west in 1683 by Dr Willen Ten Rhijn, a physician working for the Dutch East Indies Company in Japan. Dr Rhijn's report was not the first, but it was the most reliable. Usage of the English word 'acupuncture' is attributed to him.

Acupuncture was widely practised in France in the late eighteenth century with Dr Berlioz, a Parisian doctor, becoming the first western practitioner of acupuncture in the early nineteenth century. John Churchill, the first British acupuncturist, used the technique in the treatment of rheumatism in 1821. Acupuncture was even mentioned in the first edition of the *Lancet* in 1823 as being chiefly used in 'diseases of the head and lower belly'.[15]

Much interest followed the visit of President Nixon to China in 1971, especially when a reporter from the *New York Times* fell ill with appendicitis during the tour and was given acupuncture for his post-operative pain. He wrote an account of his treatment for the paper.[16] As China opened up to visitors shortly afterwards, physicians and others made visits to witness how acupuncture was being used. Indeed in 1972 I visited Nanjing and saw a surgeon directing her own abdominal operation, and observed several other minor operations and the delivery of a baby; all the procedures were performed with the aid of acupuncture needles to control the pain.

Acupuncture is now among the best-known complementary therapies in the UK. In Scotland, a random survey found that an impressive

94% of respondents in a random survey knew something about acupuncture and 25% said they would consider using it, although in practice only about 6% had actually done so.[17] It would be interesting to know why there was such a large discrepancy between the two figures.

Basics of TCM acupuncture

In addition to the classical principles of Chinese medicine outlined under the general heading TCM above, there is one key aspect of practice still to consider. This is the theory of acupuncture points. A basic 365 mapped acupuncture points (tsubos) are situated along the meridians. A further 1000 extra points and special use points may also be identified on the hand, ear and scalp. It is not known how these points were discovered – probably it was by observation over hundreds if not thousands of years – nor is it known exactly how many points were first identified. Pain points (ashi) can be located anywhere on the body where there is a pain locus (Figure 9.2).

Acupoints cannot be identified by their appearance and no consistent features of their anatomy have been found that distinguish them from other tissues. It has been suggested that the points may be sites of tenderness.[18] The methodology for investigating the tenderness of acupuncture points has been explored.[19] The study of the acupoint known as spleen 6 found that there was no strong evidence to support the hypothesis that acupuncture points were more tender than control points.

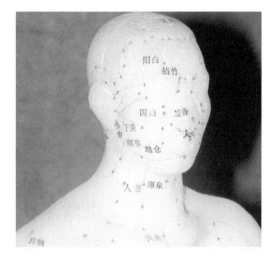

Figure 9.2 Acupuncture doll showing acupoints on the head and neck.

The practice of acupuncture

There is archaeological evidence that shows that the earliest acupuncture needles date back to the Stone Age, when instruments called bian were thought to have been used in China.[20] By the Bronze Age acupuncture was already well developed and needles were made of bronze. Needles were subsequently made of many different metals: gold, silver, copper, etc. Modern acupuncturists use solid sterile disposable needles of narrow bore, about 3 cm long (although longer needles may be used at different sites). The patient is usually treated lying down to minimise any tendency to faint. As many as 15–20 needles may be inserted superficially at the appropriate point or points. The practitioner then gently introduces the needles a little more deeply into the muscle, rotating them between finger and thumb. Qi and blood flow throughout the meridians and this is where manipulation of the needle is critical in properly moving this flow. The arrival of qi (deqi) is signified by a dull ache or tingling sensation and slight inflammation. Some practitioners may use electrical stimulation, connecting the needles to a small piece of equipment powered by batteries. Needles are left in place for up to 20 min: the patient is invited to lie back and relax. Occasionally a needle may be left in place for several days; these so-called indwelling needles should not be used in patients with heart valve disease.

Usually 10–12 sessions constitute a single course of treatment. Two or three courses may be required for the treatment of chronic conditions. Acupuncture point selection may vary at each treatment, depending on the patient's response. If significant improvement is achieved, the patient will be discharged at the end of the treatment but will normally be instructed to continue with other elements of TCM, e.g. dietary control and perhaps exercises.

Evidence of effectiveness

The reader is referred to the comments made in the general section on TCM above. Evidence of effectiveness is largely restricted to case studies, although randomised controlled trials (RCTs) are available for western acupuncture (see below).

Safety

A study that investigated the incidence and severity of acupuncture reactions has been carried out in Japan.[21] In 1441 treatment sessions involving 30 338 insertions in 391 patients, nine episodes of failure to remove the needle were reported and classified as negligence rather than an adverse reaction. The most common systemic reactions were tiredness and drowsiness (11%), aggravation of symptoms (2.8%), irritation (1%), vertigo (0.8%) and fainting (0.8%). The most common local effects were bleeding (2.6%) and pain (0.7%). The authors concluded that there were some adverse reactions associated with acupuncture, but that they were generally transient and mild. However, serious complications have been reported.[22]

There is some evidence from a lack of recent cases in the literature that the situation is improving, i.e. the incidence of adverse reactions is decreasing, particularly in the west.

Because fainting and drowsiness are commonly reported,[23] patients should be advised not to drive immediately after treatment if affected, and to exercise particular care if any prescribed or over-the-counter (OTC) medication is being taken that might enhance these effects. It has been suggested that a fall in blood sugar could be involved[24] and this might be a problem for diabetic patients using insulin or oral hyperglycaemic drugs. Advice from a pharmacist on the rescheduling of administration would be appropriate.

The adverse effects that may be attributed to acupuncture have also been catalogued.[25,26] Examples of potential dangers identified in the reviews include infection during needling and trauma.

Infection during needling

Hepatitis Re-using needles with inadequate sterilisation has been the source of hepatitis in a number of patients, although the literature refers mainly, but not exclusively, to the 1980s and before.[27–29]

HIV Human immunodeficiency virus (HIV) infection has been linked to acupuncture. In one case a patient became HIV-positive after a 6-week course of acupuncture.[30] In another case two acquired immunodeficiency syndrome (AIDS) patients were strongly suspected of contracting their condition as a result of acupuncture.[31] It must be stressed that due to lack of information a direct causal link in this case could not be established. There may also be some risk to the acupuncturist from treating a patient who already has HIV.

Other infections Other infections reported include those due to *Pseudomonas* and *Staphylococcus aureus*.[32] Two patients with staphylococcal septicaemia are reported to have died several months after receiving acupuncture.[33]

Following the adoption of disposable needles the incidence of infection during needling is likely to fall even more.

Trauma   A number of cases of damage due to acupuncture needling, including pneumothorax, cardiac tamponade and spinal cord damage, have been reviewed.[25,26] Five fatalities have been reported, although the evidence that acupuncture was solely to blame is compelling in only one of these cases,[26] that involving a 40-year-old Norwegian woman whose heart was pierced by a needle.[34] Local traumatic damage to blood vessels may produce a haematoma.

Other adverse effects   Other possible adverse reactions to acupuncture include cardiac arrhythmias,[35] the triggering of asthma[36] and the exacerbation of symptoms.[37] Allergic reactions caused by the metal of the needles, particularly chrome and nickel, are possible.[38–40] There is some evidence that it might be inappropriate to use electroacupuncture on patients with pacemakers.[41] Some concerns have been expressed about the safety issues involved with electrostimulation and the possibility of tissue damage.[42]

Accidental burns from moxibustion procedures (see below)[43] or excessively warm acupuncture needles[44] have been reported. Clinical misjudgement may give some cause for concern.

A summary of some of the complications of acupuncture is set out in Table 9.2. The table gives a simple summation of the cases of each episode computed from a literature search. The results cannot be used to make deductions of the frequency of such events.

Contraindications   Acupuncture is contraindicated or must be used with extreme care in patients who:

Table 9.2 Complications of acupuncture

Event documented	Number of cases in the literature
Drowsiness, fainting	1429
Increased pain	1129
Nausea, vomiting	540
Infections	228
Pneumothorax	129
Hepatitis	127
Psychiatric complications	112
Convulsions	80
Cardiac trauma	7

- are unwilling to be needled; they should not be pressurised to undergo treatment
- have a tendency to bleed excessively
- have a pacemaker; it might be affected by the electrical stimulation of acupuncture needles.

Precautions   A number of precautions may be suggested when practising acupuncture:

- Patients should lie down during treatment.
- Disposable sterile needles should be used.
- Needles should be counted before and after treatment so that all may be accounted for.
- Patients should be carefully observed for excessive bleeding.

Western acupuncture[45]

Some general practitioners (GPs) and physiotherapists with orthodox backgrounds find it difficult to accept the intangible nature of traditional acupuncture, which relates to the flow of qi. Many dispute the existence of meridians or acupuncture points,[46] preferring to link their practice to trigger points instead.[47,48] Trigger points are small areas in muscle that have been strained or injured and have not healed. They may remain sensitive for many years, causing pain that may be experienced some distance away from the trigger point. Interestingly, the trigger points and pain referral sites appear to be similar in all people and furthermore, many of the trigger points are identical to acupuncture points.

It is suggested that acupuncture works by stimulating the nervous system, leading to the release of opioid peptides (endorphins), compounds that are closely involved with the mechanisms by which the body controls its perception of pain. Thus, acupuncture is used in the treatment of intractable pain without the attendant traditional Chinese theory. This variant, which involves very brief needling lasting no more than a few seconds at trigger points, has been termed 'minimal acupuncture'.[49] Exponents of minimal acupuncture commonly treat musculoskeletal pain, arthritis and symptoms of stress, including tension headaches, gastrointestinal problems and nausea.

Evidence   Cautious approval of some applications of acupuncture was given by the US National Institutes of Health consensus development meeting in 1997.[50] The 12-member panel was asked to evaluate current evidence for the efficacy of acupuncture and concluded that there is 'clear evidence' of efficacy in the control of nausea and vomiting occurring in some patients postoperatively and in association with chemotherapy, and for the relief of postoperative dental pain. The panel said that acupuncture was 'probably' also effective in the control of nausea in early pregnancy. The British Medical Association reached a similar conclusion in their report on acupuncture.[51] A number of correspondents to the *British Medical Journal* criticised this support, claiming that the evidence was not sufficient to reach a positive conclusion.[52]

As already pointed out in Chapter 8, there are problems with designing trials for acupuncture associated with the control arm of an RCT.[53] The most usual placebo method is sham acupuncture, when needles are inserted outside acupuncture points with a minimum of interaction between practitioner and patient.[54] It is argued that this is an incorrect method because it leads to a study of the importance of the acupuncture point rather than of acupuncture itself.[55] Furthermore, as stated above, there are doubts about whether acupuncture points and non-acupuncture points can be identified. Even if they can, there is evidence that acupuncture at non-classical points, the so-called trigger points, may have analgesic effects. Studies of acupuncture of the back show little difference between true acupuncture at classical sites and sham acupuncture (see below). However, acupuncture has shown an advantage against a true placebo control. Notwithstanding these difficulties a number of RCT trials have been conducted, providing results that, with a few notable exceptions, are not conclusive. The evidence is briefly listed below:[56]

- **Back pain.** Many systematic reviews for back pain include trials that use different techniques and control procedures.[57] However, the balance of evidence appears to suggest that acupuncture can be useful in the treatment of back pain when compared with placebo.[58,59] A pilot study for an RCT of acupuncture in low back pain concluded that the results were 'promising' and worthy of further research.[60] According to a recent Swedish RCT, low back pain in pregnancy may also be relieved by acupuncture.[61]
- **Dental pain.** Most of the studies included in a systematic review of 16 trials of dental pain suggested that acupuncture does have a greater effect than placebo.[62]
- **Drug dependence.** In a randomised sham-controlled open trial with one active and two control arms the use of acupuncture in

cocaine dependence was investigated.[63] The primary outcome was cocaine use assessed by thrice-weekly urine analysis. A total of 52 patients completed the study. Patients who completed a course of auricular acupuncture appeared to be more likely to abstain from using cocaine than either of the other two control groups. Another study showed that acupuncture could be of use in cocaine abusers stabilised on buprenorphine as a substitute.[64]

- **Gastrointestinal disorders.** Acupuncture has a long history of use for gastrointestinal disorders, including dyspepsia, ulcers and inflammatory bowel disease.[65]

- **HIV.** Preliminary data from small numbers of participants in a pilot study using acupuncture for symptomatic relief has shown trends towards improvement in symptoms and quality of life.[66]

- **Knee pain.** Patellofemoral pain syndrome is the leading cause of chronic knee pain in young adults and may affect up to 15% of young men in the US military service.[67] The results of a controlled trial that included a total of 75 patients with patellofemoral pain led the authors to conclude that acupuncture may be beneficial as a treatment for the condition.[68]

- **Neck pain.** There is some evidence that acupuncture may be effective when it is used for neck pain,[69,70] although a systematic review of 14 RCTs of this application concluded that existing data were insufficient to make a firm judgement.[71]

- **Osteoarthritis.** In a review of acupuncture in osteoarthritis, 13 studies were identified, of which seven reported a positive result and six a negative result.[72] However, most of the positive trials were not placebo-controlled so no conclusions could be reliably drawn.

- **Nausea and vomiting.** For nausea and vomiting the P6 acupoint on the the inner wrist is usually used. In a review of 29 trials in the literature that referred to nausea and vomiting from all causes, 27 gave positive results.[73]

- **Recurrent headache.** The authors of a systematic review of 22 RCTs concluded that acupuncture may have a role in the treatment of recurrent headaches, but that the quality and volume of evidence are presently unconvincing.[74] Acupuncture may also be of assistance in migraine.[75]

- **Shoulder injury in sport.** A rigorous well-designed trial investigated the effect of treating shoulder injuries with acupuncture.[76] In a commentary on the work, White *et al.*[77] point out that this was unusual in that the authors looked at an injury rather than a disease. Results were extremely positive.

- **Smoking cessation.** A Cochrane review for smoking cessation included 18 reports, with 20 trials, that compared acupuncture with various other interventions.[77] Acupuncture did not show any advantage over sham acupuncture.
- **Stroke.** Systematic reviews and one RCT would appear to indicate that there is some effect of acupuncture on the rate of recovery of stroke patients.[78–80]
- **Temporomandibular joint dysfunction.** A small systematic review of three RCTs of acupuncture for temporomandibular joint dysfunction suggested that the treatment provided some symptomatic relief comparable with that provided by orthodox measures.[81] The normal caveat of 'more rigorous investigation needed' was expressed by the authors.
- **Weight loss.** Contrary to popular opinion, there is in fact no firm evidence that acupuncture is effective in promoting weight loss.[82]

It would appear that acupuncture can be shown to be more effective than sham acupuncture in back pain, dental pain, and nausea and vomiting. Evidence for other applications is sparse and the Scottish verdict of 'not proven' would seem to be the most appropriate in these circumstances.

Availability of acupuncture on the National Health Service   A questionnaire was sent to a random sample of 650 UK GPs selected from the British Medical Association database and representing 1.6% of the country's GP population.[83] A number of questions relating to the provision of complementary and alternative medicine were asked in the survey. The response rate was 56%. The most popular therapy arranged for patients was acupuncture (47% of respondents). In almost half these cases the service was provided within an orthodox setting such as the GP's own surgery. Pain relief and musculoskeletal disorders were the most frequently cited conditions treated; other applications included smoking cessation, stress and morning sickness.

When asked who they thought should provide acupuncture, the GPs replied strongly in favour of registered medical practitioners, followed by physiotherapists and dentists. Less than half the respondents thought that traditional Chinese medical practitioners should be involved.

Reasons for not offering acupuncture were lack of demand (63%), lack of knowledge of the services available (63%) and lack of guidelines on how to assess the competence of practitioners.

The percentage of physicians who practise acupuncture in the UK has varied widely over the last 20 years, with estimates of 1% in Scotland,[84] from 3%[85] to 21%[86] in England, and from 4%[87] to 5%[88] in the country as a whole. This compares with the USA (1%)[89] and New Zealand (Wellington 18%[90] and Auckland 21%[91]). In Australia the use of acupuncture by doctors has increased greatly since the 1984 introduction of a Medicare rebate for acupuncture. In 1996, 15.1% of Australian doctors claimed for acupuncture, with almost one million insurance claims being made.[92]

In the UK the practice of acupuncture is not legally restricted to medically qualified doctors as it is in many other European countries (e.g. France, Hungary, Italy, Poland and Portugal) so the market may be partially satisfied by non-medically qualified practitioners (NMQPs). There are more than 5500 acupuncturists in the UK, of whom 3500 are statutorily registered health professionals.

Variants of acupuncture

Acupressure (shiatsu)   Acupressure is a form of acupuncture in which fingers, thumbs and elbows are used to stimulate the body's acupuncture points. Acupressure relieves muscular tension, facilitating blood flow and therefore distributing more nutrients and oxygen throughout the body as well as removing waste products. This helps to promote both physical calmness and mental alertness. The technique involves repeatedly pressing the acupuncture points for 3–5 s and then releasing the pressure. It is believed that the practitioner's qi helps to strengthen the weakened qi of the patient. Thus it is important that the practitioner maintains a healthy body so that his or her qi is stronger than that of the recipient.[93] Because of these qi differentials, self-acupressure is not as effective as having a practitioner do it for you.

Acupressure has been used to relieve mental tension, for tired and strained eyes, headaches, menstrual cramps and arthritis as well as to promote general healthcare.[94] A trial to minimise motion sickness by intermittent pressure on the wrist point P6 with wrist bands found no reduction in symptoms.[95] However, in a later study regular pressure was applied and, under these circumstances, a clear positive outcome resulted.[96] Acupressure in sickness during pregnancy may also be helpful,[97] although the use of the P6 point with wristbands as outlined above has not been successful in this context.[98]

Acupressure should not be applied to an open wound, or to a place where there is inflammation or swelling. Areas of scar tissue, boils, blisters, rashes and varicose veins should also be avoided. Certain pressure points should be avoided during pregnancy and in patients with hyper- or hypotension.

Moxibustion (jiu)   Moxibustion is similar to both acupuncture and acupressure in its effects but uses a glowing wick instead of needles or fingertips as the source of stimulation for the acupoints. Traditionally moxa is the dried leaves of the mugwort (*Artemesia vulgaris*) made into various forms; punk is loose moxa, rather like green cotton wool, while moxa rolls are like cigars in appearance. There are also moxa cones. When lit, the moxa smoulders slowly. The glowing moxa rolls are held about 2 cm from the acupoint. Another method is for a small moxa cone to be placed on the blunt end of an acupuncture needle while it is in place. It is lit, transmitting the heat down the needle into the acupuncture point. A cone may also be placed directly on the skin over a slice of ginger. It is lit at its apex and burnt down until the patient is able to feel the heat; it is then removed. Cauterising moxibustion involves the burning of loose punk directly on the skin until blisters form.

Moxibustion tones, stimulates and supplements energy in the meridians. It is claimed to be an effective treatment for arthritis and menstrual problems.

Colourpuncture   This is a system of treating patients by focusing small coloured lamps on acupuncture points and other areas of the body.

Chinese herbal medicine (zhong yao)

In the west it is quite normal to equate the word 'herbal' with something that grows in the garden. Certainly the majority of Chinese herbal remedies are made from plant material, but others are of mineral or animal origin. For example, gypsum (shi gao) is a cooling mineral 'herb' commonly used to treat conditions characterised by much heat. Oyster shells (mu li) may be used for hypertension. The use of animal parts is a controversial issue in western communities. In China and other Asian countries the practice is still widespread, but it has been largely discontinued elsewhere following action by regulatory authorities whose enthusiasm may be occasionally misplaced. The famous highly aromatic salve marketed around the world as Tiger Balm was once the subject of a dawn raid of Chinese herbalists by police in Manchester. They thought they had uncovered the illegal use of parts from a protected wild animal. There were a few red faces when it was realised that the title merely referred to the nick name of the brand owner!

History

China's greatest materia medica (*Pen Ts'ao*) was published by Li Shih-chen in 1578.[99] The culmination of 26 years' work, it comprises 1892 species of drugs of animal, vegetable and mineral origin, and includes no fewer than 8160 prescriptions.

Secret recipes (also known as 'prepared medicines') were the equivalent of modern patent medicines. They were first produced during the Song dynasty (AD960–1234) and were dispensed by government agencies such as the Imperial Benevolence Pharmacy.[100] A variety of dose forms were available including pills, liquids and honey boluses. By the time of the Ming dynasty (1368–1644) more than 60 000 formulae had been recorded in the 1406 book entitled *Formulas of Universal Benefit* (*Pu Ji Fang*). In recent years many of these formulae have passed into public usage, but there may be as many as 5000 licensed patent medicines still circulating in China. The most famous factory is at the Tong Ren Tang pharmacy in Beijing, which has been operated by the same family since the late seventeenth century.

In the UK, Chinese herbalism is the most prevalent of the ancient herbal traditions currently being practised.[101] About 500 different herbal materials are imported into the UK and are worth several million pounds each year.[102] In addition an unquantified amount of material enters the country illegally by suitcase smuggling. There is ongoing concern about the lack of controls. In the USA legislation now allows the import of Chinese herbal materials, as the Food and Drug Administration (FDA) has lifted earlier restrictions that limited imports to ethnic groups. This has prompted the wider availability of prepared medicines.

There are now over 3000 clinics in the UK that prescribe Chinese herbal remedies for various disorders and the use of these remedies seems set to increase further, given the apparent success being reported[103] despite a lack of firm evidence of effectiveness in many cases. In the USA a survey of 575 users of CHM also showed an extremely high level of satisfaction.[104]

Like other TCM disciplines, CHM is based on the concepts of yin and yang and of qi energy. The herbs are ascribed qualities such as 'cooling' (yin) or 'stimulating' (yang) and are often used in combination according to the deficiencies or excesses of these qualities in the patient.

They may also be combined with zoological or mineral materials. Medicinal substances are combined to:

- increase therapeutic effectiveness by synergy
- reduce toxicity or adverse reactions
- accommodate complex clinical situations
- alter the actions of the substances.

CHM in practice

A Chinese herbal pharmacy and dispensing area are shown in Figures 9.3 and 9.4. A typical Chinese herbal formula usually comprises the following four main components:[105]

- the main ingredient, which treats the main disease
- the associate ingredient, which assists the main ingredient
- the adjuvant, which acts as an enhancer of the main ingredient, and moderates or eliminates the toxicity of other ingredients; it may also have an opposite effect to the main ingredient to produce supplementary benefits

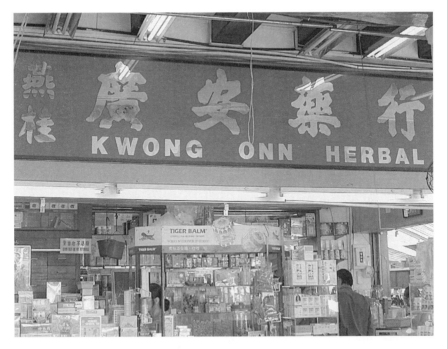

Figure 9.3 Exterior of a Chinese herbal pharmacy in Singapore.

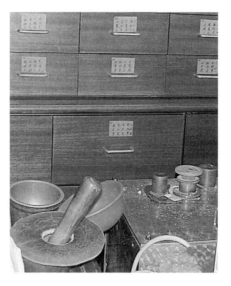

Figure 9.4 Extemporaneous dispensing area in Chinese herbal pharmacy.

- the guide ingredient (or envoy), which focuses the actions of the formula on certain meridians or areas of the body or harmonises and integrates the actions of the other ingredients.

The example of the CHM known as 'four gentleman decoction' (si jun zi tang) is quoted.[105] It is used for fatigue, reduced appetite, loose stools, pale tongue and weak pulse, which occur because of the deficiency of spleen and stomach qi and dampness in the digestive system. The formula comprises:

- main herb – *Radix ginseng* (ren shen), to enhance spleen qi
- associate – *Rhizona atiactylodis macrocephalae* (bai zhu), to strengthen the spleen and dry off the 'dampness'
- adjuvant – *Sclerotium poriae cocos* (fu ling), to assist the main and associate herbs
- guide – *Radix glycyrrhizae uralensis* (zhi gan cao), to harmonise the other three herbs and regulate spleen qi.

The use of this formula is an example of tonification, which is one of the eight general methods used in CHM. The full list of treatments is:

- cooling
- diaphoresis
- elimination
- emesis

- mediation
- purging
- tonification
- warming.

The herbs used are assigned to yin or yang categories. Herbs also have four essential energetic qualities; their corresponding actions relate to their perceived temperature, i.e. cool, warm, hot or cold. A fifth category is known as neutral. Examples of herbs from vegetable and animal origin are shown in Figure 9.5. Figure 9.6 shows a range of Chinese OTC herbs.

Evidence

As stated in the general introduction to TCM, the process of scientific validation of traditional therapies is often difficult for many reasons.

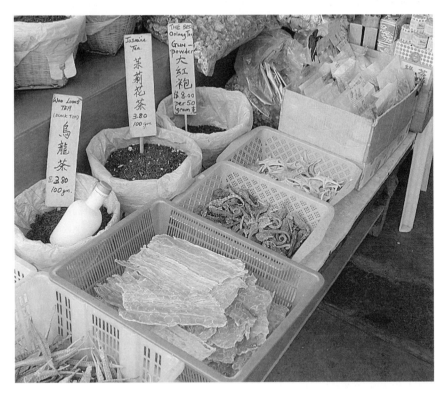

Figure 9.5 Loose herbs showing mixture of specimens from vegetable and animal origin.

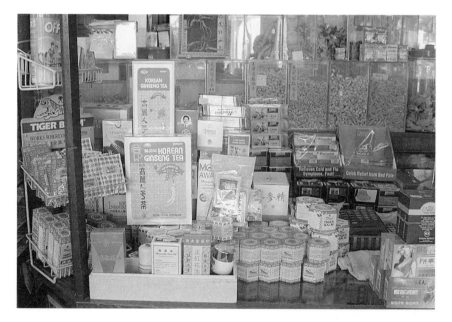

Figure 9.6 Chinese over-the-counter herbs.

However, there have been some successes. Research exists that has demonstrated the usefulness of CHM in many disorders[106] and supports its provision in state hospitals throughout China, alongside conventional medicine. It is suggested that, although the research is of variable quality, it should not be ignored.[107] Furthermore, promising trials have been carried out in the west.[108,109] Standardised oral herbal preparations that are monitored in a conventional western manner have been shown to be beneficial in eczema.[110] Unfortunately, most CHM practitioners individualise their prescriptions for every client, so the value of work on a standardised product may be limited.

In the absence of robust outcome studies of effectiveness, protagonists will continue to rely almost exclusively on circumstantial evidence obtained from case studies.

Safety

Competence of practitioners The use of CHM is increasing rapidly in the UK and relatively few patients are now Chinese. This has led to problems, as most of those who seek treatment are unable to distinguish between adequately and inadequately trained practitioners.

Practitioners fall into three broad categories:

- those who have had a full training in the discipline (available only in China)
- those who have received limited training in the UK or China
- those who have no training.

No data exist on exactly how many practitioners now offer Chinese herbal treatment in the UK, and only some of them will belong to a professional body. The main body is the Register of Chinese Herbal Medicine, which maintains minimum standards of training and practice. This body's main shortcoming is that virtually none of the fully qualified Chinese practitioners currently belongs to it.

Fully trained practitioners have a training similar to that given to orthodox doctors in the west. They receive some training in western medicine and can distinguish those conditions that would be best treated by western medicine. The main hazards of toxicity from Chinese herbs relate to unfavourable interactions with conventional pharmaceuticals and errors in identifying herbs. A few herbs may be toxic.

Intrinsic toxicity   Large amounts of traditional medicines are imported into the UK, legally and illegally, and use of such medicines is frequently not admitted on occasions when serious illness forces patients to consult western medical practitioners. These medicines carry with them a risk of adverse reactions; the risk needs to be quantified and as far as possible minimised. During the past 3 years the National Poisons Unit has taken a special interest in toxicological problems resulting from exposure to traditional medicines, and it will be publishing its findings in due course.

The herbs prescribed by practitioners of TCM in the UK are generally purchased from wholesale companies that specialise in this trade. These companies import herbs from the People's Republic of China either directly or through dealers in Hong Kong. The quality of imported herbs varies considerably, and great skill is needed to ensure that the correct herbs are provided to the practitioner. Some substitution of herbs is acceptable in China but can lead to problems if the wholesaler or practitioner is unaware of the substitution (see below). Confusion may arise over the precise identity of the herb being ordered; no standardised nomenclature exists for herbs. Fortunately, the best wholesalers and properly trained practitioners are able to make fairly reliable checks, at least visually. Unrecognised contamination by other herbs, drugs and various chemicals (including heavy metals or insecticides) is another possible hazard.

CHM has frequently been used as an alternative to orthodox therapies, especially where the latter have been considered to be ineffectual or have unacceptable side-effects. One of the most popular uses of CHM in the UK is in the treatment of atopic eczema, particularly in cases resistant to orthodox therapy. Because the herbal medicines are of natural origin, they are often perceived as being totally safe by consumers, but unfortunately many TCM remedies are potentially toxic when used in large doses and/or over extended time periods. Some examples of potentially toxic herbs are given in the following sections.[111]

For remedies readily obtainable OTC, vigilance is required to identify potentially toxic compounds. The most hazardous should be removed from circulation, and warnings should appear on packaging for the less hazardous. The Medicines Control Agency has a system for licensing such products, but this is not compulsory and potentially toxic products continue to be widely available.

Examples of toxic herbs It is estimated that there are 7000 species of medicinal plants in China and, of the 150 species most frequently used, 10 are toxic.[112] In Hong Kong most cases of serious poisoning are related to the use of the roots of caowu (*Aconitum kusnezoffiii*) and chuanwa (*Aconitum carmichaeli*). These herbs contain variable amounts of highly toxic alkaloids, including aconine, which activates sodium channels and causes widespread excitation of cellular membranes. Several other herbal preparations containing aconine alkaloids, for example monkshood (*Aconitum* spp.), are commonly used in Chinese medicine to treat arthritic, rheumatic and musculoskeletal pain. The alkaloids have analgesic, antipyretic and local anaesthetic properties but they are potentially toxic. The toxic effects include severe cardiac arrhythmias, nausea, vomiting and general debility. Unfortunately there is only a small margin between therapeutic and toxic doses.

Anticholinergic poisoning due to the flowers of yangjinhua (*Datura metel* L.) and naoyanghua (*Flos rhododendri mollis*) has been reported. These herbs, which are used to treat asthma and bronchitis and toothache, may contain scopolamine, hyoscymine and atropine, and can cause flushed skin, dilated pupils, confusion and coma.

Bajiaolian (*Dysosma pleianthum*) is a species of the mayapple that is used for the treatment of weakness and snake bites. Podophyllum resin is extracted from the plant rhizome and is thought to contain a toxin that can cause nausea, vomiting, diarrhoea and abdominal pain.[113]

Hepatotoxicity is a feature of various herbal teas, for example comfrey, also known as knitbone (*Symphytum officinalis*) and scullcap

(*Scutellaria laterflora*). A tea used for the treatment of eczema was believed to be the cause of hepatitis and acute liver failure in a 28-year-old woman. The tea contained a mixture of eight plants containing *Glycyrrhiza* and *Paeonia* spp.

Administration during pregnancy   A number of herbs, e.g. pennyroyal (*Mentha pulegium, Hedeoma pulegoides*) and valerian (*Valerian wallichi*) have abortifacient properties and should be avoided during pregnancy.[114] Their action is thought to be due to the presence of volatile oils, which can induce uterine contractions.

Administration to children   Infants are at greater risk of possible poisoning from CHM than adults because of their inadequate biotransformation processes. Chinese infants are frequently given chen-lin (*Coptis chinensus/japonicum*) by their mothers to clear up 'products of pregnancy'.[115] The main alkaloid of this herb is berberine and it can displace bilirubin from its serum-binding proteins causing a rise in free bilirubin concentration and a risk of brain damage. Yin-chen (*Artemisia scoparia*) is used for the treatment of neonatal jaundice and has a similar effect.

A fuller description of the potential toxicity of CHM has been provided elsewhere.[65]

Concurrent use with orthodox medicines   There are two problems here: an enhanced activity from the herbal medicine or the orthodox medicine, or both, and an intrinsic toxicity, real or threatened, from the allopathic ingredient.

Aristolochia is an example of a remedy whose administration concurrently with allopathic drugs in Chinese herbal preparations (albeit inadvertently) potentiates its action, causing severe adverse reactions (see below).

There are several examples of the inclusion of illegal ingredients in Chinese medicines over many years and pharmacists should be aware of this possibility. In 1975 a herbal-based preparation called Toukuwan was manufactured in Hong Kong and widely promoted in the USA for rheumatism and arthritis. It was discovered that the product contained four orthodox medicines, including the prescription drug diazepam, and its continued import was swiftly banned by the FDA. More recently, the New Zealand Director General of Health advised consumers against taking a Chinese product known as cheng kum because it contained a pharmacy-only antihistamine that could cause drowsiness.[116] The capsules have now been withdrawn from sale. They were advertised for use in the treatment of various conditions, including the promotion of joint mobility, healthy skin, as a support during menopause and of benefit while consuming alcoholic drinks. The Ministry of Health made the ruling following complaints from doctors about the product.

Another example is the intentional inclusion of steroids in oral[117] and topical preparations[118] used for the treatment of dermatological conditions. Following reports of positive clinical effects in the treatment of eczema, 11 Chinese herbal creams were analysed. Eight were found to contain dexamethasone in amounts varying from 64 to 1500 µg/g.[119] The mean of 456 µg/g approximated to a proprietary brand of 0.05% betamethasone valerate, a commonly prescribed steroid ointment in the UK. None of the patients was aware that the creams contained a steroid.

The authors[119] point out that the risk of adverse reactions with such potent steroids is increased by their inappropriate use and application to areas of thin skin such as flexures and on the face. They have called for urgent action to prevent illegal prescribing of potent steroids.

It has been suggested that exported herbal remedies have been adulterated with synthetic drugs to improve their activity, and their popularity, in western countries. A dangerous evolution in the formulation of a Chinese herbal arthritis cure, Chuifong Toukuwan, manufactured by a laboratory in Hong Kong, has been dsecribed.[120] The undeclared presence of phenylbutazone, indometacin, hydrochlorothiazide, chlordiazepoxide, diazepam and corticosteroids was reported in the product, a mixture of 23 herbs.

Inclusion of adulterants   Major problems resulting from the presence of adulterants in CHM have been experienced. It is therefore extremely important that TCM products are monitored closely. The European Agency for the Evaluation of Medicinal Products in London has a working party on herbal medicinal products, whose remit includes pharmacovigilance and the introduction of safety measures throughout member states. The Medicines Control Agency performs a similar task in the UK. Currently, Chinese herbal suppliers are engaged in agreeing guidelines to ensure that their medicines are of the highest quality and free from adulterants.

The *Aristolochia* story – a complex problem[121]   Severe concerns about the safety of the herb *Aristolochia* arose in early 1992 when two women presented with extensive interstitial renal fibrosis to doctors in a Belgian clinic that specialised in weight-loss regimens. The condition rapidly progressed to terminal renal failure.[122] The total number of patients exposed to the herb is not known exactly, but around 100 people with renal disease were eventually recorded, representing about 5% of those who took the slimming preparation.[123]

The diet regimen used by the clinic for many years without problems comprised a mixture of acetazolamide, fenfluramine and various animal and vegetable extracts. In mid 1990 the formula was supplemented by the addition of powdered extracts of Chinese herbs. A possible relationship between the renal disease and the herbs was suspected. Subsequently, it was established from an epidemiological survey that *Stephania tetrandra* was the only herb associated with all the cases of renal disease. Most unexpectedly, the alkaloid normally derived from *Stephania* – tetrandrine – could not be found in the capsules taken by the affected patients.[124] Instead, analysis revealed the presence of a series of substituted nitrophenthrene carboxylic acids, known as aristolochic acids. These were considered to be the cause of the adverse reactions.[125,126] The acids form the main active principal of various species of another Chinese herb, namely *Aristolochia*.

It was finally concluded that the *Stephania tetrandra* (han fang ji) must have been inadvertently replaced by *Aristolochia fangchi* (guang fang ji) in the powdered extracts delivered to Belgian suppliers.

Herbal ingredients are usually traded using their common Chinese names and this can lead to confusion during translation.

About 185 kg of the substituted han fang ji was distributed to practitioners throughout Belgium but it was only one particular clinic that reported problems. The intrinsic nephrotoxic effects of the *Aristolochia* may have been potentiated in this case by the combination of orthodox drugs administered concurrently. The *British National Formulary*[127] states that the use of diuretics for weight loss is inappropriate; this would seem to question the wisdom of including acetazolamide in the product. The Belgian medical authorities have also warned doctors not to prescribe slimming products composed of appetite inhibitors and diuretics. The women may have been more vulnerable to adverse reactions due to a weakening of general health caused by the calorie-controlled diet they were following.[128] In addition, the herbs were prescribed by untrained doctors and not in accordance with Chinese medical theories.

Since 1994 a total of seven cases of Chinese herb nephropathy have been reported in France. In 1998 a case of reversible acute hepatitis in a patient using a Chinese herbal tea was reported in the Netherlands.[129] *A. debilis* was identified in the tea mixture. Also around this time a case was reported in Spain of a patient with renal failure resulting from chronic intake of an infusion made with a mixture of herbs containing *A. pistolochia*. This species of the herb is native to Catalonia.[130]

The first two cases of a specific nephropathy caused by ingestion of an unlicensed Chinese herbal remedy in the UK were reported in 1999.[131] The first case was a 49-year-old woman who initially presented to her GP with headache and hypertension. Her only existing medication was a herbal preparation that she had been taking for about 2 years to treat her eczema. Renal function tests and a biopsy revealed substantial tubular atrophy and interstitial fibrosis in the cortex. The patient rapidly progressed to renal failure and dialysis was begun. Three years later she received a renal transplant.

The second patient was a 57-year-old woman who was admitted with renal failure and a 6-month history of anorexia, lethargy, nausea and weight loss. She had been taking Chinese herbal tea for eczema for 6 years. A renal biopsy showed evidence of deterioration, as in the case above. The patient was started on dialysis.

Subsequently, it was found that both patients had been exposed to aristolochic acids as a result of ingesting *A. manshuriensis* used as a substitute for mu tong in the herbal tea in place of *Clematis* or *Akebia* spp.

Following these cases the Australian Office of Complementary Medicine initiated a survey of products containing *Clematis* to determine whether inadvertent substitution with *Aristolochia* had occurred.[132] Their concern was prompted by a realisation that the Chinese name mu tong could be used to describe three different herbs, *Clematis* spp. (chuan mu tong), *Akebia* spp. (bai mu tong) and *Aristolochia manshuriensis* (guan mu tong). Of the 14 samples tested, a raw herbal material and a manufactured clematis product were found to contain *Aristolochia*. In TCM *Aristolochia* spp. are considered to be interchangeable with other commonly used herbal ingredients and substitution of one plant for another species is an established practice. Table 9.3 gives examples of common Chinese herbs.

Pharmokinetic data for aristolochic acids 1 and 11 have been studied in rats, mice, guinea pigs, dogs and humans after oral treatment.[133] The doses studied were in the range of 0.6–85 mg/kg body weight. Most of the results relate to rats. Following oral administration, aristolochic acid 1 was readily absorbed from the gastrointestinal tract. After oral administration of aristolochic acid 1 to rats, about 91% of the dose was recovered from the excreta, equally divided in the urine and faeces.

In vivo and in vitro studies have shown that aristolochic acids are both nephrotoxic and carcinogenic. Hence most European Union

Table 9.3 Species of *Aristolochia*

Species	Part used	Indication
A. fangchi	Root	Diuretic, antirheumatic
A. contorta, A. debilis	Fruit	Antitussive, antiasthmatic
A. contorta, A. debilis	Herb	Diuretic and anti-inflammatory
A. debilis	Root	Analgesic

states have taken regulatory action to protect the public from unlicensed medicines that contain *Aristolochia*. In many member states (including the UK) *Stephania tetrandra* is also being controlled because of the risk of substitution. Following the interim measures taken in July 1999 the UK Medicines Control Agency is preparing to initiate a permanent ban on the import, sale or supply of preparations containing plants of the genus *Aristolochia*. A consultation document has been issued to interested parties. It relates to proposals to make an order entitled The Medicines (*Aristolochia* and mu tong, etc.) (Prohibition) Order 2001. The new order will confirm the permanent prohibition in unlicensed medicines for human use of *Aristolochia* spp. It is unfortunate that such action is necessary and some would say that this represents another example of the government restricting consumers' choice.

There is undoubtedly a substantial risk to health from *Aristolochia* when it is improperly used. Effective control is vital to ensure that the herb is used under appropriate supervision and is of the highest quality. *Aristolochia* has been a prescription-only medicine since 1997 but currently is exempt from prescription-only medicines control when used in herbal or homeopathic medicine. It will be unaffected by the new legislation, although it is possible that the potencies (strengths) available could be restricted to those above 9c, when the dilution is of such magnitude that no molecules of drug are considered to be present.

Future measures to improve safety   The problems of TCM are not unlike those of orthodox medicine. There are both intrinsic adverse reactions resulting from the toxicity of the product and extrinsic adverse reactions arising from ancillary procedures, for example inappropriate diagnosis and prescribing. Both groups of problems need to be addressed. To minimise the chance of adverse reactions leading to a recurrence of the circumstances surrounding the use of *Aristolochia* with other herbs, the following measures should be instigated:

- Quality assurance and quality control should be put in place to ensure that unadulterated herbs are supplied to manufacturers and practitioners.
- Herbal practitioners should undergo a course of training to ensure that they provide a safe and effective service.
- Herbs with known potential to cause adverse reactions should not be mixed with orthodox drugs unless careful monitoring is carried out.
- Accurate records should be kept by all practitioners to monitor the incidence of adverse reactions. Regular audits should also be carried out. This is in any case a minimum requirement for the collection of the evidence of successful outcomes required by purchasing authorities. Effective use of the yellow card system by all disciplines of complementary medicine is long overdue. NMQPs should also be encouraged to take part. This would make sense because there are many more NMQPs than health professionals involved in TCM.

Endangered species

The conservation of rare medicinal plants is a worldwide problem affecting many cultures.[134] The issue of the usage of various endangered species, including bears and tigers, which are ingredients in the formulation of Chinese herbal patent formulae, was brought to the public eye in the USA by a World Wildlife Fund-supported report entitled *Prescription for Extinction: Endangered Species and Patented Oriental Medicines in Trade*.[135] This report was released in 1994 and resulted in widespread media attention and subsequent public concern. Researchers at Bastyr University are studying the issue of endangered species usage in depth, along with the issues of excessive toxins, drugs, adulterants and illegal and inaccurate labelling practices, which are prevalent in these formulas. Bastyr University is near Seattle, and integrates the pursuit of scientific knowledge with the wisdom of ancient healing methods and traditional cultures from around the world. Researchers plan to work with the manufacturers of Chinese herbal patent formulae toward establishing guidelines that may be implemented in the west and in Asia.

Western CHM

The use of CHM has been continued in the traditional manner by physicians and pharmacists serving Chinese communities around the world.

In many western cities the Chinatown districts support herb shops and practices with remedies imported directly from Asia, and practitioners trained by the old system of long apprenticeship. Increasingly, local western practitioners are training in their home countries to satisfy the growing interest for CHM. In particular, acupuncturists seem to be extending their practice. Many are taking a 2-year course offered by the Register of Traditional Chinese Medicine, which covers around 200 herbs and 100 classical formulae.[136]

Examples of Chinese herbs used in the UK   Examples of herbs used in TCM formulae in the UK are listed in Table 9.4.[137]

Table 9.4 Examples of common Chinese herbs[137]

Source material	Chinese name	Parts used	Main constituents	Clinical use
Agastache rugosa	Hua xiang	Herb	Essential oil	Digestive stimulant, antiemetic
Cinnamonium spp.	Rou gui	Bark	Essential oil, resin	Warms, circulatory stimulant
Clematis chinensis	Wei ling xian	Root	Anemoonin, saponins, sterols, phenols	Antirheumatic, stimulant, expels wind and damp
Glycyrrhiza uralensis	Gan cao	Root	Saponins, flavonoids	Expectorant, tonic, detoxifier
Lonicera japonica	Jin yin hua	Flowers	Luteolin, tannin	Cooling and disinfecting, anti-pyretic, detoxifier
Magnolia spp.	Xin yi hua	Bark	Essential oil, alkaloids	Digestive stimulant, expectorant
Panax ginseng	Ren shen	Root	Saponins, glycosides	Sedative, tonic
Phellodendron amurensei	Po-mu	Bark	Alkaloids, triterpenoids, sterols	Bitter digestive, diuretic, antipyretic
Taraxacum mongolicum	Pu gong ying	Whole plant	Bitters, sterol	Anti-infective, antipyretic

Other elements of TCM[138]

Chinese massage (tui na)

Massage has been an important element of TCM for at least 2000 years, featuring in the Yellow Emperor's famous text. The therapy uses hand manipulation, pushing, rolling and kneading, on specific points and parts of the body. It may be used to balance yin and yang and to regulate the function of qi, blood and the zang fu organs as well as to loosen joints and relax muscles and tendons.

Martial art therapy

This approach uses movements and exercises adapted from martial arts, such as t'ai chi chu'an, kung fu, moo doe and others.[139] A case study report has indicated that a patient suffering from severe cervical stenosis improved following martial art therapy.[140]

Mind and body exercise (qigong)

This is a meditative therapy with a history similar to that of Chinese massage. It is often combined with body movement and breathing exercises to achieve a balance of energy in the TCM meridian system. Tai ji quan, also known as tai c'hi, was created in the fourteenth century as a martial art and is practised widely in China. The term 'tai ji' refers to the balance of yin and yang. It consists of a series of slow flowing exercises inspired by the movement of animals, as reflected in the names given to the movements, e.g. 'white stork spreading wings'. Tai ji is said to reduce mental and emotional stress.

Dietary therapy

Chinese dietary therapy is an important part of life in the country as well as being included in many practitioners' prescriptions. Knowledgeable Chinese housewives often prepare special meals for common family ailments. Thus a patient suffering from insomnia due to a disharmony of heart and kidney might be advised to make a soup of lotus plumule (lian xin) to nourish the heart and include morus fruit (sang shen) to enhance kidney essence. These measures would be in addition to other TCM treatments, e.g. CHM and/or acupuncture. Nutritional interventions may be of three types:[141]

- **Supplementation:** as well as various vitamins and minerals, the range may contain animal and plant products (e.g. algae or kelp).
- **Dietary modification:** this involves changes in dietary habits to exclude elements not considered nutritious or to establish better eating patterns.
- **Therapeutic systems:** the inclusion (or exclusion) of foods considered to have a contributory role to the patient's health.

Examples of diets with properties beneficial to health include:[142]

- **White rice porridge:** this regulates the bowels (constipation and diarrhoea), for nausea and loss of appetite.
- **Sweet and sour sauce:** considered to be an important constituent of diet because of its antiseptic properties.
- **Sweet and sour crispy noodles:** noodles are a good source of nutrients for athletes and growing children. The vinegar in the sauce has antiseptic properties.

Examples of dietary remedies for common illnesses include:

- **Acne:** infusion of the flowers of peach (*Prunus persica*) or almond (*P. amygdalus*) in water daily
- **Arthritis:** cinnamon tea (*Cinnamonum cassia*); for cold arthritis, sage steeped in rice wine sipped daily and for warm arthritis infusion of purslane (*Portalaca oleracea*) in water
- **Constipation:** fig wine, stewed pears and bananas eaten cold with honey
- **Flatulence:** seeds of mandarin orange chewed
- **Haemorrhoids:** simmer a mixture of almonds, peach kernels, pine nuts and sesame seeds in water and drink as a soup
- **Halitosis:** a few leaves of peppermint or the peel of a mandarin orange chewed.

More information

British Acupuncture Council
Suite D
Park House
206/208 Latimer Road
London W10 6RE
Tel: 020 8964 0222
www.acupuncture.org.uk

British Medical Acupuncture Society
Newton House
Newton Lane
Whitley
Warrington
WA4 4JA
Tel: 01925 730727
www.medical-acupuncture.co.uk

Acupuncture Association of Chartered Physiotherapists
14 Bedford Row
London
WC1R 4ED
Tel: 020 7242 1941

The following web site will be of interest to readers:
www.demon.co.uk/acupuncture/arcc.html.

References

1. Bliss B. *Chinese Medicinal Herbs*. San Francisco: Georgetown Press, 1980: 3.
2. Harrison Nolting M. Acupuncture. In: Pizzorno J Jr, Murray M T (eds) *Textbook of Natural Medicine*, 2nd edn. Edinburgh: Churchill Livingstone, 1999: 253–256.
3. Hoizey D, Hoizey M. *A History of Chinese Medicine*. Vancouver: University BC Press, 1993: 42.
4. Williams T. *Chinese Medicine*. Shaftesbury, Dorset: Element Books, 1996.
5. Lyons A, Petrucelli R J. *Medicine. An Illustrated History*. New York: H N Abrams, 1987: 121–127.
6. Jobst K A, Shostak D, Whitehouse P J. Editorial. *J Altern Complement Med* 1999; 6: 495–502.
7. Selby A. *The Ancient and Healing Art of Chinese Herbalism*. London: Hamlyn, 1998.
8. Selby A. *The Ancient and Healing Art of Chinese Herbalism*. London: Hamlyn, 1998: 46.
9. Williams T. *Chinese Medicine*. Shaftesbury, Dorset: Element Books, 1996: 31–33.
10. Kaptchuk T J. *Chinese Medicine*. London: Rider, 2000: 105–141.
11. Fulder S. *The Handbook of Alternative and Complementary Medicine*. Oxford: OUP, 1996: 127–128.
12. Lao L. Traditional Chinese medicine. In: Jonas W B, Levin J (eds) *Essentials of Complementary and Alternative Medicine*. Baltimore: Lippincott/Williams & Wilkins, 1999: 222–223.
13. Houghton P. The role of plants in traditional medicine and current therapy. *J Altern Complement Med* 1995; 1: 131–143.

14. The State Administration of Traditional Chinese Medicine of the People's Republic of China. *Anthology of Policies, Laws and Regulations of the People's Republic of China on Traditional Chinese Medicine.* Shangdong: Shangdong University, 1997.

15. Anon. Acupunction. *Lancet* 1823; 1: 147–148.

16. Kaplan G. A brief history of acupuncture's journey to the West. *J Altern Complement Med* 1997; 3: 5–10.

17. Emslie M, Campbell M, Walker K. Complementary therapies in a local health care setting part 1: is there a real public demand? *Complement Ther Med* 1996; 4: 39–42.

18. MacDonald A J R. *Acupuncture: From Ancient Art to Modern Medicine.* Boston: George Allen & Unwin, 1982.

19. Janovsky B, White A R, Filshie J et al. Are acupuncture points tender? A blinded study of spleen 6. *J Altern Complement Med* 2000; 6: 149–155.

20. Fulder S. *The Handbook of Alternative and Complementary Medicine.* Oxford: OUP, 1996: 126.

21. Yamashia H, Tsukayama H, Hori N et al. Incidence of adverse reactions associated with acupuncture. *J Altern Complement Med* 2000; 6: 345–350.

22. Ernst E, White A R. Life threatening adverse reactions after acupuncture? A systemic review. *Pain* 1997; 71: 123–126.

23. Chen F, Hwang S, Lee H et al. Clinical study of syncope during acupuncture treatment. *Acupunct Electrother Res* 1990; 15: 107–119.

24. Brattberg G. Acupuncture treatments: a traffic hazard? *Am J Acupunct* 1986; 14: 265–267.

25. Ernst E. Adverse effects of acupuncture. In: Jonas W B, Ernst E (eds) *Essentials of CAM.* Baltimore: Lippincott/Williams & Wilkins, 1999: 172–175.

26. MacPherson H. Fatal and adverse events from acupuncture: allegation, evidence and the implications. *J Altern Complement Med* 1999; 5: 47–56.

27. Rampes H, James R. Complications of acupuncture. *Acupunct Med* 1995; 11: 26–33.

28. Boxall E H. Acupuncture hepatitis in the West Midlands. *J Med Virol* 1978; 2: 377–379.

29. Hussain K K. Serum hepatitis associated with repeated acupuncture. *BMJ* 1974; 278: 41–42.

30. Vittecoq D, Metteral J F, Rouzioux C. Infection after acupuncture treatment. *N Engl J Med* 1989; 320: 250–251.

31. Castro K G, Lifson A R, White C R. Investigations of AIDS patients with no previous identification risk factors. *JAMA* 1988; 259: 1338–1342.

32. Jeffreys D B, Smith S, Brennand-Roper D A, Curry P V L. Acupuncture needles as a cause of bacterial endocarditis. *BMJ* 1983; 287: 326–327.

33. Pierik M G. Fatal staphylococcal septicaemia following acupuncture: report of two cases. *Rhode Island Med J* 1982; 65: 251–253.

34. Halvorsen T B, Anda S S, Naess A B, Levang O W. Fatal cardiac tamponade after acupuncture through congenital sternal foramen. *Lancet* 1995; 345: 1175.

35. White A R, Abbot N C, Ernst E. Self reports of adverse effects of acupuncture included cardiac arrythmies. *Acupunct Med* 1996; 14: 121.

36. Ogata M, Kitamura O, Kubo S, Nakasono Q. An asthmatic death while under Chinese acupuncture and moxibustion treatment. *Am J Forensic Med Pathol* 1992; 13: 338–341.

37. Abbot N C, White A R, Ernst E. Complementary medicine. *Nature* 1996; 381: 361.
38. Fisher A A. Allergic dermatitis from acupuncture needles. *Cutis* 1976; 38: 226.
39. Castelain M, Castelain P Y, Ricciardi R. Contact dermatitis to acupuncture needles. *Contact Dermatitis* 1987; 16: 44.
40. Norheim A J, Fonnebo V. Acupuncture adverse effects are more than occasional case reports: results from questionnaires among 1135 randomly selected doctors and 297 acupuncturists. *Complement Ther Med* 1996; 4: 8–13.
41. Fujiwara H, Taniguchi J, Ikezono E. The influence of low frequency acupuncture on a demand pacemaker. *Chest* 1980; 78: 96–97.
42. Lyle C D, Thomas B M, Gordon E A, Krauthamer V. Electrostimulators for acupuncture: safety issues. *J Altern Complement Med* 2000; 6: 37–44.
43. Carron H, Epstein B S, Grand B. Complications of acupuncture. *JAMA* 1974; 228: 1552–1554.
44. Hung V C, Mines J S. Eschars and scarring from from hot needle acupuncture treatment. *J Am Acad Dermatol* 1991; 24: 148–149.
45. Filshie J, White A R (eds). *Medical Acupuncture, a Western Scientific Approach*. Edinburgh: Churchill Livingstone, 1998.
46. Macdonald A J R. Acupuncture and analgesia and therapy. In: Wall P D, Melzack R (eds) *Textbook of Pain*, 2nd edn. Edinburgh: Churchill Livingstone, 1989.
47. White A. The principles behind acupuncture. *Health Matters Magazine* 1999; May: 30–31.
48. Ernst E, White A. Acupuncture: safety first. *BMJ* 1997; 314: 1362.
49. Mann F. *Reinventing Acupuncture*. Oxford: Butterworth Press, 1993.
50. Marwick C. Acceptance of some acupuncture applications. *JAMA* 1997; 278: 1725–1727.
51. Silvert M. Acupuncture wins BMA approval. *BMJ* 2000; 321: 11.
52. Moore R A, McQuay H, Oldman A D, Smith L E. BMA approves acupuncture. *BMJ* 2000; 321: 1220.
53. Vincent C, Furnham A. *Complementary Medicine. A Research Perspective*. Chichester: John Wiley, 1998: 160–161.
54. Godfrey C M, Morgan P A. A controlled trial of theory of acupuncture in musculoskeletal pain. *J Rheumatol* 1978; 5: 121–124.
55. Ceccherelli F, Gagliardi G, Rossato M, Giron G. Valuables of stimulation and placebo in acupuncture reflexotherapy. *J Altern Complement Med* 2000; 6: 275–279.
56. Ernst E. Clinical effectiveness of acupuncture: an overview of systematic reviews. In: Ernst E, White A (eds) *Acupuncture. A Scientific Appraisal*. Oxford: Butterworth-Heinemann, 1999: 107–127.
57. Cummings M. Acupuncture techniques should be treated logically and methodically. *BMJ* 2001; 322: 47b.
58. Ernst E, White A R. Acupuncture for back pain: a meta analysis of randomised controlled trials. *Arch Intern Med* 1998; 158: 2235–2241.
59. van Tulder M W, Cherkin D C, Berman B *et al*. The effectiveness of acupuncture in the management of acute and chronic low back pain. *Spine* 1999; 24: 1113–1123.

60. MacPherson H, Gould A J, Fitter M. Acupuncture for low back pain: results of a pilot study for a randomised controlled trial. *Complement Ther Med* 1999; 7: 83–90.

61. Wedenberg K, Moen B, Norling A. A prospective randomised study comparing acupuncture with physiotherapy for low back pain and pelvic pain in pregnacy. *Acta Obstet Gynecol Scand* 2000; 79: 331–335.

62. Ernst E, Pittler M H. The effectiveness of acupuncture in treating acute dental pain: a systematic review. *Br Dental J* 1998; 184: 443–447.

63. Avants S K, Margolin A, Holford T R, Kosten T R. A randomised controlled trial of auricular acupuncture for cocaine dependence. *Arch Intern Med* 2000; 160: 2305–2312.

64. Margolin A, Avants S K. Should cocaine abusing, buprenorphine maintained patients receive auricular acupuncture? Findings from an acute effects study. *J Altern Complement Med* 1999; 5: 567–574.

65. Diehl D. Acupuncture for gastrointestinal and hepatobiliary disorders. *J Altern Complement Med* 1999; 5: 27–45.

66. Beal M W, Nield-Anderson L. Acupuncture for symptom relief in HIV positive adults: lessons learned from a pilot study. *Altern Ther Health Med* 2000; 6: 33–42.

67. Milgrom C, Finestone A, Eldad A, Shlamkovitch N. Patellofemoral pain caused by overactivity. A prospective study of risk factors in infantry recruits. *J Bone Joint Surg Am* 1991; 73: 1041–1043.

68. Jensen R, Gothesen O, Liseth K, Baerheim A. Acupuncture treatment of patellofemoral pain syndrome. *J Altern Complement Med* 1999; 5: 521–527.

69. Ross J, White A, Ernst E. Western minimal acupuncture for neck pain: a cohort study. *Acupunct Med* 1999; 17: 5–8.

70. Irnich D, Behrens N, Molzen H *et al*. Randomised trial of acupuncture compared with conventional massage and 'sham' laser acupuncture for treatment of chronic neck pain. *BMJ* 2001; 322: 1574–1579.

71. White A R, Ernst E. A systematic review of randomised controlled trials of acupuncture for neck pain. *Rheumatology* 1999; 38: 143–147.

72. Acupuncture as a symptomatic treatment for osteoarthritis – a systematic review. *Scand J Rheumatol* 1997; 26: 444–447.

73. Vickers A J. Can acupuncture have specific effects on health? A systematic review of acupuncture antiemesis trials. *J R Soc Med* 1996; 89: 303–311.

74. Melchart D, Linde K, Fischer P *et al*. Acupuncture for recurrent headaches: a systematic review of randomised controlled trials. *Cephalalgia* 1999; 19: 779–786.

75. Vincent C A. A controlled trial of the treatment of migraine by acupuncture. *Clin J Pain* 1989; 5: 305–312.

76. Kleinherz J, Streitberger K, Windeler J *et al*. Randomised clinical trial comparing the effects of acupuncture and a newly designed placebo needle in rotator cuff tendonitis. *Pain* 1999; 83: 235–241.

77. White A R, Rampes H, Ernst E. Acupuncture for smoking cessation. *Cochrane Library* 1999; 4: 1–10.

78. Ernst E, White A R. Acupuncture as an adjuvant therapy in stroke rehabilitation? *Wien Med Wochenschr* 1996; 146: 556–558.

79. Gosman–Hedstroem G, Cleeson L, Klingenstierna U *et al*. Effects of acupuncture

treatment on daily life activities and quality of life. *Stroke* 1998; 29: 2100–2108.

80. Johansson K, Lindgren I, Widner H *et al.* Can sensory stimulation improve the functional outcome in stroke patients? *Neurology* 1993; 43: 2189–2192.

81. Ernst E, White A R. Acupuncture as a treatment for temporomandibular joint dysfunction. *Arch Otolaryngol Head Neck Surg* 1999; 125: 269–272.

82. Ernst E. Acupuncture/acupressure for weight reduction? A systematic review. *Wien Med Wochenschr* 1997; 109: 6–62.

83. BMA. *Acupuncture: Efficacy, Safety and Practice.* Amsterdam: Harwood Academic Publishers, 2000: 66–81.

84. Reilly D T. Young doctors' views on alternative medicine. *BMJ* 1983; 287: 337–339.

85. Anderson E, Anderson P. General practitioner and alternative medicine. *J R Coll Gen Pract* 1987; 37: 52–55.

86. Wharton R, Lewith G. Complementary medicine and the general practitioner. *BMJ* 1986; 292: 1498–1500.

87. White A R, Resch K–L, Ernst E. Complementary medicine: use and attitudes among GPs. *Fam Pract* 1997; 14: 302–306.

88. Thomas K, Fall M, Parry G, Nicholl J. *National Survey of Access to Complementary Health Care via General Practice.* Department of Health report. Sheffield: Medical Care Unit, 1995.

89. Berman B M, Singh B K, Lao L *et al.* Physicians' attitudes toward complementary or alternative medicine: a regional survey. *J Am Board Fam Pract* 1995; 8: 361–366.

90. Hadley C M. Complementary medicine and the general practitioner: a survey of general practitioners in the Wellington area. *NZ Med J* 1988; 101: 765–768.

91. Marshall R J, Gee R, Dumble J *et al.* The use of alternative therapies by Auckland general practitioners. *NZ Med J* 1990; 103: 213–215.

92. Easthope G, Beilby J J, Gill G F, Tranter B K. Acupuncture in Australian general practice: practitioner characteristics. *Med J Aust* 1998; 169: 197–200.

93. Jarmey C, Tindall J. *Acupressure for Common Ailments.* London: Gala Books, 1991.

94. Marti J E. *Alternative Health Medicine Encyclopedia.* Detroit: Visible Ink Press, 1995: 3.

95. Bruce D G, Golding J F, Hockenhulkl N, Pethybridge R J. Acupressure and motion sickness. *Aviat Space Environment Med* 1990; 61: 361–365.

96. Hu S, Stritzel R, Chandler A, Stern R M. P6 acupressure reduces symptoms of vection induced motion sickness. *Aviat Space Environment Med* 1995; 66: 631–634.

97. Murphy P A. Alternative therapies for nausea and vomiting of pregnancy. *Obstet Gynecol* 1998; 91: 149–155.

98. O'Brien B, Relyea M J, Taerum T. Efficacy of P6 acupuncture in the treatment of nausea and vomiting during pregnancy. *Am J Obstet Gynecol* 1996; 174: 708–715.

99. Unschuld P U. *Medicine in China. A History of Pharmaceuticals.* Berkeley, CA: University of California Press, 2000.

100. Harrison Nolting M, Cao Q. Introduction to the clinical use of Chinese prepared medicines. In: Pizzorno J Jr, Murray M T (eds) *Textbook of Natural Medicine*, 2nd edn. Edinburgh: Churchill Livingstone, 1999: 807–814.

101. Vickers A, Zellman C. ABC of complementary medicine – herbal medicine. *BMJ* 1999; 319: 1050–1053.
102. Houghton P. Traditional Chinese medicine: does it work? Is it safe? *Chemist Druggist* 1999; 20 November: vi–vii.
103. *Complementary Medicine. Mintel Report.* London: Mintel International Group, 2001.
104. Cassidy C. Chinese medicine users in the United States part 1: utilization, satisfaction, medical plurality. *J Altern Complement Med* 1998; 4: 17–27.
105. Lao L. Traditional Chinese medicine. In: Jonas W B, Levin J (eds) *Essentials of Complementary and Alternative Medicine.* Baltimore: Lippincott/Williams & Wilkins, 1999: 215.
106. Dharmananda S. *Controlled Clinical Trials of Chinese Herbal Medicine: A Review.* Oregon: Institute for Traditional Medicine, 1997.
107. Lampert N. Letter. *Lancet* 2001; 357: 882.
108. Sheehan M P, Rustin M H A, Atherton D J *et al.* Efficacy of traditional Chinese herbal therapy in adult atopic dermatitis. *Lancet* 1992; 340: 13–17.
109. Bensoussan A, Menzies R. Treatment of irritable bowel syndrome with Chinese herbal medicine. *JAMA* 1998; 280: 1585–1589.
110. Sheehan M P, Atherton D J. A controlled trial of traditional Chinese medicinal plants in widespread non-exudative eczema. *Br J Dermatol* 1992; 126: 179–184.
111. Bateman J, Chapman R D, Simpson D. Possible toxicity of herbal remedies. *Scot Med J* 1998; 43: 7–15.
112. Chan T V K, Chan J C N, Tomlinson B, Critchley J A H. Chinese herbal medicine revisited: a Hong Kong perspective. *Lancet* 1993; 342: 1532–1534.
113. Kao W–F, Hung D–Z, Tsai W-J *et al.* Podophyllotoxin intoxication: toxic effects of Bajiaolian in herbal therapeutics. *Human Exp Toxicol* 1992; 11: 480–487.
114. Newall C A, Anderson L A, Phillipsson J D. *Herbal Medicines. A Guide for Health-care Professionals.* London: Pharmaceutical Press, 1996.
115. Chan T K Y. The prevalence, use and harmful potential of some Chinese herbal medicines in babies and children. *Vet Human Toxicol* 1994; 26: 238–240.
116. Thomson L. Chinese capsules face short shift. *NZ Pharm* 2001; 22: 8.
117. McGregoor F B, Abernethy V E, Dahabra S *et al.* Chinese herbs for eczema. *Lancet* 1989; 299: 1156–1157.
118. Hughes J R, Higgins E M, Pembroke A C. Dexamethasone masquerading as a Chinese herbal. *Br J Dermatol* 1994; 130: 261.
119. Keane F M, Munn S F, du Vivier A W P *et al.* Analysis of Chinese herbal creams prescribed for dermatological conditions. *BMJ* 1999; 518: 563–564.
120. Vander Stricht B I, Parvais O E, Vanhaelen-Fastre R J, Vanhaelen M H. Remedies may contain cocktail of active drugs. *BMJ* 1994; 308: 1162.
121. Kayne S B. Comment – *Aristolochia* – A case for exclusion. *Good Clin Pract J* 2001; 8: 9–11.
122. Vanherweghem J-L, Depierreux M, Tielmans C *et al.* Rapidly progressing interstitial renal fibrosis in young women: association with slimming regimen including Chinese herbs. *Lancet* 1993; 341: 387–391.
123. Vanherweghem J-L. Misuse of herbal remedies: the case of an outbreak of terminal renal failure in Belgium (Chinese herb nephropathy). *J Altern Complement Med* 1998; 4: 9–13.

124. Depierreux M, Van Den Houte K, Vanherweghem J-L. Pathological aspects of newly prescribed nephropathy related to prolonged use of Chinese herbs. *Am J Kidney Dis* 1994; 24: 172–180.
125. But P P. Need for correct identification of herbs in herbal poisoning. *Lancet* 1993; 341: 637.
126. Van Haelen M, Van Haelen-Fastre R, But P P H, Vanherweghem M L. Identification of aristolochic acids in Chinese herbs. *Lancet* 1994; 343: 174.
127. *British National Formulary*, vol. 41. London: British Medical Association/Royal Pharmaceutical Society of Great Britain, 2001.
128. McIntyre M. Chinese herbs: risk, side effects and poisoning: the case for objective reporting, and analysis reveals serious misrepresentation. *J Altern Complement Med* 1998; 4: 15–16.
129. Levi M, Guchelaar H J, Woerdenbag H J, Zhu Y P. Acute hepatitis in a patient using a Chinese tea – a case report. *Pharm World Sci* 1998; 20: 43–44.
130. *Working Party Report on Herbal Medicinal Products*. London: EMEA, 2000: 8.
131. Lord G M, Tagore R, Cook T *et al*. Nephropathy caused by Chinese herbs in the UK. *Lancet* 1999; 354: 481–482.
132. *Chinese Herbal Medicines in Australia found to contain Aristolochia*. Report of Therapeutic Goods Administration. Canberra: Department of Health and Aged Care, 1999.
133. *Working Party Report on Herbal Medicinal Products*. London: EMEA, 2000: 4–5.
134. Kayne S B. Plants, medicines and environmental conservation. *NZ Pharm* 1994; 14: 28–30.
135. *Prescription for Extinction: Endangered Species and Patented Oriental Medicines in Trade*. Washington, DC: Traffic USA, 1994.
136. Mills S Y. Chinese herbs in the west. In: Evans W C (ed.) *Trease and Evans' Pharmacognosy*, 3rd edn. London: W B Saunders, 1996: 506–507.
137. Mills S Y. Chinese herbs in the west. In: Evans W C (ed.) *Trease and Evans' Pharmacognosy*, 3rd edn. London: W B Saunders, 1996: 507–509.
138. Lao L. Traditional Chinese medicine. In: Jonas W B, Levin J (eds) *Essentials of Complementary and Alternative Medicine*. Baltimore: Lippincott/Williams & Wilkins, 1999: 226–227.
139. Massey P B. Medicine and the martial arts: a brief historical perspective. *Altern Complement Ther* 1998; 4: 128–133.
140. Massey P B, Kisling G M. A single case report of healing through specific martial art therapy: comparison of MRI to clinical resolution in severe cervical stenosis: a case report. *J Altern Complement Med* 1999; 5: 75–79.
141. Zollman V A. *ABC of Complementary Medicine*. London: BMJ Books, 2000: 36.
142. Windridge C. *Tong Sing, The Chinese Book of Wisdom*. London: Kyle Cathie, 1999: 211–219.

10

Indian ayurvedic medicine

Definition

The indigenous system of medicine in India is termed ayurveda (*ayu* means life or longevity and *veda* means knowledge) while that of Pakistan is called unani-tibb or unani for short. The two systems have much in common and will not be considered separately in this chapter.

Disease is considered to be an imbalance and its treatment involves diverse procedures to restore optimum function and balance. Practitioners use nutrition, yoga, exercise, complex herbal medicines and surgical techniques reactively as therapies and proactively for the preservation of health.

History

The origins of 'the science of life' have been placed by scholars of ancient Indian ayurvedic literature at somewhere around 6000 BC.[1] The teachings were orally transmitted for thousands of years and then written down in melodic Sanskrit poetic verses known as shlokas. Ayurveda in its first recorded form (literature known as vedas) is specifically called atharveda.

Indian medicine spread across the eastern world to Tibet, Central Asia, Indo-China, Indonesia and Japan, filling the same role in Asia as Greek medicine did in the west. The surgical and medical aspects of ayurveda developed separately around the eighth century BC, and were recorded in great detail in texts (samhitas). The surgical principles of ayurveda were explained by Sushruta, considered to be the father of surgery in his particular samhita. He covered a number of techniques familiar to modern-day surgery: pre- and postoperative care, asepsis, suturing and sterilisation. He also described 141 types of surgical instruments and a number of surgical procedures, including the treatment of cataracts, haemorrhoids and bone problems as well as techniques involved in cosmetic surgery.

The early medical aspects of ayurveda were collected and revised by Charak around the first century AD in his samhita and this work has provided the basis for future practice over the centuries. Charak's text described the significance of the vata, pitta and kapha doshas, elements that form the basis of tridosha physiology (see below), the seven tissues (dhatus) and the three excretions (malas) as well as giving information on the treatment of disease and the preparation of drugs. Other important compendia were written during the first and second centuries by Susruta and Vagbhata, who together with Charak are considered to be the great three fathers of ayurveda.

Eight specialities have developed within ayurveda:

- general surgery (shalya tantra)
- ear, nose and throat (shalkya)
- medicine (kaya chikitsa)
- psychiatry (bhutvidya)
- obstetrics, gynaecology and pediatrics (kumar–bhritya)
- toxicology (agada tantra)
- geriatrics (rasayans)
- fertility and sterility (vajikaran).

Theory

Ayurvedic philosophy is based on the samkhya philosophy of creation. The word *samkhya* is derived from the Sanskrit *sat* (truth) and *khya* (to know). The main beliefs are as follows:

- There is a close relationship between humans and the universe.
- Cosmic energy is manifest in all things, both living and non-living.
- There are 24 elements of the universe.
- Cosmic consciousness is the source of all existence present as male (shiva, purusha) and female (shakti, pakritt) energy.

The general ayurvedic approach is threefold:

- Determine the elemental constitution of the patient.
- Identify the cause of the illness.
- Apply therapeutic recommendations to balance any disharmonies.

Determining the constitution and the cause of illness

Ayurveda embraces certain fundamental doctrines, known as the darshnas. The body is thought of as being composed of three principal divisions:

- the three humours (or doshas), made up of the five basic elements of life

- the seven tissues (dhatus)
- the three waste products (malas).

Health is believed to comprise a balanced state of the doshas (made from five basic elements and senses), the dhatus, the malas and a gastric fire (agni), together with the clarity and balance of the mind, senses and spirit.

The five basic elements and senses of life

The five basic elements of life that join together in different combinations to make up the three doshas (or humours) are:

- ether (space), represented in the hollow spaces of the mouth, nose, gastrointestinal tract, thorax, capillaries and tissues – associated with the sense of hearing (ear and speech)
- air, represented by movement of the various organs, i.e. expansion, contraction and pulsation – associated with touch (hand)
- fire, the source of heat and represented by metabolism, digestion, body heat and intelligence – associated with sight (eyes)
- water exists as seretions of the salivary glands and mucous membranes – associated with taste (tongue)
- earth, represented by solid structures of the body, i.e. bones, cartilage and muscles – associated with smell (nose).

Ether and air are said to be the vata dosha (where dosha means a 'principal' that is protective in health or disease-producing in ill health), fire and water combine as the pitta dosha and earth and water combine as the kaph dosha. Collectively they control all biological and psychological functions of the body, mind and consciousness. They are also responsible for emotions, including anger, compassion, fear, greed and love.

The three humours (doshas)

The doshas have the following specific actions:

- Vata (air principal) is responsible for all body movement; it represents the nervous system and controls the emotions of fear and anxiety. Vata areas include the large intestine, pelvic cavity, skin and ears.
- Pitta (bodily fire principal) governs digestion, absorption, nutrition, skin colour, intelligence and understanding. It arouses hate

and jealousy. Pitta areas include the small intestine, stomach, blood, eyes and skin.

- Kapha (biological water principal) is present in the throat, chest, head, sinuses, nose, mouth, etc. It governs body resistance and biological strength, promotes wound healing and supports memory. Psychologically kapha governs greed, envy and love.

A balance of the doshas is necessary for optimal health. In childhood kapha elements associated with growth predominate; in adulthood pitta is more important, while as the body deteriorates in old age vata becomes more important. When there is an imbalance or disharmony in health more than one dosha may be present.

Physical constitution

An individual may have one of seven different constitutions, known as prakriti. It is believed that prakriti (*pra* means before and *akriti* means conception) are determined at conception and depend on the permutation and combination of the doshas. Bodily features may be characterised in terms of the doshas. For example, a person having a vata prakriti would be light-weight, tall and ill-nourished, a pitta prakriti would be characterised by moderate weight and a well-nourished appearance and a kapha prakriti would be typically associated with a heavily built person. Examples of prakriti are presented in Table 10.1.[2]

Mental constitution

Three guras or temperaments correspond to the humours that determine physical constitution, as described above, and are responsible for a person's behaviour patterns. They are, with brief examples of the main characteristics:

- Satvas: people with a satva temperament have healthy bodies and pure behaviour. They are often very religious, compassionate and loving.
- Rajas: people who are interested in business, prosperity, power and prestige. They enjoy wealth and are extroverts.
- Tamas: people who are ignorant, lazy, selfish and show little respect for others.

The seven tissues (dhatus)

The seven tissues are:

- plasma or cytoplasm (ras), which contains nutrients from digested food
- blood (rakata), which governs oxygenation
- muscles (mamsa), which maintain the physical strength of the body
- bone and cartilage (asthi), which give support to the body
- bone marrow and nerves (majja), which fill bony spaces and facilitate communication
- fat (medas) responsible for body bulk
- the sex hormones and immune system (shukra).

Each of the dhatus depends on its predecessor for good health. For good health all must function correctly.

Table 10.1 Examples of prakriti characteristics

Characteristic	Pitta	Vata	Kapha
Body size	Medium	Slim	Large
Body weight	Medium	Low	High
Eyes	Sharp, bright, grey-green	Small, sunken, black or brown	Big, blue
Nose	Long, pointed	Uneven shape	Short, round
Skin	Oily, smooth, warm	Thin, dry, cold	Thick, oily, cool
Teeth	Medium, tender gums	Protruding, thin gums	Healthy Strong gums
Appetite	Strong	Irregular, scanty	Slow, steady
Digestion	Quick with burning	Irregular with wind	Prolonged with mucus
Taste preference	Sweet, bitter	Sweet, sour, salty	Bitter, pungent
Emotions	Anger, jealousy	Anxiety, fear	Greedy
Intellect	Accurate	Quick, careless	Slow, exact
Finance	Spends on luxuries	Poor, wastes money	Thrifty, astute

The three waste products (malas)

These are sweat (svet), faeces (poorish) and urine (mutra). These must be produced in appropriate amounts and eliminated through their respective channels.

Agni

The final element important for healthy life is agni, the biological 'fire' that sustains vitality. It has been compared to the digestive enzymes but is considered to be responsible for more than just the biochemical processes for it also maintains the health of the immune system, and destroys micro-organisms and toxins in the gut.

Practice of ayurveda

Choice of treatment

After a diagnosis has been made as to the particular disfunction or disharmony present, there are several different types of treatment available to the ayurvedic practitioner. Diet, botanical, animal and mineral medicines, exercise, yoga, counselling and surgery may all be used alone or to complement each other.

An example of an ayurvedic treatment regime is known as pancha karma.[3] It consists of five very intensive and radical techniques designed to direct body toxins to specific sites for elimination. The five techniques are:

- therapeutic vomiting
- purgation
- enemas
- nasal aspiration of herbs
- therapeutic release of toxic blood.

Despite its long history, ayurveda has not been averse to change. The Indian subcontinent has been subject to countless invasions during its history, with diseases being imported from other geographic locations and techniques absorbed from other cultures.[4] During the Middle Ages, for example, heavy metals, particularly mercury, entered the ayurvedic armamentarium and were used in the treatment of syphilis, which was brought by the Portuguese. The invention of new remedies is encouraged by modern practitioners.

Indian dietary therapy

Just as with traditional Chinese medicine, Indian medicine places an importance on diet. Diet is considered to be particularly important for both its direct effect on the individual's physiological state and its influence on the medicine. Inadequate digestion will result in the formulation of intermediary products. It is suggested that a build-up of these intermediate products, collectively known as ama, might lead to disease. Ayurveda stresses the importance of avoiding this possibility through maintaining a diet appropriate to one's constitution and recommends the application of measures to ensure correct digestion. Food should be clean and fresh, taken in small quantities and chewed well before swallowing.

Ayurveda identifies six tastes and says that each taste is associated with an organ in the body and, when found in excess, will adversely affect the organ. The six tastes are:

- sweet – spleen, pancreas
- salty – kidney
- sour – liver
- pungent – lungs
- bitter – heart
- astringent – colon.

People are encouraged to take food appropriate to their constitution, for example:

- Vata is aggravated by astringent, bitter and pungent tastes, and balanced by salty, sour and sweet tastes. Generally most sweet fruit (including dates, figs and papaya) is found to be beneficial.
- Pitta is aggravated by pungent, salty and sour, and balanced by astringent, bitter and sweet. Sweet fruit (e.g. apples, cherries and ripe mangoes) is beneficial here too.
- Kapha is aggravated by salty, sour and sweet, and balanced by astringent, bitter and pungent. Cranberries and other astringent or sour fruit are beneficial.

Each person eats according to his or her own state of health in order to maintain harmony within the body. Thus an individual showing a pitta prakriti would benefit from 'cool' spices such as cardamom, mint or turmeric. Turmeric is especially beneficial to the liver as this is considered to be a pitta organ. Like their Chinese counterparts, Indian housewives choose – or perhaps 'prescribe' would be a better word –

their dinner menus carefully with reference to prevailing environmental conditions and family activities, thus ensuring that their relations are kept in the best of health, both physically and mentally. Knowing this aim, one can appreciate the origin of the delicate balance of herbs and spices so characteristic of Indian cuisine. A number of dietary incompatibilities are recognised: milk is incompatible with bananas, fish with bread, while melons are claimed to be incompatible with most other foods.

For hypertension, the instructions might be to drink one cup of mango juice, followed an hour or so later by half a cup of warm milk, a pinch of cardamom and nutmeg, and a teaspoonful of ghee. Ghee is a butter curd product that increases the digestive 'fire' (agni) and improves assimilation. Cucumber raita may also help if taken with a meal. Cucumber is a diuretic and raita is a yoghurt-based spicy condiment that often features in Indian recipes. Ayurveda prescribes specific diets for several psychiatric disorders and for different drug therapies. For anxieties almond milk may be prescribed. It is made by soaking 10 raw almonds in water overnight, then peeling and blending them with a cup of warm milk. While in the blender a small pinch of nutmeg and saffron is added.

Treatment with remedies

The type and dose of medicine chosen are influenced by the individual's constitution as well as by the nature of the disease. Other factors governing the choice of medicine include the age and strength of the patient, digestive capacity, degree of tolerance and psychological state.

The medicines are derived mainly from vegetable material and minerals (see below). There are detailed descriptions of the methods by which medicines should be prepared. One technique, known as samskara (refinement), eliminates the toxicity of the source materials, rather like the aim of serial dilution in homeopathy. Mixtures of medicines (sumyoga) may be administered to achieve a balanced preparation, one principal balancing another through synergism or antagonism, as with Chinese herbal medicine. Some ingredients enhance the action, while others reduce the toxicity. The ayurvedic formula chyavanprash combines more than 25 finely powdered herbs in a base of honey and ghee. It is taken with food as a tonic.

Herbal remedies Herbs are used by ayurvedic practitioners in a number of ways, amongst which are the following examples:

- In the treatment of a gastric disturbance in a person exhibiting a pitta prakriti the usual remedies black pepper (*Piper rotundum*) and ginger (*Zingiber officinale*) would be administered judiciously or not at all, as they are both considered to increase pitta and may exacerbate the imbalance.

- Tonification, or supplementation therapy, uses herbs and foods that build and nourish tissues. This is prescribed for individuals who are elderly, malnourished, chronically ill or emaciated. The timing of administration is also seen as being important. The particular formula given depends on the constitution of the patient.

- There is a range of herbal preparations available for treating women's problems. The Chinese herb dong quai (*Angelica sinensis*) is used in the treatment of many gynaecological ailments. It is said to regulate menstruation, 'tonify' the blood and relieve constipation. Again, there are various herbal mixtures tailored to the consitutional type. Table 10.2 illustrates remedies suitable for cramps in women.[5]

- One of the most popular herbal mixtures is known as triphala ('the three fruits'). This product is rejuvenating and strengthening for all three doshas and all seven dhatus. It is also a mild laxative. Triphala comprises three of the most popular ayurvedic herbs: amalaki, bibbitakiu and haritaki. It is normally taken alone, mixed with honey or as a tea an hour after the evening meal. However, being a mild diuretic, some people prefer to take it in the morning.

The remedies are supplied as mixtures of herbs in dried form, or more usually with a suitable vehicle (anupana) to facilitate absorption. The most usual vehicles are water, milk, honey, aloe vera and ghee. People with high cholesterol levels should be wary about taking large amounts of ghee. Herbal oils are made by introducing active principals (cloves, garlic, etc.) into a suitable oily vehicle.

Table 10.2 Example of constitutional treatments for cramping in women

Vata	Pitta	Kapha
Blue cohosh	Camomile	Black cohosh
Cramp bark	Cramp bark	Blue cohosh
Ginger	Peppermint	Camomile
Pennyroyal	Scullcap	Cramp bark
Valerian	Squaw vine	Ginger
	Yarrow	

Herbal oils, fine powders or ghee may be administered intranasally (nasya).

Until a few years ago most traditional Asian remedies used in the UK were imported from India. Only a few local hakims (traditional healers) produced their own remedies, using imported raw materials. However, there are now several companies producing ayurvedic medicines in the UK. Many of these remedies may be purchased over the counter, by mail order through Asian and English language newspapers and the internet or brought back from visits to the subcontinent. A range of ayurvedic toiletries, including soap and shampoo, has appeared on the UK market.

Animal products   There is some controversy about using animal products. However, finely ground deer horn as a paste may be applied to the thoracic region and is said to be of benefit in angina.

Metals   For medicinal use metals are traditionally taken internally after undergoing rigorous purification to neutralise any toxic effects. The metals are boiled in water that is then reduced in volume by evaporation. Typically 5 ml of this water is taken orally 2–3 times daily. Some examples of the medical uses of metals are:

- Copper is a good tonic for the liver, spleen and lymphatics.
- Gold strengthens the nervous system.
- Silver has cooling properties and is beneficial in the treatment of excess pitta.
- Iron is beneficial for bone marrow and helps in anaemia.

Precious and semiprecious stones

Gems are thought to have healing properties that can be harnessed by wearing them as jewellery or by placing them in water overnight and drinking the solution. It is believed that gems absorb the vitality of their owners, for example:

- Diamond strengthens immunity.
- Pearls have a cooling effect on wakening.
- Ruby strengthens concentration.
- Sapphire (blue) calms vata and kapha and stimulates pitta.

Aromatherapy

Sweet warming aromas such as musk and camphor can balance vata, while pitta is soothed by calming aromas such as sandalwood, jasmine and rose. Kapha is pacified by warming stimulating oils together with pungent oils such as eucalyptus, sage and thyme.

Treatment by colour therapy

Ayurvedic treatments make use of colour in their healing procedures. Because the colours of the rainbow are perceived as correlating with the body tissues (dhasus) and the doshas, the vibratory energy of the colours may be used to establish psychological harmony and peace of mind. Since colour is so important, patients are told to illuminate themselves and their environment in the appropriate coloured lighting. An appreciation of the colours of nature is also considered to be important.

Colours have particular properties:

*   Red is stimulating and warming (kapha).
*   Orange is also warming; it gives energy and strength and is stimulating (kapha).
*   Yellow relieves excess vata and kapha.
*   Gold is a warming colour beneficial to vata and kapha.
*   Silver is cooling and soothes pitta.

For further information on colour therapy, see Chapter 14.

Treatment with enema (basti)

Basti introduces medicinal remedies, including sesame oil or herbal decoctions, in a liquid medium into the rectum. Medicated enemas pacify vata and alleviate many vata disorders, such as constipation, backache, arthritis and various nervous disorders.

Treatment with massage

Nauli is a method of massaging the internal organs, particularly the colon, intestines, liver and spleen. It also helps to maintain abdominal 'fire' and keep the colon clean.

A warm ayurvedic oil massage is prescribed for anxiety. Vatas should use sesame oil, pittas sunflower or coconut oil and kaphas corn oil.

Treatment with meditation

Meditation, the art of bringing harmony to body, mind and consciousness, is used to soothe the body and reduce stress. Meditation is not concentration, quite the opposite. There should be no conscious effort – the mind should be allowed to relax completely ('float') as one listens to every sound.

Safety concerns

Intrinsic toxicity[6]

The following examples illustrate the toxicity problems of certain herbs used in traditional Indian medicine.

Khat (*Catha edulis*)   It has been claimed that the fresh or dried leaves of *Catha edulis*, popularly known as khat, can be used to treat depression, but it is unclear whether it has this function in the UK. The herb is chewed, smoked or drunk as an infusion by Asian immigrants. There is some concern that this practice may cause psychological problems and carcinoma of the oral cavity.

Khat produces a feeling of well-being and lessens fatigue. The active principals are two alkaloids, norpseudoephedrine (cathinine) and cathinone. Although users say that the herb is not addictive, withdrawal has been known to cause lethargy and nightmares.

Betel (*Piper betle*)   A betel quid comprises tobacco, areca catechu, saffron and lime wrapped in a leaf from the plant *Piper betle*. The quid is placed in the buccal cavity, where it stimulates salivation. It is considered to have beneficial digestive properties. A number of the ingredients are reported to be carcinogenic.

An associated practice involves chewing betel nuts, often together with tobacco, and this too is known to cause buccal carcinoma.

Heavy metals   Practitioners of traditional medicine from the Indian subcontinent have generally received 5 years' training in academic establishments. They understand well their patients' beliefs about disease, and great benefits undoubtedly arise from their practice. However, their medicines – and some cosmetics too[7] – may be hazardous due to the presence of heavy metals or other adulterants, by accident or by design.

Ayurvedic medicine uses arsenic, mercury[8] and lead[9] as active ingredients. Lead is regarded as an aphrodisiac, and has been used to counteract impotence in the diabetic male. Other examples are:

- The product al kohl is applied as an eye cosmetic; its main ingredient is lead sulphide.
- Suma powders contain over 80% lead and are applied as a cosmetic to the conjuctival surface of infants and children, from where they may be transferred to the mouth by the hands.
- Sikor is rich in lead and arsenic; it is used as a remedy for indigestion.

Drugs   Some years ago a report appeared of a patient presenting at a hospital in Birmingham with powders from the Punjab individually wrapped in newspaper that he was using to self-treat psoriasis.[10] High-performance liquid chromatography analysis of the powders revealed the presence of prednisolone, a prescription medicine which is potentially dangerous.

Concurrent treatment

There is a substantial risk that patients will receive simultaneous western and traditional treatments. Patients seldom volunteer information concerning any traditional medicines being taken. A case has been reported in which a woman receiving chemotherapy for Hodgkin's disease supplemented her treatment with at least nine different ayurvedic medicines.[11] She suffered a thrombosis thought to result from an interaction between the orthodox and traditional medicines. Pharmacists can provide an extremely valuable function in this respect by intervening with advice whenever they consider it to be appropriate.

An interaction between the fruit karela (*Momordica charantia*), an ingredient of curries, and chlorpropamide has been reported.[12] Although this particular drug has been superseded, it serves to flag up a possible difficulty with concurrent treatment. Karela improves glucose tolerance and is therefore hypoglycaemic. There are a number of other close relatives of this plant that are also used by hakims to treat diabetes, including crushed seed kernels of the marrow (*Curcubita pepo*) and the honeydew melon (*Cucumis melo*). There is a danger that some patients may be treating their diabetes with both allopathic and traditional remedies without realising the risk of interaction.

Betel nut (see above) is prescribed by hakims either alone or in mixtures. There may be a risk of interactions between this herbal medicine and orthodox drugs.

Safety of surgical and manipulative procedures

The inclusion of surgical techniques adds another potential danger from non-sterile instruments and consulting environments, and incompetent procedures. There is also a risk from undue pressure or incorrect manipulation by inexperienced practitioners.

Difficulties for pharmacists

A number of problems that pharmacists may experience in identifying ingredients and assessing their potential toxicity in Asian remedies have been identified:[13]

- typographical errors on the label
- phonetic transliteration
- changes in nomenclature
- absence of generic names on the label
- undeclared ingredients and adulterants
- assessing the literature and finding information – *Trease and Evans' Pharmacognosy*,[6] to which frequent references are made in this chapter, provides an excellent and readily available source of information for traditional medicine practices.

Evidence of effectiveness

As stated in Chapter 9, there are difficulties in applying western methods to proving the effectiveness of traditional therapies. The best that can be said is that ayurveda has stood the test of time and appears to have some impressive successes. Its complex nature means that practitioners require extensive training, and a proper integrated ayurvedic treatment is not something that can be bought off-the-shelf in a health store or, for that matter, a pharmacy.

In the past 12 years the Indian Council of Medical Research has set up a unique network throughout India for carrying out controlled clinical trials of herbal medicines.[14] The programme is monitored by a scientific advisory group consisting of people from the ayurveda, unani and modern allopathic systems of medicine. This group contains experts in pharmacognosy, toxicology, pharmacology and clinical pharmacology as well as clinicians and experts in standardisation and quality control. Trials are planned and protocols prepared by the whole group. All trials are comparative, controlled, randomised and double-blind unless there is a reason for carrying out a single-blind study. The trials are planned by the whole group but carried out at the centres of allopathic medicine with established investigators. There are over 20 clinical trial centres throughout the country for carrying out the multicentred studies. Using this network the council has shown the efficacy of several traditional medicines, including *Picrorhazia kurroa* in hepatitis and *Pterocarpus marsupium* in diabetes.[15] As a result of these trials these traditional medicines can be used in allopathic hospitals.

The Central Council of India systems of medicine oversees research institutes, which evaluate treatments. The government is adding 10 traditional medicines into its family welfare programme, funded by the World Bank and the Indian government. These medicines are for anaemia, oedema during pregnancy, postpartum problems such as pain, uterine and abdominal complications, difficulties with lactation, nutritional deficiencies and childhood diarrhoea.[16]

New regulations were introduced in July 2000 to improve Indian herbal medicines by establishing standard manufacturing practices and quality control. The regulations outline requirements for infrastructure, labour, quality control and authenticity of raw materials, and absence of contamination. Of the 9000 licensed manufacturers of traditional medicines, those who qualify can immediately seek certification for good manufacturing practice. The remainder have 2 years to comply with the regulations and to obtain certification.

The government has also established 10 new drug-testing laboratories for Indian systems of medicine and is upgrading existing laboratories to provide high-quality evidence to the licensing authorities of the safety and quality of herbal medicines. This replaces an ad hoc system of testing that was considered unreliable. Randomised controlled clinical trials of selected prescriptions for Indian systems of medicine have been initiated. These will document the safety and efficacy of the prescriptions and provide the basis for their international licensing as medicines rather than simply as food supplements.[17]

A recently published randomised double-blind placebo-controlled parallel group monocentre trial with 182 patients investigated the efficacy and toxicity of an orally administered ayurvedic formulation for rheumatoid arthritis.[18] It was concluded that the preparation was not significantly superior to a strong placebo response except for joint swelling, although improvement in the velum group was numerically superior at all evaluation time points.

Integration with western medicine

The Indian Medicine Central Council was established by a 1970 act to oversee the development of Indian systems of medicine and to ensure good standards of training and practice. Training for Indian medicine is given in separate colleges, which offer a basic biosciences curriculum followed by training in a traditional system. Recently the Department of Indian Systems of Medicine has expressed concern over the substandard quality of education in many colleges, which in the name of integration have produced hybrid curricula and graduates, unacceptable to either modern or traditional standards. The department has made it a priority to upgrade training in Indian systems of medicine.[19]

Purists in ayurveda and unani oppose this trend to modernise their systems, particularly when such integration is carried out by experts in allopathy.[20] They have no objection to the use of modern concepts of the methodology of clinical trials in evaluating the efficacy and side-effects of herbal preparations used in the traditional systems. Such clinical evaluation is essential because the remedies used in these systems will not be used in allopathic hospitals in a country such as India unless these have shown efficacy in well-controlled trials. However, carrying out randomised, double-blind, multicentred trials with standardised extracts is a slow and laborious process. Furthermore, not all herbal medicines need to undergo this rigorous trial because these preparations are already in use. The situation is still further complicated because the randomised trial may not be totally appropriate for the evaluation of medicines from the traditional systems, where the prakriti (ayurveda system) or mijaj (unani system) of the individual determines the specific therapy to be used.

Examples of common ayurvedic medicines

Some examples of herbal ingredients used in the preparation of common ayurvedic medicines in the UK are provided in Table 10.3.[21] Information on the chemical characteristics may be found in Chapters 5 and 6.

Examples of common ayurvedic treatments[22]

By the very nature of the philosophy surrounding the practice of ayurvedic it should not really be possible to treat conditions purely symptomatically. However, Table 10.4 gives a brief list of treatments to illustrate the general approach to herbal treatment.

Table 10.3 Examples of herbs used in the UK for ayurvedic medicines

Source material	Indian name	Parts used	Main constituent	Example of use
Azadirachta indica	Neem	Seeds, oil	Alkaloids, glycosides	Anthelmintic, antiseptic, astringent
Abrus precatorius	Ghunghi rati	Root, seeds	Alkaloids	Abortifacient, eye inflammation, oral contraceptive
Allium cepa	Tukhm piyaz	Seeds	Volatile oils (allyl sulphate)	Diuretic, expectorant, poultice
Artemesia absinthium	Afsentin roomi	Leaves	Sesquiterpines, lactones, bitters	Anthelmintic, tonic
Artemesia indica	Nagdoona			
Bombax celba	Mush simbhal	Gum, root	Glycosides, tannins	Hepatic dysfunction, menorrhagia
Cassia absus	Chaksu	Seeds	Alkaloids	Astringent, eye inflammation, ringworm
Crocus sativus	Zafran (saffron)	Flower styles	Volatile oil	Catarrh, enlarged liver
Cyperus rotundus	Nutgrass	Root, seeds	Sesquiterpenes	Antiemetic, anti-inflammatory, antipyretic
Ferula galbaniflua	Jawashir	Oleo-gum-resin	Sesquiterpenes	Asthma, bronchitis, dysentery, menstrual irregularities
Ficus benghalensis	Anjir jangli	Root	Glycosides	Bark: Tonic, diuretic
		Bark	Triterpenes	Root: Diarrhoea and hypoglycaemic
Hedera nepalense	Bikh tablab	Fruit	Triterpenoid saponins	Rheumatism
Mallotus philippensis	Kamala	Fruit	Resin	Anthelmintic, oral contraceptive, red dye
Mentha piperita	Paparaminta	Leaves	Volatile oil	Cough and fever, diarrhoea, flatulence, nausea and vomiting
Quercus infectoria	N/A	Galls	Tannins	Haemorrhoids – ointments and suppositories
Rosmarinus officinalis	Rusmari	Leaves	Volatile oil	Pulmonary infections
				Oil: toothache, rheumatism
Salvia officinalis	Bahaman surkh	Leaves	Volatile oil	Gargle, gingivitis, treatment of thrush
Solanum indicum	Bari-khatai, barhanta	Fruiting plant	Steroidal alkaloids	Chest and urinary infections, skin conditions (paste)
Tephrosia purpurea	Sarphunkha	Whole plant	Flavonoids	Cystitis, dysentery, facial oedema
Vitex agnus-castus	Remuka	Fruit	Flavonols	Diuretic, stimulant
Zingiber officinalis	Zanjibil	Rhizome	Oleo-resin	Antiemetic, bronchitis, rheumatism

Table 10.4 Examples of ayurvedic treatments for common conditions

Condition	Typical herbal treatment	Other treatments
Acne	a. Herbs: kutki, guduchi, shatavari b. Aloe vera juice c. Tea: cumin, coriander and fennel	a. Apply melon to the skin b. Yoga postures c. Breathing exercises
Anxiety	Calming tea: valerian, musta	a. Relaxing bath b. Almond milk c. Acupressure
Athlete's foot	a. Tea tree oil b. Aloe vera gel and turmeric	a. Wash with neem soap b. Neem oil applied
Boils	a. Neem powder paste b. Triphala wash c. For diabetics: neem, turmeric, kutki taken orally	a. Cooling, healing paste of sandalwood and turmeric b. Poultice of cooked onions to draw c. Liver cleanser (aloe vera gel)
Diarrhoea	a. Ghee, nutmeg, ginger, sugar b. Ginger powder with sugar. Mix and chew	
Eye problems		a. Cool water wash b. Gaze into the flame of a traditional ghee lamp
Jet lag	a. One hour before flight – ginger b. On flight – drink water c. After flight – rub warm sesame oil on scalp	
Sore throat	a. Gargle – turmeric and hot water b. Ginger–cinnamon–liquorice tea	a. Avoid dairy produce b. Yoga postures c. Breathing exercises

More information

The Ayurvedic Medical Association
59 Dulverton Road
South Croydon CR2 8PJ
Tel: 020 8657 6147

The Ayurvedic Institute
PO Box 23445
Albuquerque

New Mexico 87192-1445
USA
Tel: 505 291 9698

References

1. Sodhi V. Ayurveda: the science of life and mother of the healing arts. In: Pizzorno J Jr, Murray M T (eds) *Textbook of Natural Medicine*, 2nd edn. Edinburgh: Churchill Livingstone, 1999: 257–258.
2. Lad V. *The Complete Book of Ayurverdic Home Remedies*. London: Patkus, 1999: 18–19.
3. Packard C C. *Pocket Guide to Ayurvedic Healing*. Freedom, CA: Crossing Press, 1996: 111.
4. Glazier A. A landmark in the history of ayurveda. *Lancet* 2000; 356: 1118–1122.
5. Jonas W B, Ernst E. *Essentials of CAM. Introduction: Evaluating the Safety of Complementary and Alternative Products and Practices*. Baltimore: Lippincott/Williams & Wilkins, 1999: 89–107.
6. Aslam M. *Asian Medicine and its Practice in Britain*. In: Evans W C (ed.) *Trease and Evans' Pharmacognosy*, 14th edn. London: W B Saunders, 1996: 489–491.
7. Aslam M, Davis S S, Healy M A. Heavy metals in some Asian medicines and cosmetics. *Public Health* 1979; 93: 274–284.
8. Kew J, Morris C, Athie A *et al*. Arsenic and mercury intoxication due to Indian ethnic remedies. *BMJ* 1993; 306: 306–307.
9. Keen R W, Deacon A C, Delves H T *et al*. Indian herbal remedies for diabetes as a cause of lead poisoning. *Postgrad Med* 1994; 70: 113–114.
10. Barnes A R, Paul C J, Secrett P C. Adulteration of Asian alternative medicines. *Pharm J* 1991; 247: 650.
11. Fletcher J, Aslam M. Possible dangers of Ayurvedic herbal remedies. *Pharm J* 1991; 247: 456.
12. Aslam M, Stockley I H. Interaction between curry ingredient (Karela) and a drug (chlorpromamide). *Lancet* 1979; I: 607.
13. Aslam M. Problems of identity with traditional Asian remedies. *Pharm J* 1992; 248: 20–21, 23.
14. Indian Council of Medical Research. *Annual Report of Council 1998–99*. New Delhi: Indian Council of Medical Research.
15. Atherton D J. Towards the safer use of traditional remedies. *BMJ* 1994; 308: 673–674.
16. Kumar S. India's government promotes traditional healing practices. *Lancet* 2000; 335: 1252.
17. Hoizey D, Hoizey M. *A History of Chinese Medicine*. Vancouver: University BC Press, 1993: 42.
18. Chopra A, Lavin P, Patwardhan B, Chitre D. Ayurvedic medicine reduces joint swelling in patient with rheumatoid arthritis. *J Rheumatol* 2000; 27: 1365–1372.

19. Department of Indian Systems of Medicines and Homoeopathy. *Annual Report 1999–2000*. Department of Indian Systems of Medicines and Homoeopathy, 2000. http://mohfw.nic.in/ismh/ (Data accessed 25 October, 2000.)

20. Chaudhury R R. Commentary: challenges in using traditional systems of medicine. *BMJ* 2001; 322: 167.

21. Aslam M. Asian medicine and its practice in Britain. In: Evans W C (ed.) *Trease and Evans' Pharmacognosy*, 14th edn. London: W B Saunders, 1996: 491–504.

22. Lampert N. Letter. *Lancet* 2001; 357: 802.

Part Four

Other CAM disciplines

11

Naturopathy

Naturopathy is not widely practised in the UK, but the therapy is very popular in many other English-speaking countries, including Australia, New Zealand, South Africa and the USA.

Definition

Naturopathy is a multidisciplinary approach to healthcare that recognises the body's innate power to heal itself. It is primarily a preventive discipline with education in the basics of healthcare as one of its most important goals. The philosophy of naturopathic medicine also includes the treatment of disease through the stimulation, enhancement and support of the inherent healing capacity of the person.

History

Naturopathy can trace its origins back to doctors Bernard Lust and Robert Foster, who worked in the USA around the turn of the nineteenth century. American doctors disillusioned with contemporary procedures were joined by a number of European immigrants involved in natural cures. In the following years the popularity of naturopathy became cyclical, with periods of intense interest and scepticism. At one time there were thousands of practitioners, numerous journals and much informed debate. In recent years the discipline has enjoyed a revival, particularly in the countries stated above. In the UK there are currently around 400 practitioners, with qualifications recognised by the the General Council and Register of Naturopaths.

Theory

Naturopaths work from the premise that the body needs certain basics to function properly: the correct nutrients, adequate rest and relaxation, appropriate exercise, fresh clean air, clean water and sunlight. They are skilled in adapting natural health programmes to patients' unique requirements.

There are considered to be six important principles for naturo-pathic practice:[1]

- The healing power of the body (*vis medicatrix naturae*) has the ability to establish, maintain and restore health.
- The cause of the illness must be identified and treated (*tolle causam*) – underlying causes of a disease must be discovered and removed; symptoms are not the cause of a disease, and the causes of diseases include physical, mental, emotional and spiritual factors, which all must be dealt with.
- First do no harm (*primum no nocere*) – therapeutic action should be complementary to and synergistic with the healing process.
- Treat the whole person.
- The physician as teacher (*docere*) – he or she should create a healthy interpersonal physician–patient relationship.
- Prevention is the physician's aim and the best cure; naturopathy is the building of health rather than fighting the disease.

Professor Hans Selye of Montreal was the first to postulate the concept of a general adaptation syndrome, by which an individual reacts positively to an episode of injury or disease. According to Selye the body's response to any physical or emotional stress initiates a three-phase sequence:

- alarm – there is pain from an injury
- shock – from bad news
- inflammation – due to friction.

Naturopaths attach great importance to the body's adaptive capacity and recognise that symptoms such as inflammation, fever or pain are signs of the defences at work and should not be suppressed. Furthermore, the process of recovery from chronic ailments may necessitate a return to the stage of resistance, known in natural therapy as the healing crisis. As the body adjusts to the crisis, there is a stage of resistance in which the body adapts to withstand the stimulus. If the stresses are prolonged and the body is no longer able to adapt, it becomes exhausted and collapse or degeneration occurs.

The contribution of emotions to the cause of physical illness is considered carefully by many naturopaths, with a variety of counselling and psychological approaches being adopted.

Practice of naturopathy

While recognising the limitations of our modern world, the naturopath seeks to assist patients to create a healthier diet and lifestyle that will help their health return. Thus, a cold might be considered as being self-limiting and not treated directly, but the patient will be supported in a return to good health using various naturopathic measures. In degenerative disease the body may be supported in its compensatory reorganisation of function.

Information is gathered during a consultation by the usual complementary techniques of listening, observing, questioning and physical examination so that an overall impression of the patient and his or her particular requirements may be obtained. Factors such as hereditary tendencies, constitution and previous treatments are considered to be particularly important in choosing an appropriate course of action.

Naturopaths use a variety of treatments, including dietary advice, nutritional supplements, detoxification, hands-on work (such as osteopathy and massage), herbs, homeopathic remedies and hydrotherapy, which can be summarised as follows:

- nutrition – dietetics, nutritional supplements and the maintenance of optimum health through good wholesome food (see below)
- hydrotherapy – hot and cold water treatments to encourage circulation (see below)
- detoxification – cleansing programmes that allow healing to take place (see below)
- physical therapy – to restore structural balance and improve tissue tone; may include gentle manipulation, massage and ultrasound and exercise (Chapter 13)
- administration of homeopathic or herbal medicines (Chapters 4 and 5)
- minor surgery – in some countries naturopaths may perform simple surgical procedures, e.g. removal of warts.

The particular portfolio of therapies chosen will depend on factors other than those found during the consultation process.

The time spent with a naturopath is variable. Typically a first consultation can take 1–2 h. Subsequent repeat sessions may last only half an hour.

Evidence

Because of the complex nature of naturopathy, research on its practice as a complete therapy has rarely been studied. Elements of naturopathic practice have been considered but naturopaths claim that the overall benefit from their therapy is more than the sum of individual disciplines, so the application of these results is limited.

Qualifications

Membership of the British Naturopathic Association is open to any practitioner who has a Naturopathic Diploma after completing a course in naturopathy accredited by the General Council and Register of Naturopaths and who is registered with that body. Such courses are currently offered by the British College of Naturopathy and Osteopathy and the College of Osteopaths Educational Trust. There is also a modular postgraduate course available from the British Naturopathic and Osteopathic Association.

Therapies used in naturopathy

Detoxification therapy

Naturopathy believes that a common cause of all diseases is the accumulation of waste and poisonous matter in the body resulting from overeating. Most people eat too much and follow sedentary occupations that do not permit sufficient and proper exercise for the utilisation of this large quantity of food. The surplus food overburdens the digestive and assimilative organs and clogs up the system with impurities or poisons. Digestion and elimination become slow and the functional activity of the whole system is deranged. The onset of disease is merely the process of ridding the system of these impurities. Fasting is recognised as the cornerstone of natural healing. The duration of the fast depends on the age of the patient, the nature of the disease, and the amount and type of drugs previously used, but can be 1 or 2 days or even, in stages, up to a week.

Practice[2]

Detoxification programmes are often used to assist a transition from an unhealthy lifestyle to a healthier one. There are a number of stages involved:

- initiating the cleansing process through elimination of the offending substances and application of a formal cleansing procedure through dietary modification and fasting
- facilitating elimination through normal excretion (e.g. colonic cleansing and increased fluid intake to stimulate urine flow)
- nutritional supplementation
- return to healthier lifestyle and diet.

Safety

Detoxification over extended periods can lead to a risk of nutritional deficiencies.

Chelation therapy

Chelation therapy is used to rid the body of toxic metals (e.g. arsenic, cadmium, lead, mercury and nickel), which can cause disruption of basic cell function. Signs of metal poisoning include headaches, dizziness, memory impairment, irritability and weight loss. Chelation is the incorporation of a metal ion into a heterocyclic ring structure. More than 10 000 chelating agents exist, but only seven or eight are available for administration to humans by intravenous infusion.

Lead, cadmium and nickel may be removed with calcium disodium ethylenediaminetetraacetic acid (a synthetic amino acid with chelating properties), meso-2,3-dimercaptosuccinic acid (DMSA) or D-penicillamine. DMSA is also used for removing arsenic and mercury. Treatment is usually associated with the administration of various supplements (vitamins, minerals, etc.).

Chelation therapy may be useful in various coronary and vascular diseases.[3]

Hydrotherapy[4]

Water has been used as a valuable therapeutic agent since time immemorial. In all major ancient civilisations, bathing was considered an important measure for the maintenance of health and prevention of disease. It was also valued for its remedial properties.

History

The ancient vedic literature in India contains numerous references to the efficacy of water in the treatment of disease. In modern times, the therapeutic value of water was popularised by Vincent Priessnitz, Father Sebastian Kneipp, Louis Kuhne and other European water-cure pioneers. They raised water cure to an institutional level and employed it successfully for the treatment of almost every known disease. There are numerous spas and *Bads* in most European countries where therapeutic baths are used as a major healing agent.

Water exerts beneficial effects on the human system. It is claimed to have beneficial effects on circulation, to boost muscular tone and to aid digestion and nutrition. Hydrotherapy may also be of great value in restoring a better range of joint motion through a combination of pain relief, muscle relaxation and stretching exercises.[5]

Practice of hydrotherapy

The main methods of water treatment that can be employed in the healing of various diseases in a do-it-yourself manner are described below.

Enema   Rectal irrigation or enema involves the injection of 1–2 l of warm water into the rectum and is used for cleaning the bowels. After 5–10 min, the water can be ejected together with the accumulated morbid matter.

A cold-water enema is helpful in inflammatory conditions of the colon, especially in cases of dysentery, diarrhoea, ulcerative colitis, haemorrhoids and fever.

A hot-water enema is beneficial in relieving irritation due to inflammation of the rectum and painful haemorrhoids. It also benefits women in leucorrhoea.

Compress

Cold compress   A cold compress is claimed to be an effective means of controlling inflammatory conditions of the liver, spleen, stomach, kidneys, intestines, lungs, brain and pelvic organs. It is also advantageous in cases of fever and heart disease. It is generally applied to the head, neck, chest, abdomen and back.

Heating compress   A heating compress consists of three or four folds of linen cloth wrung out in cold water, applied to the affected area, and then completely covered with a dry flannel or blanket to prevent the circulation of air and help accumulation of body heat. A compress is sometimes applied for several hours. A heating compress can be applied to the throat, chest, abdomen and joints. A throat compress relieves sore throat, hoarseness, tonsillitis, pharyngitis and laryngitis. An abdominal compress helps those suffering from gastritis, hyperacidity, indigestion, jaundice, constipation, diarrhoea, dysentery and other ailments relating to the abdominal organs. A chest compress, also known as a chest pack, relieves cold, bronchitis, pleurisy, pneumonia, fever, cough and so on, while a joint compress is helpful for inflamed joints, rheumatism, rheumatic fever and sprains.

Baths   The common water therapy temperature chart is: cold 10–18°C, neutral 32–36°C and hot 40–45°C. Above 45°C, water loses its therapeutic value and is destructive.

Hip baths   A hip bath involves only the hips and the abdominal region below the navel. A special type of tub is used for this purpose. A cold hip bath (10–18°C) is a routine treatment in many diseases. It relieves constipation, indigestion, obesity and helps the eliminative organs to function properly.

A hot hip bath (40–45°C) is generally taken for 8–10 min. A hot hip bath helps to relieve painful menstruation, pain in the pelvic organs, painful urination, inflamed rectum or bladder and painful piles. It also benefits an enlarged prostatic gland, painful contractions or spasm of the bladder, sciatica and neuralgia of the ovaries and bladder. It is recommended that a cold shower be taken immediately after the hot hip bath.

A neutral hip bath (32–36°C) is generally taken for 20–60 min. It helps to relieve all acute and subacute inflammatory conditions, such as acute catarrh of the bladder and urethra and subacute inflammations in the uterus, ovaries and tubes. It also relieves neuralgia of the fallopian tubes or testicles, painful spasms of the vagina. It is used as a sedative treatment for sexual hyperactivity in both sexes.

In an alternate hip bath, also known as a revulsive hip bath, the patient sits in a hot tub for 5 min and then in a cold tub for 3 min. The duration of the bath is generally 10–20 min. The head and neck are kept cold with a cold compress. The treatment ends with a dash of cold water to the hips. This bath relieves chronic inflammatory conditions of the pelvic viscera such as salpingitis, ovaritis, cellulitis and various neuralgias of the genitourinary organs, sciatica and lumbago.

Spinal bath   A spinal bath is another important form of hydrotherapy treatment. This bath provides a soothing effect on the spinal column and thereby influences the central nervous system. It is given in a specially designed tub with a raised back in order to provide proper support to the head. The bath can be administered at cold, neutral and hot temperatures. The water level in the tub should be 4–5 cm and the patient should lie in it for 3–10 min.

A cold spinal bath relieves irritation, fatigue, hypertension and excitement. It is beneficial in almost all nervous disorders, such as hysteria, fits, mental disorders, loss of memory and tension. The neutral spinal bath is a soothing and sedative treatment, especially for the hyperactive or irritable patient. It is the ideal treatment for insomnia and also relieves tension of the vertebral column. The duration of this bath is 20–30 min.

A hot spinal bath, on the other hand, helps to stimulate the nervous, especially when they are in a depressed state. It also relieves vertebral pain in spondylitis and muscular backache. It relieves sciatic pain and gastrointestinal disturbances of gastric origin.

Foot baths   In this method, the patient keeps his or her legs in a tub or bucket filled with hot water at a temperature of 40–45°C. Before taking this bath, a glass of water should be taken and the body should be covered with a blanket so that no heat or vapour escapes from the foot bath. The head should be protected with a cold compress. The duration of the bath is generally 5–20 min. The patient should take a cold shower immediately after the bath.

A hot foot bath stimulates the involuntary muscles of the uterus, intestines, bladder and other pelvic and abdominal organs. It also relieves sprains and ankle joint pains, headaches caused by cerebral congestion and colds. In women it helps restore menstruation, if suspended, by increasing the supply of blood, especially to the uterus and ovaries.

For a cold foot bath, 7–10 cm of cold water is placed in a small tub or bucket and the patient's feet completely immersed in the water for 1–5 min. Friction is continuously applied to the feet during the bath, either by an attendant or by the patient by rubbing one foot against the other. A cold foot bath, taken for 1–2 min helps in the treatment of sprains, strains and inflamed bunions when taken for longer periods.

Steam bath   A steam bath is one of the most important time-tested water treatments and induces perspiration in a natural way. The patient first takes one or two glasses of water and then sits on a stool inside a specially designed cabinet. The duration of the steam bath is generally

10–20 min or until perspiration takes place. A cold shower is taken immediately after the bath.

A steam bath helps to eliminate morbid matter from the surface of the skin. It also improves the circulation of the blood and tissue activity. It relieves rheumatism, gout, uric acid problems and obesity. A steam bath is helpful in all forms of chronic toxaemias. It also relieves neuralgias, chronic nephritis, infections, tetanus and migraine.

Immersion bath An immersion bath, also known as a full bath, is administered in a bath tub that can be neutral, hot, graduated or alternate.

A cold immersion bath may last from 4 s to 20 min at a temperature ranging from 10 to 23.8°C. This bath helps to bring down fever. It also improves the skin when taken for 5–15 s after a prolonged hot bath, by exhilarating circulation and stimulating the nervous system. This bath should not be given to young children or very elderly persons, nor be taken in cases of acute inflammation of some internal organs such as acute peritonitis, gastritis, enteritis and inflammatory conditions of uterus and ovaries.

In a graduated bath the patient enters the bath at a temperature of 31°C. The water temperature is gradually lowered at the rate of 1°C/min until it reaches 25°C. The bath continues until the patient starts shivering. A graduated bath is intended to avoid the nervous shock caused by a sudden plunge into cold water. This bath is often administered every 3 h in cases of fever. It effectively brings down the temperature, except in malarial fever. It also produces a general tonic effect, increases vital resistances and energises the heart.

A neutral bath is given for 15–60 min at a temperature of 26–28°C. It can be given over a long duration, without any ill effects, as the water temperature is akin to body temperature. A neutral bath diminishes the pulse rate without modifying respiration. Since a neutral bath excites activity of both the skin and the kidneys, it is recommended in cases relating to these organs. It helps those suffering from chronic diarrhoea and chronic afflictions of the abdomen.

A hot bath can be taken for 2–15 min at a temperature of 36.6–40°C. Before entering the bath, the patient should drink cold water and also wet the head, neck and shoulders with cold water. A cold compress should be applied throughout the treatment. This bath can be advantageously employed to relieve capillary bronchitis and bronchial pneumonia in children. It is also invaluable in the treatment of chronic rheumatism and obesity.

Epsom salt bath The immersion bath tub should be filled with about 135 l of hot water at 40°C. Epsom salts (1–1.5 kg) should be dissolved in this water. The patient should drink a glass of cold water, cover the head with a cold towel and then lie down in the tub, completely immersing the trunk, thighs and legs for 15–20 min. The best time to take this bath is just before retiring to bed. It is useful in cases of sciatica, lumbago, rheumatism, diabetes, neuritis, cold and catarrh, kidney disorders and other uric acid and skin affections.

Evidence

The literature reveals three randomised controlled trials of the use of hydrotherapy in the treatment of chronic venous insufficiency.[6] Two applied cold-water stimuli alone, or in combination with warm water, and suggested beneficial effects for the condition.

Safety

Certain precautions are necessary while taking therapeutic baths.

- A cold foot bath should not be taken in cases of inflammatory conditions of the genitourinary organs, liver and kidneys.
- Very weak patients, pregnant women, cardiac patients and those suffering from high blood pressure should avoid steam baths.
- Full baths should be avoided within 3 h of a meal and 1 h before it; however, local baths, such as hip and foot baths, may be taken 2 h after a meal.

Women should not take any of the baths during menstruation. They can take only hip baths during pregnancy until the completion of the third month.

Nutritional therapy

> Your food shall be your medicine.
>
> Hippocrates

Diet plays a vital role in the maintenance of good health and in the prevention and cure of disease. As seen in Part Three, it is extremely important in traditional Chinese medicine and ayurvedic medicine.

The human body builds up and maintains healthy cells, tissues, glands and organs only with the help of various nutrients. The body cannot perform any of its functions, be they metabolic, hormonal, mental, physical or chemical, without specific nutrients. The food that provides these nutrients is thus one of the most essential factors in building and maintaining health.

Nutrition can be important in the cure and prevention of disease. Naturopaths believe that the primary cause of disease is a weakened organism or lowered resistance in the body, arising from the adoption of a faulty nutritional pattern. There is an elaborate healing mechanism within the body but it can only perform its function if it is abundantly supplied with all the essential nutritional factors.

Nutrition can also be the cause of disease. Environmental factors, including diet and lifestyle, are thought to play a role in the development of most kinds of cancer. Some forms of cancer are more common in some countries than others, and people who migrate from one country to another eventually assume the cancer risks linked to their new neighbours. For example:

• Stomach cancer in parts of Japan is associated with diets that contain substantial amounts of salt, particularly salted dried fish.
• Colorectal cancer is more common in Australia and New Zealand; red meat and alcohol are possible causes.

An expert panel convened by the World Cancer Research Fund and the American Institute for Cancer Research estimated that 40% of cancer cases worldwide could be prevented by taking an appropriate diet.[7]

It is possible that at least 45 chemical components and elements are needed by human cells. Each of these 45 substances, called essential nutrients, must be present in adequate diets. These nutrients include oxygen and water. The other 43 essential nutrients are classified into five main groups: carbohydrates, fats, proteins, minerals and vitamins. All 45 of these nutrients are vitally important and they work together, therefore the absence of any of them will result in disease and eventually death.

It has been found that a diet that contains liberal quantities of (i) seeds, nuts, and grains; (ii) vegetables; and (iii) fruits will provide adequate amounts of all the essential nutrients. These foods have, therefore, been aptly called basic food groups and a diet containing these food groups is the optimum diet for vigour and vitality.

Seeds, nuts and grains

These are the most important and the most potent of all foods and contain all the important nutrients needed for human growth. They contain the germ, the reproductive power that is of vital importance for the lives of human beings and their health. Millet, wheat, oats, barley, brown rice, beans and peas are all highly valuable in building health. Wheat, mung beans, alfalfa seeds and soya beans make excellent sprouts. Sunflower seeds, pumpkin seeds, almonds, peanuts and soya beans contain complete proteins of high biological value.

Vegetables

Vegetables are an extremely rich source of minerals, enzymes and vitamins. Faulty cooking and prolonged careless storage, however, destroy these valuable nutrients. Most vegetables are, therefore, best consumed in their natural raw state in the form of salads.

Fruits

Like vegetables, fruits are an excellent source of minerals, vitamins and enzymes. They are easily digested and exercise a cleansing effect on the blood and digestive tract. They contain high alkaline properties, a high percentage of water and a low percentage of proteins and fats. Their organic acid and high sugar content have immediate refreshing effects. Apart from seasonable fresh fruits, dry fruits, such as raisins, prunes and figs, are also beneficial.

Fruits are at their best when eaten in the raw and ripe states. In cooking, they lose portions of the nutrient salts and carbohydrates. They are most beneficial when taken as a separate meal by themselves, preferably for breakfast in the morning.

Other items

Milk is an excellent food. It is considered to be nature's most nearly perfect food. Practitioners advise that the best way to take milk is in its soured form, that is, yoghurt and cottage cheese. Soured milk is superior to sweet milk as it is a predigested form and more easily assimilated. Milk helps maintain a healthy intestinal flora and prevents intestinal putrefaction and constipation.

It is recommended that high-quality unrefined oils be added to the diet. They are rich in unsaturated fatty acids, vitamins C and F, and lecithin. The average daily amount should not exceed two tablespoons. Honey is also an ideal food. It helps increase calcium retention in the system, prevents nutritional anaemia and is beneficial in kidney and liver disorders, colds, poor circulation and complexion problems. It is one of nature's finest energy-giving foods.

A diet of the three basic food groups and the special foods mentioned above will ensure a complete and adequate supply of all the vital nutrients needed to satisfy the requirements of any complementary disciplines for maintaining health and vitality, and preventing disease.

Animal proteins such as egg, fish or meat, are not mandatory in the diet as they may have a detrimental effect on the healing process. Many complementary practitioners believe that a high animal protein intake is harmful to health and may be responsible for many of our common ailments.

Nutraceuticals[8]

Increasingly, opportunities are arising for pharmacists to offer assistance in the maintenance of health using a group of food supplement products collectively known as nutraceuticals. The term was invented in 1989 by Stephen De Felice of the American Foundation for Innovation in Medicine, who defined a nutraceutical as being a 'food, or part of a food, that provides medical or health benefits, including the prevention and treatment of disease'.[9]

Nutraceuticals have also been called medical foods, designer foods, phytochemicals, functional foods and nutritional supplements, and include such everyday products as bio-yoghurts and fortified breakfast cereals, as well as vitamins, herbal remedies and even genetically modified foods and supplements such as fatty acids.[10] In the UK the idea is still comparatively new, but in many traditional healing therapies, for example ayurvedic and traditional Chinese medicine, nutrition has been used medicinally for centuries.

Not all fats are bad for you

One example of a nutraceutical that at the time of writing is of topical interest is nutritional supplementation using essential fatty acids (EFAs). Food-labelling regulations do not allow food labels to carry health claims. This makes it hard for companies marketing nutraceuticals to advertise the exact benefits of their products and may result in some confusion among consumers as to how such products should be used. Furthermore, there is a general perception that one should avoid any food that has the word 'fat' associated with it because it will cause weight gain, disrupt cholesterol readings and generally have an injurious effect on health. In fact there are good fats and bad fats, with consumption of the former often helping to reduce desire for the latter. Fats help balance the body's chemistry and provide 'padding' as protection for vital organs. They also act as a source of energy for body processes and help with the transportation of vitamins such as A, D, E and K, as well as providing a source of vital nutrients known as EFAs.[11]

Types of fatty acid

Saturated fats   These are found in red meat, butter, cheese and certain oils. They contain single bonds between all the carbon atoms in a chain saturated with hydrogen. They are usually solid at room temperature. When a person's diet is high in saturated fats, these tend to clump together and form deposits with protein and cholesterol that tend to lodge in blood vessels and organs.

Unsaturated fats   These are said to be either monounsaturated (e.g. oleic acid found in olive and sesame oils) or polyunsaturated (found in corn, soyabean and sunflower oils). The molecules have one or more positions with double bonds between the carbon atoms and have less hydrogen. The lower the number of hydrogen atoms, the more fluid the fat. Included in this group are the EFAs.

Essential fatty acids

EFAs are vital nutritional components that are required for good health. They are found in the seeds of plants and in the oils of cold-water fish. EFAs cannot be synthesised by the body and must be supplied externally.

There are two main types of EFA: the omega-3 oils and the omega-6 oils; the numbers refer to the position of the first double-carbon link in the chain. The importance of nutritional omega-3 oils was realised by UK researchers in 1970.[12] Omega-3 oils are more unsaturated than omega-6 oils.

The following are usually recognised as EFAs; some are precursors for others:

- **Linoleic acid** – an omega-6 fatty acid found in evening primrose, sunflower and sesame oils; symptoms such as acne, arthritic pain and skin disorders, which are regularly seen in the pharmacy environment, may be due to a deficiency of linoleic acid.
- **Gamma-linolenic acid** – found in small amounts in evening primrose, blackcurrant and borage oils.

- **Alpha-linoleic acid** – an omega-3 fatty acid found in flax and walnut oils.
- **Arachidonic acid** – a long-chain unsaturated fatty acid found in beef, pork, chicken and turkey; both arachidonic and docosahexanoic (see below) acid are present in brain and eye membranes, and play an important role in vision and brain cell function.
- **Docosahexanoic acid** – a long-chain omega-3 unsaturated fatty acid comprising 22 carbon atoms with six double bonds bent in a U shape. It is found in anchovies, herring, mackerel, salmon, sardines and tuna. It is necessary for normal function of both the eye and the cerebral cortex, which is responsible for higher functions such as reasoning and memory. A lack of this acid may lead to attention deficit hyperactivity disorder (ADHD: see below).

The EFAs are claimed to have many vital functions, including:

- lowering dietary triglyceride levels in the blood, thus improving mental state
- assisting in the eradication of plaque from artery walls
- lowering blood pressure
- construction of cell membranes
- prolonging clotting time
- nourishing skin, hair and nails
- acting as precursors to the production of prostaglandins, hormone-like substances that act as catalysts for many physiological processes, including neurotransmission
- regulating the body's use of cholesterol.

Fatty acids and diet

The dietary balance of fatty acids is important, and is usually expressed in terms of ratios, comparing one type to another. It has been suggested that the most beneficial ratio for human brain function is a 1:1 mixture of omega-6 to omega-3 oils. In 1990 the Canadian Minister of National Health and Welfare recommended a daily 6:1 ratio of omega-6 to omega-3 fatty acids for people between the ages of 25 and 49.[13] Today the ratio for most people in industrialised nations is estimated to be from 20:1 to 30:1 in favour of omega-6 oils. In breast milk the ratio may be as high as 45:1. Infant feeds are estimated to have a ratio of about 10:1.

There is another difficulty affecting fatty acid ingestion, even if a correct balance of food is being achieved. The production of the appropriate oils in plant material is affected by climate. Northern plants, in response to cold weather, produce more omega-3 fats while in southern, warmer areas more omega-6 oils are produced. Thus, depending on the source of foodstuffs, the ratio of oils in a person's diet may vary.

Many factors, including stress, allergies, disease and a diet high in fried foods, such as that found in the west of Scotland, may increase the body's nutritional need for EFAs. Because solid saturated fats are more stable than liquid unsaturated fats when they are exposed to light, heat and air, they are more desirable than oils for commercial frying. The Chinese method of stir-frying is preferred.

The changing ratio of fatty acids appears to have significant implications for brain function and forms a basis for supplementation with nutraceuticals. Modern lifestyle demands mean that optimal diets are not always followed. Advice offered in the pharmacy on nutritional issues is consistent with the extended role and development of pharmaceutical care programmes, which are gaining acceptance throughout the profession.

Evidence

The difficulty for pharmacists is to know when to recommend EFA supplementation. Published studies cover a wide range of conditions but the validity of some of the work is questionable, either because the preparations used were inadequately standardised or because the influence of confounding dietary factors was not recognised. Notwithstanding this criticism, there is both scientific and circumstantial evidence that EFA supplementation can be of benefit in both the treatment and prevention of disease. The following examples of research provide evidence of effectiveness in a number of conditions commonly seen in the pharmacy environment.

A pilot study of 44 patients started in the 1980s demonstrated that conditioms such as dry skin dermatosis, fatigue, bursitis and irritability appeared to respond to omega-3 supplementation as flax seed oil.[14]

Evening primrose oil has been shown to relieve the distressing itching of atopic eczema in most subjects taking Efamol over several months.[15] It contains gamma-linolenic acid, which converts to arachidonic acid.

Other controlled trials have demonstrated the benefit of evening primrose oil[16] and fish oil[17] administered to patients with rheumatoid arthritis. Evening primrose oil has been used in the treatment of premenstrual syndrome.[18]

Linoleic acid has been shown to stimulate fat utilisation and decrease body fat content in mice, but has not yet been tested in humans.[19]

A recent prospective study found that a higher consumption of fish and omega-3 polyunsaturated fatty acids is associated with a reduced risk of stroke, primarily among women who do not take aspirin regularly.[20]

Population studies have shown that frequent consumption of small amounts of omega-3 oils protects against the development of type 2 diabetes.[21] Gamma-linolenic acid supplementation in diabetes has been shown to improve nerve function and prevent diabetic nerve disease.[22]

A short attention span, inattentiveness and hyperactivity are diagnostic features of the syndrome now called ADHD, first described 100 years ago and suffered from by up to 16% of young children.[23] A connection between omega-3 deficiency and ADHD has been suggested by studies in which youngsters with the condition, when compared with non-ADHD children, had much lower blood levels of DHA.[24] Children with ADHD may have trouble converting the short EFAs into omega-3 and omega-6 fats; thus these patients will benefit from receiving ready-made decosahexanoic acid, a long-chain fat, in the form of fish oil. Evening primrose oil can provide the omega-6 fat gamma-linolenic acid, bypassing a blocked omega-6 conversion stage. As a combination product these EFAs offer a healthier balance of omega-3 and omega-6 to the brain and body tissue.[25]

There is considerable debate as to how ADHD should be recognised and whether it should be treated.[26] It has been suggested that a specific diagnosis should be deferred until pediatricians are certain that a problem exists. Under these circumstances EFA supplementation may provide parents with a temporary solution to the problem of an apparently overactive child. Children under the age of 2 years should be referred to their general practitioner.

Safety

Tolerance of EFAs is usually satisfactory. However, some allergic skin reactions have been reported. Patients with epilepsy or who are taking phenothiazine should be advised to consult their physician before self-treating with EFAs.

EFA supplementation in the pharmacy

EFAs offer the opportunity for pharmacists to become involved in improving and/or maintaining health through offering advice on nutrition, especially in the following situations:

- Patients with acne, alcoholism, cardiovascular disease, premenstrual syndrome and rheumatoid arthritis may use EFAs with safety to complement orthodox drug treatment.
- Patients with substantial risk factors of developing type 2 diabetes are likely to benefit from taking EFAs.
- EFAs may be of benefit to patients suffering from anxiety, general lethargy and premenstrual syndrome.
- ADHD may respond to EFA supplementation, although this should be an interim measure pending referral for further investigation.

Ingestion of EFAs may be required over extended periods – months rather than weeks – and to improve concordance patients should be informed as fully as possible of the aim of the supplementation.

More information

The British Naturopathic Association
Goswell House
2 Goswell Road
Street
Somerset
BA16 0JG
Tel: 01458 840072
www.naturopathy.org.uk

References

1.   Oumeish O. The philosophical, cultural and historical aspects of complementary alternative unconventional and integrative medicine in the Old World. In: Fontanarosa P B (ed.) *Alternative Medicine*. Washington, DC: American Medical Association, 2000: 136–137.
2.   Haas E, Novey D. Detoxification therapy. In: Novey D (ed.) *Clinician's Complete Reference to Complementary and Alternative Medicine*. St Louis, MO: Mosby, 2000: 705–707.
3.   Casdorph H R. EDTA chelation therapy, efficacy in arteriosclerotic heart disease. *J Hol Med* 1981; 3: 53–57.
4.   Shri H K. Bakhru. *A Complete Handbook of Naturocare*. www.healthlibrary.com/reading/ncure/index.htm.
5.   Dieppe P. Fortnightly review: management of hip osteoarthritis. *BMJ* 1995; 311: 853–857.
6.   Pittler M. Complementary therapies for chronic venous insuifficiency. *Focus Altern Complementary Med (FACT)* 2001; 6: 3–5.
7.   *Food, Nutrition and the Prevention of Cancer*. New York: World Cancer Research Fund/American Institute for Cancer Research, 1997.

8. Kayne S B. Getting to know the bad guys. *Chemist Druggist* 2001; 255: 22–23.

9. Mannion M. Nutraceutical revolution continues at Foundation for Innovation in Medicine conference. *Am J Nat Med* 1998; 5: 30–33.

10. Bull E, Rapport L, Lockwood B. What is a nutraceutical? *Pharm J* 2000; 265: 57–58.

11. Lee D. *Essential Fatty Acids*. Pleasant Cove, UT: Woodland Publishing, 1997: 5–6.

12. Fiennes R N, Sinclair A J, Crawford M A. Essential fatty studies in primates: linoleic acid requirements of Capuchins. *J Med Primatol* 1973; 2: 155.

13. *Report on Nation's Health*. Ottawa, Canada: Canadian National Ministry of Health and Welfare, 1990.

14. Rudin D, Felix C. *Omega-3 Oils. A Practical Guide*. New York: Avery Publishing Group, 1996: 39–49.

15. Burton J L. Dietary fatty acids in inflammatory skin disease. *Lancet* 1989; i: 27.

16. Belch J J. Effects of altering dietary essential fatty acids on requirements for non-steroidal anti-inflammatory drugs in patients with rheumatoid arthritis: a double blind placebo controlled study. *Ann Rheum Dis* 1988; 47: 96.

17. Fortin P R, Lew R A, Liang M H *et al.* Validation of a meta-analysis: the effect of fish oil in rheumatoid arthritis. *J Clin Epidemiol* 1995; 49: 1379–1390.

18. Burdeiri D, Li Wan Po A, Dornan J C. Is evening primrose oil of value in the treatment of premenstrual syndrome? *Controlled Clin Trials* 1996; 17: 60–68.

19. Dyck D J. Dietary fat intake, supplements and weight loss. *Can J Appl Physiol* 2000; 25: 495–523.

20. Iso H, Rexrode K M, Stampfe M J *et al.* Intake of fish and omega-3 fatty acids and risk of stroke in women. *JAMA* 2001; 285: 304–312.

21. Feskens E J, Bowles C H, Kromhout D. Inverse association between fish intake and risk of glucose intolerance in normoglycemic elderly men and women. *Diabetes Care* 1991; 14: 935–941.

22. GLA Multicenter Trial Group. Treatment of diabetic neuropathy with GLA. *Diabetes Care* 1993; 16: 8–15.

23. Naveem S, Chaghary B, Collop N. Attention deficit hyperactivity disorder in adults and obstructive sleep apnea. *Chest* 2001; 119: 294–296.

24. Colquhoun I, Bunday S. A lack of EFAs as a possible cause of hyperactivity in children. *Med Hypoth* 1981; 7: 673.

25. Rudin D, Felix C. *Omega 3 Oils*. New York: Avery Publishing Group, 1996: 97–98.

26. Blackman J A. Attention-deficit/hyperactivity disorder in preschoolers. Does it exist and should we treat it? *Pediatr Clin North Am* 1999; 46: 1011–1025.

12

Diagnostic therapies

Iridology

'Iri' and 'iris' are derived from the Greek name for the goddess of the rainbow, Iris. 'Ology' also comes from the Greek, meaning 'study of'. Literally translated, therefore, iridology means the study of the coloration of the eye. It is a diagnostic tool, relying on a perceived link between ill health and changes in the iris. It offers practitioners a foresight of certain abnormalities in the body long before symptoms manifest themselves. The prevention of disease is thus seen as a crucial aspect of the iridologist's work. The number of specialist iridologists in western Europe is small – probably fewer than 2000 – although iridology is used quite widely by German *Heilpraktikers*. The discipline is more popular in Russia, where it is restricted to medically qualified doctors, around 5000 of whom may use the technique. Iridology may be used by specialists who subsequently refer on as appropriate or it may be used by naturopaths and other practitioners as a diagnostic tool prior to treatment.

Definition

Iridology is the diagnosis of medical conditions and predisease states through the study of abnormalities of pigmentation on the iris. It may also yield information on general consitutional and genetic features of individuals.

History[1]

The first reference by a physician to iridology was made by Philipus Meyens in his book *Chiromatica Medica*, published in Dresden in 1670. Meyens accurately mapped out the segments of the iris and described how they represent certain organs and tissue systems. The method was further refined by a Hungarian monk Ignaz (Edmund) von Peczely (1822–1911). He is said to have accidentally broken the leg of his pet owl as a child and noticed a black shadow on the bird's eye that slowly changed in texture as the leg healed.[2] In a book published in 1880 he describes a method linking the site of certain iridic phenomena to the site of organic disease.[3] Other workers in this field were von Peczely's contemporary, the Swedish naturopath Liljequist, and Felke in the early 1900s.

Modern iridology owes its development to several Germans, including Angerer[4] and Deck.[5] In the USA Jensen, a chiropractor from California, is an active proponent of iridology.[6]

Theory

Iridologists believe that the iris reveals the changing conditions of every part and organ of the body. Every organ and part of the body is represented in the iris in a well-defined area. In addition, through various marks, signs and discoloration in the iris, nature reveals inherited weaknesses and strengths.

Typically, an iridology map may comprise 60 different sectors for the right and left irises, each being related to an organ to which it is connected by multiple nerve connections, or a body function.[7] The exact nature of the manner in which the segments are subdivided is still under discussion.

Iridologists also believe that the pigment deposits indicate that the body is in a defensive state and that the colour, density and position of pigmentation may offer clues to the identification of pathogenesis and specific organ involvement. Iridology cannot detect a specific disease, but can tell an individual if he or she has over- or underactivity in specific areas of the body. For example, an underactive pancreas might indicate a diabetic condition. Ophthalmologists, on the other hand, see no significance in the diversity of iridic pigmentation, attributing it to an individual's normal characteristics.

Practice

Iridologists investigate the iris by hands-on clinical examination with an illuminated magnifier or study high-definition colour photographs taken with special cameras. Thorough analysis of the results and referral to charts or maps lead to a diagnosis and treatment or referral as appropriate.

Evidence

A systematic review identified eight tests of iridology, of which four were not evaluator-blind or not controlled or both and were therefore excluded from the evaluation.[8] One of the remaining four studies involved 23 patients and reported significant differences in the photometric values in the iris of patients with mitral stenosis.[9] However, there were concerns about the methodology. The other three studies were close to random. It was concluded that the validity of iridology as a diagnostic tool was not supported by scientific evaluations and that patients and therapists should be discouraged from using the method.

Kinesiology

A key diagnostic component of kinesiology is its use of muscle testing as part of an interactive neurological assessment process that helps the practitioner determine areas of structural, chemical and mental dysfunction. There are around 50 methods of muscle-testing kinesiology in the world today. Applied kinesiology is described in this section.

The treatment phase that follows diagnosis incorporates procedures from many other complementary disciplines including acupressure, chiropractic and osteopathic manipulation, and nutritional therapy.

Definition

Applied kinesiology comprises both a diagnostic tool and a holistic therapeutic modality that, in much the same way as Chinese or Indian medicine, focuses on bodily dysfunction rather than directly on the disease itself.

History

All the different kinesiologies use the same basic muscle-testing principle and a treatment model based on traditional acupuncture theory. Each variant reflects the interests and personality of its developer. For example, applied kinesiology, created in 1964 by George Goodheart Jr, a chiropractor, has an emphasis on correcting structural problems. Using chiropractic knowledge of the trigger or reflex points on the body and of acupuncture meridians and their relationship to organs and muscle groups, Goodheart developed a consistent diagnosis and treatment system.[10]

Theory[11,12]

The theoretical basis of applied kinesiology rests on the assumption that muscle weakness is the result of the functional state of the nervous system, expressed in the muscle–nerve connections. The organs express their function via nerves to specific muscle groups. Applied kinesiologists believe that structural, chemical and mental dysfunction is associated with secondary muscle imbalance, usually inhibition. The application of appropriate therapy results in normalisation of the inhibited muscle. The therapy may include manipulation of cranium, spine and extravertebral joints.

Practice

Applied kinesiology is used to detect incorrect joint function, spinal lesions, muscle weakness, psychological problems and allergies. Gentle pressure is applied to a muscle and the response monitored. The normal muscle response is to lock. By placing a limb in a particular position it is possible effectively to isolate an individual muscle (often an arm muscle) and test its response to this pressure. If the muscle gives way or is spongy, it indicates an energy disturbance in the meridian system. If, for example, this occurs when a muscle is tested in the presence of a food, it may mean that the person is allergic to that food. If the muscle unlocks after a question is asked, it indicates a negative answer to that question.

Some branches of kinesiology do not accept the use of muscle testing to obtain yes/no answers to verbal questions, but rely on a system of reflex points and finger modes to identify current stressors. A wide range of applications is listed in applied kinesiology textbooks.[13] These include allergies, arthritis, asthma, constipation, diarrhoea, hypertension, insomnia and musculoskeletal problems.

Evidence

A number of papers that discuss the use and efficacy of applied kinesiology may be found in the literature. The most recent deal with the neurological basis of applied kinesiology.[14]

More information

National Council and Register of Iridologists
40 Stokewood Road
Winton
Bournemouth
Dorset
BH3 7NE

British Society of Iridologists
998 Wimborne Road
Bournemouth
Dorset
BH9 2DE
Tel: 01202 518078

Guild of Naturopathic Iridologists
94 Grosvenor Road
London
SW1V 3LS
Tel: 020 7834 3579

International Association of Clinical Iridologists
Orchard Villa
Porters Park Drive
Shenly
Radlett
Herts
WD7 9DS
Tel: 01923 856222

Association for Systematic Kinesiology
39 Browns Road
Surbiton
Surrey
KT5 8ST
Tel: 020 8399 3215

Health Kinesiology
Sea View House
Long Rock
Penzance
TR20 8JF
Tel: 01736 719030

International College of Applied Kinesiology
Tel: 913 384 5336
www.icak@usa.net

Kinesiology Federation
30 Sudley Road
Bognor Regis
Sussex
PO21 1ER

References

1. Wolf H. Iridology. In Novey D (ed.). *Clinician's Complete Reference to Complementary and Alternative Medicine*. St Louis, MO: Mosby, 2000: 756–757.
2. Fulder S. *The Handbook of Complementary and Alternative Medicine*. Oxford: OUP, 1996: 245.
3. Peczely I. *Discoveries in the Field of Natural Science and Medicine: Instruction in the Diagnosis from the Eye*. Budapest: KgL, 1880.
4. Angerer J. *Handbook of Iridiagnosis*. Saulgen: Haug, 1953.
5. Deck J. *Fundamentals of Iris Diagnosis*. Karlsruhe: Institute for Fundamental Research in Iris Diagnostic, 1965.
6. Jensen B. *The Science and Practice of Iridology*, 14th edn. Escondido, CA: Jensen's Nutritional and Health Products, 1985.
7. Sharan F. *Iridology: A Complete Guide to Diagnosing Through the Iris and to Related Forms of Treatment*. Wellingborough: Thorson's, 1989.
8. Ernst E. Iridology: a systematic review. *Forsch Komplemed* 1999; 6: 7–8.
9. Popescu M P, Waniek D A. Perfectionarea metodei iridodiagnostica; posibilitati de computerizare a iridologei. *Oftalmologia* 1996; 30: 29–33.
10. Birdwhistle R L. *Kinesics and Context: Essays on Body Motion Communication*. Philadelphia: University of Philadelphia Press, 1970.
11. Fulder S. *The Handbook of Complementary and Alternative Medicine*. Oxford: OUP, 1996: 226–227.
12. Maffetone P. Applied kinesiology. In: Novey D (ed.) *Clinician's Complete Reference to Complementary and Alternative Medicine*. St Louis, MO: Mosby, 2000: 639–640.
13. Valentine T, Valentine C. *Applied Kinesiology*. Rochester, VT: Healing Arts Press, 1987: 28–35.
14. Schmitt W, Yanuk S. Expanding the neurological examination using functional neurologic assessment. Part 2: neurologic basis of applied kinesiology. *Int J Neurosci* 1999; 97: 77–108.

13

Manual therapies

Alexander technique[1-3]

> Every man, woman and child holds the possibility of physical perfection; it
> rests with each of us to attain it by personal understanding and effort.
>
> F.M. Alexander[1]

Definition

The Alexander technique is an educational and therapeutic method of
encouraging an individual to expend a minimum of effort to achieve the
maximum efficient use of muscles and movement with the aim of relieving pain and improving posture and overall health.[4] Put more simply, it
is a practical method for finding out what habits of body use a person
has and how best he or she can promote the most beneficial actions and
prevent the most harmful actions.

History

Born in Tasmania in 1869, Frederick Mathias Alexander found the
development of his promising career as a young Shakespearean actor
hampered by respiratory and vocal troubles.[5,6] None of the local doctors
seemed able to offer much help other than to suggest that he rested his
voice. FM, as he was known, suffered from poor health for much of his
life and had to give up acting in favour of teaching at home.

Alexander eventually concluded that his problems lay within his
own body. He discovered that the principles of physical coordination
do not work in isolation from the rest of our functioning. Specifically,
the quality of muscle tone and the way we are supported at rest and in
movement is only one aspect of a whole that includes our thought processes and emotional states. In trying to unravel and understand the
interrelationship between these different aspects of his organism,
Alexander realised that they were inextricably linked with habit patterns that were deep-rooted and connected with his 'intention to act' or
his 'will to do'. During several years of painstaking self-observation

with the aid of a mirror, he noted that while reciting prose he tended to adopt a posture that depressed his larynx and vocal cords, and shortened his spine. He realised that he needed to train himself into adopting a more appropriate posture if he was going to improve his delivery. His own success prompted him to teach other actors how to improve their technique. Alexander's improvements in voice and general health led him to propose a new approach to the use of the body as a whole. Encouraged by doctors he moved to London at the turn of the twentieth century and expounded his ideas in England and the USA until his death in 1955.

The thespian origins of Alexander's technique have been reinforced over the years and the method has received the acclaim of many theatrical people, including such diverse personalities as playwright George Bernard Shaw and actor John Cleese.

Theory

When Alexander first tried to apply his observational findings to his own behaviour during public performances, he found that he slipped back into his old habits very quickly. Seeking an explanation for this action, he found three fundamental reasons:

- **End gaining and the means whereby.** Alexander used the term 'end gaining' to describe the tendency to follow some course of action almost automatically without first thinking through one's intended actions carefully. He called the opposite process of waiting, thinking and assessing the most appropriate activity the 'means whereby'.
- **Faulty sensory appreciation.** With this term Alexander acknowledged the presence of habits of proprioception or feeling underlying habitual actions. This can result in a feeling of uneasiness during the correction of a long-standing incorrect posture because it represents a change from what has been regarded as normal behaviour in the past.
- **Inhibition.** The third idea is linked to the second. It represents a natural self-control of unwanted and inappropriate reactions without any sense of suppressing sponteneity.

When Alexander discovered a way of integrating these concepts he found the solution to his problems. By recognising the strength of his old habits and the inappropriateness of end gaining, he was forced to consider the 'means whereby' he could secure the necessary improvements in posture.

To do this he had to overcome the faulty sensory perception of how his body should be. This he did by inhibiting his end-gaining behaviour.

Practice

The technique involves a process of psychophysical re-education that engages both mind and body. This learning process is best achieved through a series of one-to-one lessons with a qualified teacher who, using very gentle non-manipulative touch, gives the pupil the necessary new experiences. Modern practitioners recommend up to an hour to enable changes to be made. In group classes the emphasis is more on experiment and observation. Pupils are also encouraged to observe the thought processes and tensions associated with their activities in daily life. As the principles are assimilated, the pupil begins to develop the tools necessary to make his or her own discoveries and can continue to learn independently.

Evidence

Research into the Alexander technique was pioneered by Frank Pierce-Jones, who used photographic, mechanical and electromyographical methods to demonstrate that when a person is guided by its teachings the muscles work more effectively and there is less tiredness.[7] Respiratory function has been investigated in a control group and an active group that had received 20 lessons in Alexander technique.[8] A significant, though relatively small, increase of 6–9% in peak flow of the active group was recorded.

By reorganising body function in a general way, many specific difficulties are claimed to be alleviated or eliminated. These include chronic pain,[9] repetitive strain injury, back pain[10] and many conditions related to stress, including those related to performing. The technique has gained some support amongst nurses and other workplace groups involved in carrying and lifting activities.

Feldenkrais technique

In recent years a technique similar to Alexander's has been promoted by Moshe Feldenkrais.[11] He synthesised his ideas from eastern and western body concepts, combining some aspects of the Alexander technique with knowledge of oriental body training in the martial arts. The result is a series of exercises that facilitate awareness of the body in movement.

Chiropractic

Chiropractic is gaining in popularity and in the USA its practitioners are third in number to physicians and dentists. The discipline is the most popular example of complementary and alternative medicine (CAM) in that country, with as many as one in three patients with lower back pain being treated in this way.[12] A review of the use of CAM in the UK states that four of five studies considered placed the popularity of CAM disciplines in the order acupuncture, chiropractic, herbalism, homeopathy and osteopathy.[13] The remaining study, by MORI in 1989, did not ask about herbalism and recorded faith healers as third choice but was otherwise identical.

A survey of the 481 primary-care groups in England and Wales[14] showed that in 58% of the 60% of groups that responded, CAM was available through primary-care services. Chiropractic (available in 23% of respondents) was among the most commonly used therapies.

Definition

A rather wordy definition for chiropractic has been provided:[15]

> Chiropractic is a complementary discipline that focuses on the spine as being integrally involved in maintaining health, providing primacy to the nervous system as the primary coordination for function and thus health in the body. Maintenance of optimal neurophysical balance in the body is accomplished by correcting structural or biomechanical abnormalities or disrelationships through the use of manipulation and adjustment.

Chiropractors specialise in the diagnosis, treatment and prevention of biomechanical disorders of the musculoskeletal system, particularly those involving the spine and their effects on the nervous system.

History[16]

Although manipulation dates back to ancient times, its popularity in modern times is attributed to Daniel David Palmer (1845–1913), a self-educated scientist from Iowa. In 1895 Palmer was waiting in his office for a client when his janitor, Harvey Lillard, who had been deaf for 17 years, walked by. Noticing a small bump on the back of Lillard's neck, Palmer pushed it in. Lillard felt a snap in his back and suddenly declared that he could hear again. This led Palmer to deduce that the nervous system was the ultimate control mechanism of the body and that even minor misalignments of the spine, which he termed subluxations, could significantly impact on a person's health.

In the closing years of the nineteenth century, Palmer produced his theory of musculoskeletal effects on the central nervous system and developed the first manipulative techniques to relieve them. He asked his friend, the Rev. Samuel H. Weed, for advice. Weed turned to classic Greek and chose the words *chieri*, meaning hand, and *praktikos*, meaning performed, thus chiropractic means performed or done by hand.

Palmer is reputed to have opened his own school in the 1890s; some texts quote 1895 and others 3 years later. The profession celebrated its centenary in 1985 so the earlier date would seem to be the more appropriate!

Daniel's son, Bartlett Joshua (1882–1961) promoted chiropractic enthusiastically, helped by a number of his father's contemporaries and his own students.

Theory

There are four aspects of chiropractic philosophy:

- **The importance of the nervous system.** The basis of Palmer's technique is that as many as 31 different pairs of spinal nerves travel through openings in the vertebrae to and from the brain. If one of the vertebrae is partly displaced from its correct position, it can cause an impingement and pressure, or irritate the surrounding nerves. As a result, essential nerve messages are distorted, causing damage to the surrounding tissues.
- **The body's inherent ability to heal itself.** This is embodied in the phrase *vis medicatrix naturae*.
- **The effect of subluxation or joint dysfunction.** Such abnormalities are believed to interfere with the ability of the neuromuscular system to act in an optimal fashion, in turn contributing to the presence of disease.
- **The identification and treatment of subluxations.**

Practice

Examination

As spinal manipulation is of such importance to the chiropractor, examination of this area of the body is of particular interest, following an initial history-taking. The acronym PARTS has been suggested as an appropriate way to proceed with this inspection:[17]

- **Pain:** pain and tenderness are identified using observation, palpation and percussion.
- **Asymmetry:** this may be identified by palpation, radiographic analysis or observation of gait.
- **Range of motion:** this includes assessment of different types of motion, including stability of joints using palpation and radiography.
- **Tissue characteristics:** these include tone, texture and temperature abnormalities; a range of diagnostic techniques may be employed.
- **Special procedures:** electromyography, ultrasound and kinesiology may be considered to augment information obtained from previous tests.

Treatment[18]

Procedures used during chiropractic treatment may include gentle massage, ultrasonic treatment and adjustment. The chiropractic adjustment (often also called manipulation) to joints in the spine or extraspinal regions entails placement of the practitioner's hands on appropriate contact points. This is followed by positioning of the joint, during which the patient may feel tension of the muscles and ligaments; a popping sound may occur. A short sharp thrust may then be delivered. Chiropractors use different parts of the hand to direct the thrust, depending on the joint being adjusted. For example, the middle or base of the index finger may be used to adjust the neck whereas an area of the wrist bone may be used to adjust the lumbar spine. In cases of injury an indirect thrust may be used. The joint to be manipulated may be gently stretched over a pad or wedge-shaped block until realignment is accomplished.

A typical course of treatment for uncomplicated cases may involve six sessions over a 2–3-week period.

Evidence

In the UK 22 million people suffer from some form of back pain and 310 000 people are absent from work with the complaint every day of the year. Most people who consult chiropractors do so for low back pain, and it is to this application that much of the literature applies.

The literature contains a variety of low back pain research studies, including sham-controlled randomised controlled trials (RCTs), comparative RCTs and meta-analytic reviews. A selection of research information is presented here. For a fuller account the reader is referred to a comprehensive text published by *JAMA*.[19]

Some authors emphasise the distinction between spinal manipulation therapy (SMT) and chiropractic while others use the terms interchangeably.[20] This complicates the situation for the casual observer who wishes to research the literature. In fact chiropractic is much more than SMT alone, for it includes massage techniques such as myofascial muscle stimulation, and rehabilitative medicine procedures such as exercise, bracing, taping, splinting and casting. Herbal medicines are also often prescribed. This confusion may explain the wide range of results obtained from trials; they may not be comparing like with like.

Many US health agencies have endorsed chiropractic treatments and many insurance companies now pay for it. Workmen's compensation commissions have provided an opportunity to compare the efficiency of chiropractic and medical treatment in occupational terms. In Oregon, albeit 30 years ago, it was found that 82% of claimants with certain injuries treated by chiropractors returned to work within 7 days – twice as many as those with similar injuries who were treated by conventional doctors.[21]

Thirty-five RCTs of back and neck pain that compared spinal manipulation with other treatments have been evaluated.[22] Unfortunately the methodology was generally of a poor standard (e.g. low numbers, high drop-out rates, doubtful outcome measures, etc.) but 51% showed favourable results.

In the UK there are national guidelines on the treatment of low back pain that recommend chiropractic manipulation as a symptomatic treatment for acute uncomplicated cases where pain fails to resolve spontaneously within the first months.[23] However, the evidence base for such advice, largely derived from a meta-analysis of nine studies,[24] has been questioned in a *BMJ* editorial.[25] It was pointed out that there were no chiropractic studies included in the clinical trials that generated favourable data for the treatment of back pain. Other trials systematically reviewed in another paper revealed substantial methodological flaws.[26] The authors (Assendelft *et al.*) concluded that the trials did not provide convincing evidence for the effectiveness of chiropractic in the treatment of low back pain.

The editorial generated a substantial correspondence, much of it from North America. Some correspondents accused the editorial of excluding important papers. For example, one study claimed that significantly more of those patients who were treated by chiropractic expressed satisfaction with their outcome after 3 years than those treated in hospital: 84.7% (127/150) versus 65.5% (76/116) for those referred by chiropractors ($P < 0.0001$) and 79.2% (103/130) versus 60.2% (71/118) for those recruited from hospitals ($P = 0.001$). The outcome was assessed 3 years after entry to the trial.[27] It was also asserted that 'There is substantial scientific evidence that the manipulation that chiropractors (and indeed osteopaths and some physiotherapists) do for back pain is both effective and safe'.[28]

Other contributors claimed that the editorial was 'misleading'[29] and ignored patients' expressions of satisfaction.[30] One correspondent acknowledged that in various studies patient satisfaction with chiropractic was indeed relatively high.[31] On balance some benefit seems to accrue from using chiropractic to treat low back pain.

In other applications evidence is similarly rather less than robust. There appears to be some evidence that chiropractic may be beneficial for neck pain,[32,33] migraine,[34,35] tension headaches (examples of both positive[36] and inconclusive[37] evidence may be found in the literature) and headaches resulting from neck dysfunction.[38] Other applications include menstrual pain,[39] asthma[40] and colic,[41] but evidence of effectiveness is mixed. Sports applications are growing in usage. For example, the New Zealand olympic team appointed a chiropractor some years ago and found his involvement to be beneficial.[42]

A qualitative review that evaluated the direct analgesic effect of spinal manipulation on spinal or referred pain has been published.[43] A total of 11 studies were considered and they were largely consistent with the theory that the sensory input from spinal manipulation results in some form of pain inhibition.

Safety

Potential risks exist from inappropriate or unskilled manipulation (particularly cervical manipulation[44] and to a lesser extent lumbar spine manipulation[45–47]). A review of the literature to compare the risk of severe complication from non-steroidal anti-inflammatory drugs (NSAIDs) with cervical manipulation concluded that 'cervical manipulation for neck pain is much safer than the use of NSAIDs, by as much as an estimated factor of several hundred times'.[48] Notwithstanding this conclusion, severe complications, even death, have been reported, although the incidence of adverse reactions is relatively low when trained personnel are involved.[49] A small prospective study concluded that many so-called adverse reactions are really only an initial mild discomfort that may be reasonably expected from spinal manipulation and that this should be set against the long-term benefits of the treatment.[50] The methodology of this study was subsequently heavily criticised.[51]

The overuse of radiography by chiropractors has been cited as a potential hazard, but this is disputed by many practitioners.[52]

Chiropractic is contraindicated in certain vascular complications, arteriosclerosis, traumatic injuries and arthritis.

Statutory regulation

Osteopathy and chiropractic are the only two complementary therapies that are regulated by statute. An act of parliament passed in the mid 1990s established a General Chiropractic Council with the aim of regulating the profession. The organisation operates in a similar way to the General Medical Council and has the authority to remove practitioners from the register in disciplinary hearings.

Training

At the Anglo-European College in Bournemouth a 5-year full-time course leads to a BSc (Honours) degree in human sciences after 4 years, followed by a further year leading to a postgraduate diploma in chiropractic, validated by the University of Portsmouth and recognised by the European Council for Chiropractic Education.

Most of the chiropractors in the UK are trained in the McTimoney school in Abingdon (identifiable by the letters AMCA, MMCA or FMCA) and the Oxford College of Chiropractic (previously the Witney School). The two schools teach a similar whole-body approach, although there are differences in technique. Both schools are committed to providing a training equivalent to the European standards on chiropractic education, and to complying with the requirement for UK national registration. The approach to treatment varies in that the Anglo-European graduates tend to treat only subluxations whereas their colleagues from the McTimoney school tend to treat the whole spine at every session.

In the USA there are 16 chiropractic colleges and there are two in Canada.

Massage

Although remedial massage has its own methods and procedures, at its simplest it may be considered as being the age-old response to a painful stimulus, i.e. rubbing the bit that hurts! Massage is now used in a variety of health professions, including therapeutic massage, body work, physical therapy, sports medicine, nursing and, as an adjunct to chiropractic, osteopathy and naturopathy. Its aims are to:

- relieve pain and reduce swelling
- relax the muscles
- encourage the healing process following strain and sprain injuries.

Contrary to popular opinion, it cannot prevent loss of muscle strength nor reduce fat deposits.

Definition

Massage is the systematic manipulation of body tissues, performed primarily (but not exclusively) with the hands for therapeutic effect on the nervous and muscular systems, and on systemic circulation. The primary characteristics of massage are touch and movement. It may be performed in association with another therapy or alone.

History

Massage is reputed to have been used more than 3000 years ago by the Chinese. Later, the Greek physician Hippocrates used friction in the treatment of sprains and dislocations, and kneading to treat constipation. Early in the nineteenth century, Per Henrik Ling (1776–1839) of Stockholm devised a system of massage to treat ailments involving joints and muscles. Ling believed that vigorous massage could bring about healing by improving the circulation of the blood and lymph. In the past 20–30 years complementary therapists have adapted Swedish massage so as to place greater emphasis on the psychological and spiritual aspects of the treatment. The benefits of massage are now described more in terms such as 'calmness' or 'wholeness' than in terms of loosening stiff joints or improving blood flow. In contrast to the vigorous and standardised treatment recommended by Ling, current massage techniques are more gentle, calming, flowing and intuitive.

Ling's Swedish system was popular at European spa towns in the nineteenth century, when it was used in conjunction with hydrotherapy. It was taken to the USA in 1854 by Dr George Taylor and his brother Dr Charles Taylor.[53] Others later extended the treatment to relieve deformities of arthritis and to re-educate muscles following paralysis.

In the 1940s and 1950s massage became associated with the sex industry, and its use in serious medicine fell into decline, a trend exacerbated by the social conservatism of the day, which questioned the propriety of allowing practitioners to touch an unclothed body. Furthermore, there was a growing scepticism at its effectiveness. However, in the 1960s massage regained its popularity, particularly with sports trainers and later physiotherapists. A decade later the 'wellness' movement gained support, and health professionals began to reassess the benefits of therapies involving touch. The use of massage in UK hospital physiotherapy departments is currently less than in the past, but for the aromatherapist it has always maintained a high profile. For the sports person massage is also important, as part of the preparation for competition.

Theory

Massage involves two main components: touch and pressure. Attaining a balance between the two is an important skill. Touch with appropriate sensitivity allows the practitioner to gather information about the body. While giving a standard massage, practitioners gather palpatory information, which helps to adapt treatment to individual needs. For example, a practitioner will devote extra time to massaging an area of increased muscle tension. Touch can also communicate a sense of caring and relaxation, essential elements in the therapeutic process. Pressure and manipulation stimulate blood circulation and reduce muscular tension.

Practice

The most commonly used therapeutic massage is known as Swedish massage, although many other variants exist, including deep-tissue massage (used to release chronic patterns of muscular tension), sports massage (similar to both Swedish and deep-tissue massage) and acupressure (Chapter 9). Craniosacral massage is designed to deal with cranial and spinal imbalance.

Treatment often involves several different procedures and may last between 15 and 90 min.[13] It commences with the case history, although this is usually relatively short compared with other complementary therapies.

The patient is ideally treated unclothed on a specially designed massage couch. This normally incorporates soft but firm padding and a hole for the face. The treatment room is kept warm and quiet. Soft music may sometimes be played.

Practitioners generally treat the whole body, using oil, lotion or talc to help their hands move over the patient's body smoothly. A variety of strokes are used:

- Effleurage is a deep stroking movement in the direction of the venous flow that relaxes muscles, improves circulation to the small surface blood vessels and is thought to increase the flow of blood towards the heart.
- Pétrissage is a compression procedure that includes kneading, squeezing and friction; it is useful in stretching scar tissue, muscles and tendons so that movement is easier.
- Friction or rubbing is carried out with a slow elliptical or circular movement to increase blood flow and muscle movement.
- Tapotement or percussion uses the sides of the hands to strike the surface of the skin in rapid succession to improve circulation.
- Vibration or shaking is used on the extremities and is said to lower muscle tone.

Massage practitioners who treat sports injuries and musculoskeletal disorders may incorporate techniques derived from physiotherapy, osteopathy and chiropractic. These include deep massage, passive and active stretching, and muscle energy techniques (in which the patient moves against resistance from the practitioner).

Therapeutic uses

Massage is used by practitioners as a method of treatment for many common ailments. The various forms of massage and their usefulness in various diseases are described here in brief.

Massage of the joints

Stiff and swollen joints can be cured by massage combined with mechanical movements. Massage is, however, not recommended in serious inflammatory cases of the joints and in tubercular joints. Sprains and bruises can be cured by massage. In these cases, affected parts should first be bathed with hot water for 15–30 min. Next the massage should be done for a few minutes. Gentle stroking and kneading are recommended on and around the injured tissues. Fractures can also be treated through massage.

Massaging the nerves

Massage benefits many nerve problems. In cases of acute inflammation of the nerves, massage should be done carefully. Light and gentle stroking is recommended. Deep pressure should not be used on swollen nerves because it will increase the inflammation. All that is needed is a gentle tapotement or beating of the nerve.

Abdominal massage

This form of massage is beneficial in constipation. It stimulates peristalsis of the small intestines, tones up the muscles of the abdomen walls and mechanically eliminates the contents of both large and small intestines.

Chest massage

Chest massage is helpful in many ways. It strengthens the chest muscles, increases circulation and tones up the nervous system of chest, heart and lungs. It is especially recommended in weakness of the lungs, palpitation and organic heart disorders. Bust and mammary glands can be developed by proper massage.

Massage of the back

The purpose of massage of the back is to stimulate the nerves and circulation for treating backache and rheumatic afflictions of the back muscles, and for soothing the nervous system. The patient is made to lie down with the arms at the sides.

Massage of the throat

This helps to overcome headache, sore throat and catarrh of the throat.

Evidence

Anxiety

There is some good evidence from RCTs that massage can reduce anxiety in the short term in child and adolescent psychiatric patients,[54] and palliative care.[55] In one study of cancer patients suffering from pain, 60%

of the respondents reported a reduction in pain after half an hour's massage.[56] Massage has been beneficial in intensive care following cardiac surgery,[57] although some concerns about its effect on critically ill patients have been expressed.[58] Long-term elderly hospital patients are reported to have responded to massage with a reduction in anxiety, tension and heart rate.[59]

Premenstrual syndrome

Massage therapy may be an effective long-term aid for pain reduction and water retention, and a short-term aid for decreasing anxiety and improving mood for women with premenstrual dysphoric disorder.[60]

Low back pain

An RCT with four parts sought to compare the effectiveness of massage therapy with other interventions for the treatment of low back pain.[61] The massage provided a benefit to patients in excess of the other interventions.

AIDS

There is some evidence that massage may improve the immune function and quality of life of acquired immunodeficiency syndrome (AIDS) patients.[62]

Massage for children

A critical review of the use of massage therapy in children concluded that there was insufficient evidence to support its use without qualification.[63] None the less it is used in both neonates and older children with a variety of medical conditions. Benefits include improved mood (less crying and salivation), increased sleep and reduced pain in children with juvenile rheumatoid arthritis.

Sports massage; muscular fatigue

Statistics from the Great Britain team at the Atlanta Olympics in 1996 revealed that massage formed 47% of all treatments to athletes from all sports. The demand for massage in Albertville (1992) for the winter Olympics and Barcelona (1992) was also significant. Despite its popular appeal, a consensus as to its benefit is difficult to obtain from the literature because of the wide range of techniques employed and the outcome measures chosen.[64]

Some clinical trials do exist that are appropriate to mention within the sports context, and a selection have been considered in a review.[65]

Pre-exercise massage   Athletes often use massage prior to exercise but there is little evidence to support the hypothesis that it will enhance athletic performance. A whole range of liniments and rubs for use with accompanying massage are available. Many have the characteristic 'go faster' pungent aroma of wintergreen, turpentine or other popular essential oils instantly recognisable in a typical changing-room environment. Some of these products are rubifacients, containing constituents that are irritant to the skin (e.g. salicylates and capsicum) and cause dilation of superficial blood vessels, creating a pleasant warm sensation. There is a risk of an allergic reaction to these chemicals.

The effects of pre-exercise massage, warm-up and stretching movements on the joint range of movement and quadriceps and hamstring strength have been investigated.[66] The results showed that warm-up and stretching produced significant increases in all ranges of movement. The only other significant finding was that massage and warm-up, both separately and in combination, appeared to increase the range of movement on the calf. It was concluded that general warm-up and stretching were a better way of increasing flexibility, with the added advantage of being performed by the athlete without the need for expensive equipment or operators.

A psychological evaluation of pre-exercise massage was undertaken in 10 healthy men.[67] Each subject was assigned to a group receiving massage or a group receiving no massage before 10 min submaximal exercise. Various parameters were measured, including V_{O_2}, and cardiac output. No difference in performance was detected between the two groups. The very low numbers of subjects is a major criticism. The difficulty of eliminating bias in the placebo group, who obviously knew they were not receiving treatment, is always a potential problem in this type of study.

Although massage is widely used, there is no firm scientific evidence that it confers either physical or mental benefits.

Post-exercise massage   Post-exercise massage is often applied in the belief that it will help overcome fatigue and aid recovery.

Delayed-onset muscle soreness   Delayed-onset muscle soreness is a frequent problem after strenuous exercise, particularly among those persons unaccustomed to such activity. The condition usually subsides after 3–4 days but can hamper athletes in that it curtails training and can cause a lack of performance. A number of treatments have been tried, including ultrasound, NSAIDs, homeopathic Arnica and steroids. Massage therapy has also been suggested, but once again considerable uncertainty exists as to its effectiveness.[68] One study evaluated the effects of manual and mechanical massage on recovery from overall muscular and physiological fatigue.[69] It was concluded that there were definite recuperative benefits from the two types of massage, but not from rest alone. The study had several limitations, however. The numbers involved were low, the results were not treated statistically and most importantly, it was not made clear whether or not the types of massage delivered by the masseur and the machine were comparable.

If one of the reasons for fatigue is a restriction of blood flow to active muscles due to muscle contractions then it is reasonable to suppose that any action that increases blood flow to allow transport of metabolic byproducts would be beneficial. Increased blood flow was thought to be a major advantage of vibratory massage, yet when this type of massage was studied, it was not shown to help recovery.[70]

Another study was conducted involving nine athletes.[71] Having completed a maximal run, all participants were rested or manually massaged for 17 min or invited to warm down by exercising at a moderate level. Delayed-onset muscle soreness was less pronounced in the massaged individuals, who also showed a more rapid decline in muscle lactate levels. This was encouraging, but the small sample size hampered its conclusiveness.

A systematic review of seven studies on delayed-onset muscle soreness and massage found that most of the methodology described was seriously flawed.[72] However, it was concluded that massage therapy may be a promising treatment for the condition. Further study is warranted.

Muscle fatigue The effects of various massage techniques on muscle soreness and fatigue following intense muscular activity have been studied. Twenty female volunteers received electrical vibration massages for 40 min after maximal muscular activity.[73] The control group received no treatment following the same physical effort. A pain-rating scale and dynamometric measurements were used as end points. Compared to controls there appeared to be less loss of muscular strength in the massaged thighs after 1 and 3 days. However, in the upper limbs no such difference could be demonstrated; the pain was not significantly different in the control or massage groups.

In a similar study 12 male volunteers performed quadriceps contractions up to the point of exhaustion.[70] Percussive vibratory massage bouts lasting 4 min did not alter the degree of fatigue in repeated series with or without massages.

A group of 16 volunteers were randomised into two groups receiving massage or placebo massage (near-zero applied force), or no massage at all.[74] Dynamometric measurements and soreness perception were evaluated before, 24 h and 48 h after work. There were no effects of massage on any of the variables measured. The use of so-called placebo massage has to be questioned. The subject must be aware that true massage is not being applied and therefore could be biased. On the basis of these findings the effectiveness of massage in preventing muscle soreness and fatigue remains unproven.

In another study 46 patients suffering from fibrositis were treated 19 times in 4 weeks by massage lasting 30–40 min.[75] Effectiveness was evaluated by a fibrositis score during the treatment period. This parameter decreased significantly following massage therapy. Unfortunately, this trial did not include a control group. Thus, one is left to speculate whether the improvement was due to the treatment per se, a placebo effect, or would have occurred spontaneously anyway.

Several studies have compared massage as a therapy applied in the control group when evaluating treatments such as exercise or manipulation for back pain. Results are mixed, with both positive and negative outcomes being reported.[76,77] Unfortunately, there appears to be little convincing evidence of the effectiveness of manipulation with which to make a meaningful comparison.[78]

The effect of treatment with ultrasound, massage and exercises on myofascial trigger points in the neck and shoulder was assessed in an RCT.[79] The patients were randomised to three groups. The first group was treated with ultrasound, massage and exercise, the second group with sham ultrasound, massage and exercise, while the third group was a control group. The study lasted 6 weeks. The outcome measures were pain at rest and on daily function using a visual analogue scale, analgesic usage, global preference and index of myofascial trigger points. The long-term effect of the treatment and control groups was assessed after 6 months using a questionnaire. No difference was detected between the groups given ultrasound but minor improvement was noted in both test groups over the control. The combined massage and exercise regime conferred a slight benefit. It is not possible to say whether the exercise or massage element was the more effective.

Sports specificity   Different sports or even different disciplines within the same sport require a different massage regime. Cycling has traditionally regarded the masseur as an important member of the team, yet the rationale for this is doubtful. In one study six elite cyclists performed a 4-day stage race by race simulation.[80] After each stage the cyclists were given either massage for 20 min or 30 min blind placebo microwave. The race simulation was repeated 18 days later but the post-race treatments were altered. Serum muscle and liver enzymes were measured to detect muscle damage and recovery status. There were no significant differences between massage and placebo at any time during the study. It was concluded that post-event massage did not expedite muscle recovery or improve performance. A second study to test the effect of massage on the cyclists' psychological profiles also revealed no benefit.[81]

Conclusion

It seems that much work is required to establish whether or not massage is as effective as people believe. Much of the existing evidence is contradictory and invalidated to some extent by poor methodology. There may be psychological benefit from massage with essential oils.

Safety

Most massage techniques have a low risk of adverse effects. Adverse effects reported in the literature are rare and have usually involved extremely vigorous massage techniques that are highly unusual in the UK. Certain aromatherapy oils may pose a risk (Chapter 6).

Baby massage is becoming popular and it has been suggested that the oils used in this procedure may pose a hazard.[82] Special-care baby units, such as those serving Queen Charlotte's and Chelsea Hospitals, recommend arachis oil for massage of premature babies.[83] However, if tiny babies suck their hands after a hand massage with arachis (peanut) oil they may ingest large quantities of nut products, with potentially serious consequences.[84,85] It could be argued that the potential risks should be indicated on the labels of massage oils and in baby massage books and at classes. Alternative products could also be used to minimise the risk of reaction.

Osteopathic medicine

The name 'osteopathy' stems from the Latin words *osteon* and *pathos*, which translates to 'suffering of the bone'. This name has caused confusion in the sense that it makes people believe that an osteopath only treats conditions of the bones. However, the name was chosen because its founder, Dr Andrew Still, recognised that a well-balanced, properly functioning body relies on both the muscular and skeletal systems of an individual being healthy and well.

The World Health Organization recognises the osteopathic concept of somatic dysfunction as being scientifically proven, and the British Medical Association also recognises osteopathy as a discrete medical discipline. In Australia, osteopaths are statutorily registered practitioners who have a 5-year, full-time university training.

Definition

Osteopathy is a medical discipline that is based primarily on the manual diagnosis and treatment of impaired function resulting from loss of movement. Its philosophy has an emphasis on internal relationships of structure and function, with an appreciation of the body's ability to heal itself. It uses a wide range of techniques to treat musculoskeletal problems and other functional disorders of the body.

History

Osteopathy was developed in the USA in the 1870s by an American frontier doctor, Andrew Taylor Still (1828–1917). Still used his extensive knowledge of anatomy and physiology to develop a method to diagnose and treat the body through palpation and manipulation. He founded the American School of Osteopathy at Kirksville, Missouri in 1892.

Theory

The philosophy of osteopathic medicine is based on the idea that the human body constitutes an ecologically and biologically unified whole. Body systems are united through the neuroendocrine and circulatory systems. In the study of health and disease, therefore, no single part of the body can be considered autonomous. Osteopaths believe that the problems of health and the treatment of disease can only be rationally considered through the study of the whole person in relation to both internal and external environments. The following key principles are involved:[86]

- The body comprises interrelated organs and systems, and functions as a whole unit; disease results from an imbalance in overall health.
- The body has an ability to heal itself and may be assisted in this function by the practitioner; disease represents a breakdown in this capability.
- The body is much more than the sum of its individual parts; nothing exists in isolation and the totality must be considered, for example, dysfunction in the musculoskeletal system frequently contributes to pain, poor circulation and changes in function leading to constipation, headache, fatigue, etc.
- Treatment is based on the three basic principles of body unity, self-regulation and the interrelationship of structure and function, as stated above.

Practice

Osteopathic treatment is purely and solely based on manual techniques, which are used to adjust and correct mechanical problems in the whole body. The osteopath does not prescribe any medicines, nor does he or she use any invasive techniques (injections, surgery, etc.), although in the USA the scope of treatment may be wider than this. Diagnostic techniques are as for chiropractic and may include radiology.

The aim is not to treat the illness itself but to stimulate the patient's natural healing processes. There are four phases to treatment:

- detection of changes in muscles and tissues (by palpation)
- observation of any body asymmetry (e.g. leg length), posture and respiratory function
- testing of mobility and sensitivity
- application of treatment.

Usually, a patient will be asked to be passive during this phase. However, at times there are some techniques for which the patient must actively participate in the movements. The following treatments are examples of the direct and indirect techniques employed by osteopaths:

- Counterstrain techniques achieve release of restriction by placing the affected joint or muscle in a position of comfort, while applying a counter-stretch to the antagonists of the tight muscles.
- Functional techniques involve gentle mobilisation of joints so that

barriers to normal movement are identified until a way is found through the restriction.

- Osteopathic manipulations are carried out using minimum force levels in order to maximise safety and minimise patient discomfort; manipulation is not the mainstay of most osteopathic treatments.
- Craniosacral techniques are very gentle release techniques particularly suited to young children and the physically frail; this therapy was evolved by the Swiss practitioner William Garner Sutherland (1873–1954) and depends on the suggestion that cranial sutures have the ability to move slightly and their manipulation is thought to improve the circulation of cerebrospinal fluid, which in turn may relieve certain local symptoms.[87]
- Visceral techniques are used in the management of conditions affecting internal organs and involve gentle and rhythmical stretching of the visceral areas.

A treatment session lasts approximately half an hour.

Apart from low back pain,[88,89] other conditions treated by osteopathy are similar to those addressed by chiropractors and include neck and shoulder pain, sports injuries, repetitive strain disorders and headache. In addition, practitioners also treat arthritis; although they cannot affect disease pathology or progression, they claim to be able to treat secondary symptoms such as pain from associated muscle spasm. Cranial osteopathy has a particular reputation for treating children with conditions such as infantile colic, constant crying and behavioural problems.[90] Osteopathy has been introduced by some general medical practitioners in the UK to a limited extent.[91,92] Referral to registered osteopaths under the National Health Service (NHS) is also possible in some areas and a few NHS hospital trusts have taken on osteopaths to work within hospital physiotherapy departments.

Comparison with other manual disciplines

Chiropractic

Chiropractic always looks for the cause of the complaint in the vertebral column and treats it by means of manipulations, while osteopathy considers all the other body systems. Chiropractors are more likely to push on vertebrae with their hands, whereas osteopaths tend to use the limbs to make levered thrusts. Osteopathic and chiropractic techniques appear to be converging, and much of their therapeutic portfolio is shared.

Physiotherapy

Physiotherapy principally deals with rehabilitation and local treatment while osteopathy approaches the patient as a whole. Many physiotherapists use osteopathic and chiropractic techniques.

Manual therapy

Manual therapy is a method of detecting and treating loss of movement in the locomotor system. Osteopathy goes much further by also subjecting all the other tissues to a thorough examination.

Evidence

Although many people have osteopathic manual therapy, few trials have evaluated this therapy – most patients improve within a month, even without treatment, so assessment of any therapy for low back pain is difficult. Because of the convergence of chiropractic and osteopathy, the evidence for the former (see above) is often applied to the practice of the latter.

In a commentary[93] on a trial it was reported that a total of 1193 patients were screened to find 178 individuals who had had back pain for at least 3 weeks but less than 6 months.[94] Twenty-three patients later dropped out, leaving 72 patients in the allopathic treatment group and 83 patients in the osteopathic treatment group. Standard treatment included analgesics, anti-inflammatory drugs, active physical therapy and ultrasonography but no manual therapy. Physicians from the Chicago College of Osteopathic Medicine treated the other group with a number of osteopathic techniques. At the end of a 12-week period, all the patients had improved, but there were no significant differences between treatment groups, except in medication use. In the allopathic group, NSAIDs and muscle relaxants were prescribed at 54.3% and 25.1% of patient visits, respectively. In the osteopathy group, these drugs were prescribed at only 24.3% and 6.3% of visits.

The General Osteopathy Council website states that, following a year-long clinical trial at Salford University, researchers have revealed that an osteopathic approach has demonstrated up to a 40% improvement in the very severe symptoms of chronic fatigue syndrome.[95] Two groups took part. One group of patients received osteopathy for 12 months, while a control group was allowed any therapy of their choosing, with the exception of osteopathy. A 40% improvement in all symptoms – severe depression, chronic fatigue, back pain, headaches and sleeplessness – in the patient group was registered by the end of the year. Nine patients recorded an improvement of over 50% while two felt completely symptom-free. Only seven members of the patient group improved by less than the 23% improvement scored by the best result of the control group. The control group's mean result was 1% worse after the 12 months, with one sufferer worsening by 36%.

Osteopathic manipulation has been used as a complementary modality for treating musculoskeletal problems during postoperative surgery. In a prospective single-blinded two-matched group outcome study involving a total of 76 patients, patients receiving osteopathic treatment in the early postoperative period negotiated stairs earlier and walked further distances than did control group patients.[96]

Safety

Safety considerations are similar to those for chiropractic (see above). It is contraindicated in patients with brittle bones.

Statutory regulation

Osteopathy and chiropractic are the only two complementary therapies regulated by statute. The Osteopaths Act 1993 established a General Osteopathic Council with the aim of regulating the profession. The act may be accessed on the internet at the following address: www.hmso.gov.uk/acts/summary/01993021.htm.

The General Osteopathic Council is responsible for regulating, developing and promoting osteopathy in the UK. It has taken over the functions of previous voluntary bodies whose regulatory functions have now ceased. The legislation was fully enacted in May 2000, and it is now an offence for anyone practising in the UK to claim expressly or by implication to be any kind of osteopath unless registered with the General Osteopathic Council. The General Osteopathic Council operates in a similar way to the General Medical Council and has the authority to remove practitioners from the register in disciplinary hearings.

Training

In the UK most osteopaths now take a 4-year full-time course leading to a Bachelors degree (BOst or BSc) and must register with the General Osteopathic Council (see above). In the USA the original qualification offered by Still was a Diploma in Osteopathy, although under state law he could have conferred the degree of MD. Today the degree is Doctor of Osteopathic Medicine, which allows the holder to practise all branches of medicine.

Reflexology

The word 'reflexology' comprises 'reflex', in this case meaning one part reflecting another part, and 'ology', meaning study of. Put together, we get the study of how one part reflects another. However, the discipline involves much more than simply a study of parts. Reflexology is the most popular complementary discipline in Denmark.

Definition

Reflexology may be defined as 'the scientific theory that maps out the reflexes on the feet and hands to all the organs and the rest of the body'. It involves the application of pressure to reflex areas of the hands or feet to produce specific effects in other parts of the body.

History

A pictograph in the tomb of Ankhmahar, a physician of particularly high esteem, discovered at Saqqara in 1979, revealed that the ancient Egyptians were aware of the benefits of foot and hand reflexology. The pictograph, dating back to around 2500 BC, shows a therapist working on a patient's foot and a second therapist working on another patient's hand. The inscription reads: 'Don't hurt me'. The practitioner's reply is: 'I shall act so you praise me'. Reflexology is also said to have been practised in Chinese and North American Indian cultures.

While working in Vienna in the early 1900s an American ear, nose and throat specialist, Willam Fitzgerald (1872–1942), observed that applying pressure to specific areas of hands and feet caused an anaesthetising effect on other areas of the body and was useful in the treatment of pain. When he returned to the USA he divided the body into five longitudinal zones on each side of the body. These terminated in the toes and fingers. Fitzgerald suggested that a direct link existed between the areas and organs within each of the zones. This idea was developed by Eunice Ingham (1879–1974), who charted reflex areas in the foot that appeared to correspond to areas of the entire body. Several other charts have been produced since this early work, incorporating various refinements.

Theory

It is suggested that when the reflexes are stimulated, the body's natural electric energy works along the nervous system and meridian lines to clear any blockages on those lines and in the corresponding zones. A treatment seems to break up deposits (felt as gritty areas under the skin) that may interfere with the natural flow of the body's energy.[97]

Practice

Unlike some other complementary disciplines, reflexologists do not seek to diagnose medical conditions, nor do they prescribe medicines, although the topical use of oils or herbal preparations is often recommended.[98] Dietary advice may also be given.

Most reflexologists work on the feet, although the hands may also be involved. A treatment session lasts around 40 min. Practitioners usually advise their patients that the effects of a treatment may last up to a week. The need for further treatment will vary according to the severity of the condition and the patient.

The following benefits are possible:

• improved urination
• improved digestion
• heightened sense of energy
• reduction in pain.

Evidence

A review of literature on the effectiveness of reflexology splits the evidence into anecdotal and scientific evidence.[99] Examples of each are presented below. They do not add up to much more than just an impression that reflexology is of benefit.

Anecdotal evidence

There are a number of conditions for which case study reports are available. These include stress-related conditions (anxiety, migraine), back pain, gastrointestinal complaints and arthritis. As well as these specific conditions, patients report an improvement in their ability to relax and this may encourage self-healing.[100] Other benefits include a pleasant warming sensation in an injured area and improved sleep patterns.

Whilst acknowledging that there was no scientific evidence to support the statement, it has none the less been suggested that reflexology may provide some relief from postnatal problems following caesarean section and forceps delivery.[101] Cases have also been presented that demonstrate the apparent benefit of reflexology in midwifery.[102] Reflexology may also be of use during labour.

Scientific data

The first placebo-controlled RCT was reported in an investigation of the use of reflexology in premenstrual syndrome.[103] The trial began with 83 patients but, due to a high drop-out rate, only 35 completed the 6-month protocol. Treatment comprised eight weekly reflexology or placebo treatments. The verum was application of pressure to areas of the hands and feet appropriate to the condition being treated, while placebo reflexology was uneven light or heavy pressure to areas considered to be inappropriate to the conditions being treated. The results were in favour of reflexology. However, the type of reflexology used was not stated. This is significant because a number of different schools of thought on reflexology practice have been proposed. These reflect variations in the exact location of some of the reflexes and the methods of treatment. It is thus important that when outcomes from any particular set of treatments are discussed, the researcher states exactly which approach has been employed. Furthermore, the placebo points chosen in the study were acupressure points and may have been stimulated by the pressure applied to them.[104]

Low back pain was investigated in a double-blind RCT using a total of 91 patients assigned to treatment and placebo groups.[105] The authors report a statistically significant positive outcome with reduction in pain and improvements in muscular contractibility and mobility.

A number of other small-scale studies of reflexology used in the treatment of anxiety states, back pain and chest pain have been reported.[99]

Safety

Concerns may be expressed over the use of reflexology in diabetic patients due to the possibility of damage to the feet that will not be noticed by the patient. Furthermore, it is theoretically possible that stimulation of the reflexes could lead to the increased release of insulin from the pancreas in type 1 diabetes, upsetting patients' calculations as to how much insulin they need to administer. Other common foot diseases may preclude the use of reflexology.

Areas of injury, for example fractures and areas corresponding to internal organs that are diseased (e.g. the heart or gastrointestinal system), should be avoided.

Reiki

> Just for today, I will let go of anger.
> Just for today, I will let go of worry.
> Just for today, I will give thanks for my many blessings.
> Just for today, I will do my work honestly.
> Just for today, I will be kind to my neighbour and to every living thing.
>
> Dr Mikao Usui[106]

Reiki (pronounced ray-key) is another healing discipline with its origins in the east. It involves the laying-on of hands.

Definition

The Japanese compound word *reiki* may be translated simply as 'healing'. However, to followers of the practice it stands for far more than this one English word can imply. *Rei* means 'universal' or 'spiritual' and *ki* is 'life force energy'. Thus, more correctly it should be translated as 'universal life force energy'. It is the coming together of the spiritual dimensions and living energies to awaken a dynamic healing process and release the cause of stress in the body, mind, emotions and spirit.[107] Despite having these religious connotations, reiki is not a religion.

History

It is commonly believed that the origins of reiki may be traced back to early Tibetan teachings from around 3000 BC. It has also been suggested that the method was used by Buddha and Jesus Christ. The methodology employed in modern reiki is known as the Usui natural healing system (sometimes written as Usui shiki ryoho) from the name of Dr Mikao Usui of Kyoto, a Christian theologian who developed the system towards the end of the nineteenth century. Dr Usui spent many years on a quest for the secret of the ancient healing traditions. He went to a mountain top in Japan and underwent a 21-day purification, fasting and meditation, at the end of which he received enlightenment and the power of healing. He came down from the mountain and spent the rest of his life practising and teaching reiki. He took reiki to the USA in 1936.

Theory

The reiki therapist body's channels ki energy through his or her hands to the recipient, activating the body's natural ability to heal itself. Reiki energy goes to the deeper levels of a person's being, where many illnesses have their origins. It works wherever the recipient needs it most, releasing blocked energies, cleansing the body of toxins, relieving stress, alleviating pain and working to recreate the natural state of balance.

Practice

Reiki practitioners are said to be attuned to the reiki energy, and develop their abilities in conformance with Usui's original system. The procedures are very simple and non-intrusive. A treatment session lasts about an hour. It is usually carried out with the recipient remaining fully clothed, lying on a therapy couch. The practitioner places his or her hands on to the patient's body at a number of strategic points. Each position is held for up to 3 min. There is no pressure exerted. Energy is said to flow into the body and move to the source of the imbalance, not just to the manifesting symptoms.

Evidence

The use of reiki in chronic pain management as an adjunct to opioid therapy has been investigated.[108] Twenty patients collectively experiencing pain at 55 sites were subjected to reiki treatment by a certified therapist. Pain was measured using a visual analogue scale and the Likert scale before and after treatment. A significant reduction in pain was recorded following treatment.

There is some circumstantial evidence from case studies that reiki may be beneficial in stress, tension, sinusitis, menstrual problems, cystitis, migraines, asthma, psoriasis, myalgic encephalomyelitis, constipation, eczema, arthritis, menopausal problems, back pain, anxiety, depression, insomnia and sciatica. Chronic ailments also respond well.

Rolfing

When the body gets working appropriately the force of gravity can flow through then, spontaneously, the body heals itself.

Dr Ida P. Rolf

Definition

Rolfing is a comprehensive system of hands-on, connective tissue manipulation and movement education that releases stress patterns in the human organism.

As with other similar techniques (Hellerwork, Aston patterning, Feldenkrais, etc.), rolfing seeks to organise and integrate the body in relation to gravity by manipulating the soft tissues or by correcting inappropriate patterns of movement.[109] The final goal is that the client can move and function with greater freedom, and effortlessly maintain a more upright posture.

History

Rolfing is the creation of Dr Ida Rolf, a biochemist and physiologist who established the Rolf Institute for Structural Integration in 1970. She believed that, for optimum health, the body must be in alignment with gravity: any deviation from the norm requires extra energy for movement and imposes unnecessary strain on the muscles. She contended that, as the muscles work to compensate for failing efficiency over the passing years, the fascia surrounding them tend to bunch up and harden, creating even more strain. Ultimately, she said, the cumulative stress can interfere with normal breathing and impair circulation, digestion and the nervous system.

Theory

The deep massage techniques employed in rolfing seek to loosen and relax the fascia – the membranes that surround the muscles. (Rolfers believe that the fascia toughen and thicken over time, subtly contorting the body and throwing it out of healthy alignment.)

Practice

To break up knots in the fascia and 'reset' the muscles, rolfers apply slow, sliding pressure with their knuckles, thumbs, fingers, elbows and knees. The treatments are not mild and relaxing – indeed, they can cause a degree of pain. However, practitioners view this temporary discomfort as a sign that the treatment is achieving the changes necessary to bring the body back into proper alignment. During each session, the rolfer will concentrate on a different set of muscles, starting with those nearest the surface and moving on to those deep within the body. To maximise the benefits of treatment, the therapist may also teach self-help exercises known as movement integration. Sessions usually last 60–90 min. The basic sequence of rolfing consists of 10 sessions through which a new structural order and a more efficient movement pattern are developed.

Evidence

Rolf published a total of 13 papers, mainly on the subject of children with poor coordination and disorganised movement patterns.[110] The children established improved muscle tone, improved language skills and social responsiveness after rolfing. A study of neurologically compromised subjects with cerebral palsy found significant improvements in locomotion after rolfing.[111] The facilitation of greater ease of motion has also been shown after rolfing.[112]

More information

Alexander technique

Society of Teachers of the Alexander Technique
20 London House
266 Fulham Road
London
SW10 9EL
Tel: 020 7352 0828
www.stat.org.uk

Chiropractic

British Chiropractic Association
Blagrave House
17 Blagrave Street
Reading
Berks
RG1 1QB
Tel: 0118 950 5950
Fax: 0118 958 8946
www.chiropractic.org.uk/

British Association of Applied Chiropractic
The Old Post Office
Cherry Street
Stratton Audley
Nr Bicester
Oxon
OX6 9BA
Tel/fax: 01869 277111

McTimoney Chiropractic Association
21 High Street
Eynsham
Oxon
OX8 1HE
Tel: 01865 880974
Fax: 01865 880975

The Oxford College of Chiropractic
(formerly the Witney School)
c/o The Old Post Office
Cherry Street
Stratton
Audley
Nr Bicester
Oxon
OX6
www.lifesciences.napier.ac.uk/courses/projects/backpain/chircar.htm

Scottish Chiropractic Association
16 Jenny Moores Road
St Boswells
TD6 0AL
Tel: 01835 823645
Fax: 01835 823930
E-mail: Carlahow@scotborders.co.uk

American Chiropractic Association
1701 Clarendon Blvd
Arlington
VA 22209
USA

Tel: 800 986 4636
www.amerchiro.org

Massage

British Massage Therapy Council
17 Rymers Lane
Oxford
OX4 3JU
Tel: 01865 774123
www.bmtc.co.uk

Osteopathic medicine

The General Osteopathic Council
Osteopathy House
176 Tower Bridge Road
London
SE1 3LU
Tel: 020 7357 6655
www.osteopathy.org.uk

British Osteopathic Association
Langham House East
Luton
Bedfordshire
LU1 2NA
Tel: 01582 488455
www.osteopathy.org

American Osteopathic Association
142 East Ontario Street
Chicago
IL 60611
USA
Tel: 800 621 1773
Fax: 312 202 8200
www.am-osteo-assn.org

Reflexology

Association of Reflexologists
27 Old Gloucester Street
London
WC1N 3XX
Tel: 0870 5673320
E-mail: aor@reflexology.org

British Association of Reflexology
Monks Orchard
Whitbourne
Worcester
WR6 5RB
Tel: 01886–821207
E-mail: bra@britreflex.co.uk

Research sites:

www.pacificreflexology.com/res.htm
www.reflexology-research.com
www.internethealthlibrary.com/Therapies/Reflexology-Research
% 20.htm#top

Reiki

Reiki 4 All UK
Tel: 01283 716465
info@reiki4all.co.uk
www.psinet.co.uk/reikiuk

Center for Reiki Training
www.reiki.com

Rolfing

The Rolf Institute
205 Canyon Blvd
Boulder
CO 80302
USA
Tel: 303 449 5903
www.rolf.org

UK contact:
Simon Wellby
PO Box 14793
London
SW1 V2WB
Tel: 020 7834 1493

References

1. Alexander F M. *The Use of the Self*. London: Gollancz, 1985.
2. Stevens C. *Alexander Technique*. London: Vermilion, 1966.
3. McDonald G. *The Complete Illustrated Guide to the Alexander Technique*. Boston: Element Books, 1998.
4. Jonas W, Levin J S (eds). *Essentials of Complementary and Alternative Medicine*. Baltimore: Lippincott/Williams & Wilkins, 1999: 576.
5. Fulder S. *The Handbook of Complementary and Alternative Medicine*. New York: OUP, 1996: 143.
6. Heaton J, Fisher V. Alexander technique. *Health Which?* 1999; April: 26–27.
7. Jones F P. *Freedom to Change: The Development and Science of the Alexander Technique*. London: Mauritz, 1997.
8. Austin J H M, Ausubel B A. Enhanced respiratory muscular function in normal adults after lessons in proprioceptive musculoskeletal education without exercise. *Chest* 1992; 162: 486–490.
9. Fischer K. Early experience of a multi-disciplinary pain management programme. *Holistic Med* 1988; 3: 25–29.
10. Caplan D. *Back Trouble: A New Approach to Prevention and Recovery Based on the Alexander Technique*. Gainesville, FL: Triad Communications, 1987.
11. Feldenkrais F. *Awareness Through Movement: Health Exercises for Personal Growth*. New York: Harper & Row, 1972.
12. Deyo R A, Tsui-Wu Y J. Descriptive epidemiology of low-back pain and its related medicinal care in the United States. *Spine* 1987; 12: 264–268.
13. Zollman C, Vickers A. *ABC of Complementary Medicine. Massage Therapies*. London: BMJ Books, 2000: 32–35.
14. Bonnet J. *Complementary Medicine in Primary Care – What are the Key Issues?* London: NHS Executive, 2000.
15. Jonas W, Levin J S (eds) *Essentials of Complementary and Alternative Medicine*. Baltimore: Lippincott/Williams & Wilkins, 1999: 577.
16. Maeri J E. *Alternative Health Medicine Encyclopedia*. Detroit: Visible Ink Press, 1995: 6–7.
17. Bergmann T F, Peterson D, Lawrence D J. *Chiropractic Technique*. New York: Churchill Livingstone, 1993.
18. Freeman L W, Lawlis G F. *Mosby's Complementary and Alternative Medicine. A Research-based Approach*. St Louis, MO: Mosby, 2001: 297.
19. Kaptchuk T, Eisenberg D M. Chiropractic. In: Fontanarosa P B (ed.) *Alternative Medicine. An Objective Assessment*. Washington, DC: *JAMA*, 2000: 514–515.

20. Wright G T. Confusing a profession with a treatment modality again. *BMJ* online 1999; 20 July.
21. Martin R A. A study of time loss back claims: workmen's compensation boards (Medical Director's report, State of Oregon). *Arch Calif Chiropractors' Assn* 1975; 4: 83–97.
22. Koes B W, Assendelft W J J, van der Heijden J *et al.* Spinal manipulation and mobilisation for back and neck pain: a blinded review. *BMJ* 1991; 303: 1298.
23. Waddell G, Feder G, McIntosh A *et al. Clinical Guidelines for the Management of Acute Low Back Pain: Low Back Pain Evidence Review.* London: Royal College of General Practitioners, 1996.
24. Shekelle P G, Adams A H, Chassin M R *et al.* Spinal manipulation for back pain. *Ann Intern Med* 1997; 117: 590–598.
25. Ernst E, Assendelft W J J. Chiropractic for low back pain. *BMJ* 1998; 317: 160.
26. Assendelft W J J, Koes B W, van der Heijden G J, Bouter L M. The effectiveness of chiropractic for treatment of low back pain: an update and attempt at statistical pooling. *J Manipulative Physiol Ther* 1996; 19: 499–507.
27. Meade T W, Dyer S, Browne W, Frank A O. Randomised comparison of chiropractic and hospital outpatient management for low back pain: results from extended follow up. *BMJ* 1995; 311: 349–351.
28. Breen A. Chiropractic for low back pain. *BMJ* 1999; 318: 261.
29. Leerberg E. Efficacy of spinal manipulation for low back pain has not been reliably shown. *BMJ* 1999; 318: 261.
30. Meade T W. Patients were more satisfied with chiropractic than other treatments for low back pain. *BMJ* 1999; 319: 57.
31. Ernst E, Assendelft W J J. Reply to correspondence. *BMJ* 1999; 318: 261.
32. Jordan A, Bendix T. Intensive training, physiotherapy or manipulation for patients with chronic neck pain. A prospective single-blinded randomised clinical trial. *Spine* 1998; 23: 311.
33. Rogers R G. The effects of spinal manipulation on cervical kinaesthesia in patients with chronic neck pain: a pilot study. *J Manipulative Physiol Ther* 1997; 20: 80.
34. Nelson C F, Bronford G. The efficacy of spinal manipulation, amitriptyline and the combination of both therapies for the prophylaxis of migraine headache. *J Manipulative Physiol Ther* 1998; 21: 511.
35. Tuchin P J, Pollard H, Bonello R. A randomised controlled trial of chiropractic spinal manipulative therapy for migraine. *J Manipulative Physiol Ther* 2000; 23: 91–95.
36. Boline P D, Kassak K. Spinal manipulation vs amitriptyline for the treatment of chronic tension type headaches: a randomised clinical trial. *J Manipulative Physiol Ther* 1995; 18: 148.
37. Bove G, Nilsson N. Spinal manipulation in the treatment of episodic tension-type headaches. *JAMA* 1998; 280: 1576.
38. Nilsson N H, Christiansen H W, Hartvigsen J. The effect of spinal manipulation in the treatment of cervicogenic headache. *J Manipulative Physiol Ther* 1997; 18: 435.
39. Kokjohn K, Schmid D M, Triano J J, Brennan P C. The effect of spinal manipulation on pain and prostaglandin levels in women with primary dysmenorrhoea. *J Manipulative Physiol Ther* 1992; 15: 279.

40. Balon J, Aker P D, Crowther E R *et al.* A comparison of active and simulated chiropractic manipulation as adjunctive treatment for childhood asthma. *N Engl J Med* 1998; 339: 1013.

41. Klougart N, Nilsson N, Jacobsen J. Infantile colic treated by chiropractors: a prospective study of 316 cases. *J Manipulative Physiol Ther* 1989; 12: 281.

42. Hill C L. Barcelona Olympics – chiropractic report. *NZ J Sp Med* 1993; 21: 8.

43. Vernon H. Qualitative review of studies of manipulation-induced hypoalgesia. *J Manipulative Physiol Ther* 2000; 23: 134–138.

44. Powell F C, Hanigan W C, Olivero W C. A risk/benefit analysis of spinal manipulation for relief of lumbar or cervical pain. *Neurosurgery* 1993; 33: 73–78.

45. Halderman S, Rubinstein S M. Cauda equina syndrome following lumbar spine manipulation. *Spine* 1992; 17: 1469–1473.

46. Assendelft W, Bouter L, Knipschild P G. Complications of spinal manipulation – a comprehensive review of the literature. *J Fam Pract* 1996; 42: 475–480.

47. Triano J, Schultz A B. Loads transmitted during lumbosacral manipulative therapy. *Spine* 1997; 22: 1955–1964.

48. Dabbs V, Lauretti W J. A risk assessment of cervical manipulation vs NSAID for the treatment of neck pain. *J Manipulative Physiol Ther* 1995; 18: 530–553.

49. Terrett A G. Misuse of the literature by medical authors in discussing spinal manipulative therapy injury. *J Manipulative Physiol Ther* 1996; 18: 203–210.

50. Barrett A J, Breen A C. Adverse effects of spinal manipulation. *J R Soc Med* 2000; 93: 258–259.

51. Ernst E. Commentary. *Focus Altern Complement Ther* (FACT) 2000; 6: 206.

52. Wright G T. Confusing a profession with a treatment modality again. *BMJ* (electronic edition) 1999; 20 July.

53. Freeman L W, Lawlis G F. *Mosby's Complementary and Alternative Medicine. A Research-based Approach.* St Louis, MO: Mosby, 2001: 363–366.

54. Field T, Morrow C, Valdeon C. Massage reduces anxiety in child and adolescent psychiatric patients. *J Am Acad Child Adolesc Psychiatry* 1992; 31: 125–131.

55. Wilkinson S. Aromatherapy and massage in palliative care. *Int J Palliat Nurs* 1995; 1: 21–30.

56. Ferrel-Tory T, Glick O J. The use of therapeutic massage as a nursing intervention to modify anxiety and the perception of pain. *Cancer Nurs* 1993; 16: 93–101.

57. Stevenson C. The psychophysiological effects of aromatherapy massage following cardiac surgery. *Complement Ther Med* 1994; 2: 27–35.

58. Hill C F. Is massage beneficial to critically ill patients in intensive care units? A critical review. *Intensive Crit Care Nurs* 1993; 9; 116–121.

59. Fraser J, Kerr J B. Psychological effects of back massage on elderly institutionalised patients. *J Adv Nurs* 1993; 18: 238–245.

60. Hernandez-Reif M, Martinez A, Field T *et al.* Premenstrual symptoms are relieved by massage therapy. *J Psychosom Obstet Gynaecol* 2000; 21: 9–15.

61. Preyde M. Effectiveness of massage therapy for subacute low-back pain: a randomised controlled trial. *Can Med Assoc J* 2000; 162: 1815–1820.

62. Birk T J, McGrady A, MacArthur R D, Khuder S. The effects of massage

therapy alone and in combination with other complementary therapies on immune system measures and quality of life in human immunodeficency virus. *J Altern Complement Med* 2000; 6: 405–414.

63. Ireland M, Olson M. Massage therapy and therapeutic touch in children: state of the science. *Altern Ther Health Med* 2000; 6: 54–63.

64. Callaghan M J. The role of massage in the management of the athlete. A review. *Br J Sports Med* 1993; 27: 28–33.

65. Ernst E, Fialka V. The clinical effectiveness of massage. *Forsch Komplementärmed* 1994; 1: 226–232.

66. Wiktorsson-Moller M, Oberg B, Eksrand J, Gillquvist J. Effects of warming up, massage and stretching on range of motion and muscle strength in the lower extremity. *Am J Sports Med* 1983; 11: 249–252.

67. Boone T, Cooper R, Thompson W R. A psychological evaluation of the sports massage. *Athletic Training* 1991; 26: 51–54.

68. Cafarelli E, Flint F. The role of massage in preparation for and recovery from exercise: a review. *Sports Med* 1992; 14: 1–9.

69. Baike B, Anthony J, Wyatt F. The effects of massage treatment on exercise fatigue. *Clin Sports Med* 1989; 1: 189–196.

70. Carafelli E, Sim J, Carolan B, Libesman J. Vibratory massage and short term recovery from muscular fatigue. *Int Sports Med* 1990; 11: 474–478.

71. Bale P, James H. Massage, warmdown and rest as recuperative measures after short term intense exercise. *Physiotherapy Sport* 1991; 13: 4–7.

72. Ernst E. Does post-exercise massage treatment reduce delayed onset muscle soreness? A systematic review. *Br J Sports Med* 1998; 32: 212–214.

73. Eltze Ch, Hildebrandt G, Johansson M. Über die Wirsankeit der Vibrationsmassage beim Muskelkater. *Z Phys Med Bain Klimatol* 1982; 11: 366–376.

74. Ellison M, Goehrs C, Hall L *et al*. Effects of retrograde massage on muscle soreness and performance. *Phys Ther* 1992; 72: 100.

75. Danneskiold-Samsoe B, Christianen E, Bach-Anderson R. Myofascial pain and the role of myoglobin. *Scand J Rehabil Med* 1983; 15: 174–178.

76. Hoehler F K, Tobis J S, Buerger A A. Spinal manipulation for low back pain. *JAMA* 1981; 245: 1835–1838.

77. Godfrey C M, Morgan P P, Schatzker J. A randomized trial of manipulation for low back pain in a medical setting. *Spine* 1984; 9: 301–304.

78. Ernst E. Spinal manipulation for low back pain. *Eur J Phys Med Rehabil* 1998; 8: 1–2.

79. Gam A N, Warming S, Larsen L H *et al*. Treatment of myofascial trigger points with ultrasound with massage and exercise – a random controlled trial. *Pain* 1998; 77: 73–79.

80. Drews T, Knieder B, Drinkard D *et al*. Effects of post event massage therapy on repeated endurance cycling. *Int J Sports Med* 1990; 11: 407.

81. Drews T, Krieder R B, Drinkard B, Jackson C W. Effects of post event massage therapy on psychological profiles of exertion, feeling and mood during a four day ultraendurance cycling event. *Med Sci Sport Exerc* 1991; 23: 91.

82. Joyce R, Frosh A. Baby massage oils could be a hazard. *BMJ* 1996; 313: 299.

83. Vickers A, Ohlsson A, Lacy J B, Horsley A. Massage therapy for premature and/or low birth-weight infants to improve weight gain and/or to decrease hospital length of stay. Oxford: Cochrane Library, 1998: issue 3.

84. Sampson H A. Managing peanut allergy. *BMJ* 1996; 312: 1050–1051.

85. Ewan P W. Clinical study of peanut and nut allergy in 62 consecutive patients: new features and associations. *BMJ* 1996; 312: 1074–1078.

86. Kappler R, Ramey K A, Heinking K P. Osteopathic medicine. In: Novey D (ed.) *Clinician's Complete Reference to Complementary and Alternative Medicine*. St Louis, MO: Mosby, 2000: 326.

87. Holmes P. Cranial osteopathy. *Nurs Times* 1991; 87: 36–37.

88. MacDonald R S. An open controlled assessment of osteopathic manipulation in non-specific low back pain. *Spine* 1990; 15: 364–370.

89. MacDonald R S. Osteopathic diagnosis of back pain. *Manual Med* 1988; 3: 110–113.

90. Vickers A, Zollman C. ABC of complementary medicine. The manipulative therapies: osteopathy and chiropractic. *BMJ* 1999; 319: 1176–1179.

91. Pringle M, Tyreman S. Study of 500 patients attending an osteopathic practice. *Br J Gen Pract* 1993; 43: 15–18.

92. Williams N. Managing back pain in general practice – is osteopathy the new paradigm? *Br J Gen Pract* 1997; 47: 653–655.

93. Senior K. Is osteopathy the best way to treat low back pain? *Lancet* 1999; 354: 1705.

94. Andersson G, Lucente T, Davies A M. A comparison of osteopathic spinal manipulation with standard care for patients with low back pain. *N Engl J Med* 1999; 341: 1426–1431.

95. GOC website. www.osteopathy.org.uk/goc/links/research.shtml.

96. Jarski R, Loniewski E G, Williams J *et al.* The effectiveness of osteopathic manipulative treatment as complementary therapy following surgery: a prospective match-controlled outcome study. *Altern Ther Health Med* 2000; 6: 77–91.

97. Bisson D A. Reflexology. In: Novey D (ed.) *Clinician's Complete Reference to Complementary and Alternative Medicine*. St Louis, MO: Mosby, 2000: 437.

98. Wolfe F A. *Reflexology*. New York: Alpha Books, 1999: 50.

99. Botting D. Review of literature on the effectiveness of reflexology. *Complement Ther Nurs Midwifery* 1997; 3: 123–130.

100. Shaw J. Reflexology. *Health Visitor* 1987; 60: 367.

101. Evans M. Reflex zone therapy for mothers. *Nurs Times* 1990; 86: 29–32.

102. Tiran D. The use of complementary therapies in midwifery practice: a focus on reflexology. *Complement Ther Nurs Midwifery* 1996; 2: 32–37.

103. Oleson T, Flocco W. Randomised controlled study of premenstrual symptoms treated with ear, hand and foot reflexology. *Obstet Gynecol* 1993; 82: 906–911.

104. Vickers A. *Massage and Aromatherapy – A Guide for Health Professionals*. London: Chapman & Hall, 1996.

105. Kovaks F M, Abraira V, Lopez-Abente G, Pozo F. Neuro-reflexology intervention in the treatment of non-specified low back pain. In: *Reflexology Research Report*, 2nd edn. London: Association of Reflexologists, 1994.

106. Reiki4All UK website. http: //www.geocities.com/reiki4alluk/reiki_inf.htm# HISTORY.

107. Fairblass J. Reiki. In: Novey D (ed.) *Clinician's Complete Reference to Complementary and Alternative Medicine*. St Louis, MO: Mosby, 2000: 435.

108. Olson K, Hanson J. Using reiki to manage pain: a preliminary report. *Cancer Prevent Control* 1997; 1: 108–111.
109. Freeman L W, Lawlis G F. *Mosby's Complementary and Alternative Medicine. A Research-based Approach*. St Louis, MO: Mosby, 2001: 363.
110. Freeman L W, Lawlis G F. *Mosby's Complementary and Alternative Medicine. A Research-based Approach*. St Louis, MO: Mosby, 2001: 448.
111. Perry J, Jones M H, Thomas L. Functional evaluation of Rolfing in cerebral palsy. *Dev Child Neurol* 1981; 23: 717–729.
112. Weinberg R, Hunt V. Effects of structural integration on state–trait anxiety. *J Clin Psychol* 1979; 35: 319–322.

14

Mind and body therapies

In this chapter a number of mind and body therapies are discussed in sufficient detail for readers to understand the basic concepts involved.

Colour therapy

Definition

Colour therapy (also called aura soma) is a natural and non-invasive form of healing using pure light/colour energy for the well-being of mind, body and spirit. According to colour therapy, the seven rainbow colours relate to the seven main energy centres (chakras) of the body. Colour has an effect on perception and this therapy seems to have a place in complementary practice, although the attachment of the sobriquet 'therapy' might be questioned by many.

History

Colour was of great importance to the Egyptians. They built temples for colour healing where people would gather to be revitalised and renewed.

It is interesting to look at the different phases in history and how those phases have been reflected in the colours generally worn at those times. During times of severity and propriety the code of dress was dominated by black and grey. The Victorians mainly wore black – influenced by Queen Victoria's long period of mourning, no doubt – and were, in many ways, quite austere and not very colourful. The Puritans too, of course, dressed in black.

Wearing black with another colour can enhance that other colour's energy. Black can also give the space sometimes needed for reflection on an inner searching. It can indicate inner strength and the possibility for change.

Theory

Relationships between various colours and areas of the body, glands or organs (known as chakras) are identified by practitioners. Some of the most common colours and their associated chakras are given below.

- Violet/purple relates to the crown chakra, which is at the top of the head. The related organ to this chakra is the brain and the endocrine gland is the pineal gland. Violet relates to our spiritual awareness.
- Indigo relates to the brow chakra or third eye, which is in the centre of the forehead. The related organs to this chakra are the eyes, lower head and sinuses and the endocrine gland is the pituitary gland. Indigo relates to self-responsibility, that is to say trusting our own intuition.
- Blue relates to the throat chakra. Organs associated with this chakra are the throat and lungs and the endocrine gland is the thyroid gland. The upper digestive tract can be affected by imbalance in this area. This chakra relates to self-expression.
- Green relates to the heart chakra. Associated organs to this chakra are the heart and breasts. The gland is the thymus gland. Allergies and problems related to the immune system can also be connected with this chakra. This chakra relates to love/self-love.
- Yellow relates to the solar plexus chakra, situated below the ribs. Associated organs are the liver, spleen, stomach and small intestine. The endocrine gland is the pancreas. This chakra relates to self-worth.
- Orange relates to the sacral chakra, which is situated in the abdomen. The organs to which this chakra relates are the uterus, large bowel and prostate. The endocrine glands are the ovaries and testes. This chakra relates to self-respect.
- Red relates to the base chakra, which is situated at the base of the spine. The organs to which this chakra relates are the kidneys and bladder. The vertebral column, hips and legs are also related to this chakra. The endocrine gland is the adrenal gland. This chakra relates to self-awareness.

Practice

An aura soma treatment begins with an examination of the responses triggered by a selection of colours made by the patient. These responses highlight areas of the physical body that are holding a negative pattern.

Colour therapy healing can be used in many ways, for example, using a light box with the appropriate colour/colours, wearing silk colour scarves. Light box therapy is also very helpful for those suffering from seasonal affective disorder.

Evidence

Before the Second World War it was noted that a lot of red was being worn. Red in its most positive aspect is the colour for courage, strength and pioneering spirit, all of which were much needed by the men and women fighting that war. However, in the most negative aspect, it is the colour of anger, violence and brutality. As the war came to an end, pale blue became a popular colour – an omen of the peace to come, perhaps, and also giving everyone the healing they must have needed so badly. More recently, in a systematic review of 12 published studies, it was shown that colours affect the perceived action and effectiveness of drugs.[1] Moreover, a relation exists between the colouring of drugs that affect the central nervous system and the indications for which they are used. Red, yellow and orange appeared to be associated with a stimulant effect, while blue and green were related to a tranquillising effect. Furthermore, hypnotic, sedative and anxiolytic drugs were more likely than antidepressants to be green, blue or purple.

Businesses are accepting that their employees may work better given a certain environment and hospitals and prisons are also becoming aware of the effect that the colour around them can have on patients and prisoners respectively. Paint companies have introduced new colour cards with the therapeutic aspects of colour in mind.

Crystal therapy[2]

This is a healing method similar to colour therapy in that it uses crystals and gems for physical, emotional and spiritual balance and healing. The crystals are worn or placed near the body. The body needs seven colour rays, red, orange, yellow, green, blue, indigo and violet, for balanced health (as in colour therapy). Each colour ray is associated with one or more of the chakras. By using crystals associated with the colour ray that supports a particular chakra, one can speed healing of the associated areas and organs. For example, emerald is the carrier of the green ray.

Examples of the uses of some crystals are:

- Amber is great at lifting the heaviness of burdens, allowing happiness to come through.
- Aquamarine can help one understand difficult situations and may be helpful for people who are experiencing a lot of grief.
- Coral protects and strengthens one's emotional foundation.
- Emerald may help in physical and emotional healing.
- Jade helps cure a sore shoulder or back and is useful in relaxation.
- Opal helps one see possibilities and discover a broader view.
- Ruby opens the heart and allows one to overcome fear.

Dance and movement therapy

Dance and movement therapy depends on the ability to perform various actions, not necessarily on the skill or talent apparent in doing so.

Definition

Dance and movement therapy are basic forms of authentic communication, and as such are an especially effective medium for therapy. Based on the belief that the body, mind and spirit are interconnected, dance/movement therapy is defined by the American Dance Therapy Association as 'the psychotherapeutic use of movement as a process that furthers the emotional, cognitive, social and physical integration of the individual'.[3]

History

Dance and movement was first practised as a separate therapy in the 1940s in the USA.

Theory

Dance and movement therapy, a creative art therapy, is rooted in the expressive nature of dance itself. Dance is the most fundamental of the arts, involving a direct expression and experience of oneself through the body. Changes that occur during therapy relate directly to the brain's interactive function, physical exercise and neural interplay between motion and emotion.[4]

Practice

Dance and movement therapists work with individuals of all ages who have social, emotional, cognitive and/or physical problems. They work in settings that include psychiatric and rehabilitation facilities, schools, nursing homes, drug treatment centres, counselling centres, medical facilities, crisis centres and wellness and alternative healthcare centres. They focus on helping their clients to improve self-esteem and body image, develop effective communication skills and relationships, expand their movement vocabulary, gain insight into patterns of behaviour, as well as to create new options for coping with problems.

Dance and movement therapy is claimed to be a powerful tool for stress management and the prevention of physical and mental health problems.

A novel use of dance was employed by Dr Pamela Garlick, a biochemist and senior lecturer at the Guy's, King's and St Thomas' School of Medicine, London. She won a Millennium Award for an innovative dance project about sickle-cell anaemia. The aim of the project was to increase the awareness and understanding of sickle-cell anaemia in her local borough of Haringey, London, by making the video entitled *Sickle Cell Anaemia – An Exploration through Dance*, for use in secondary schools. In the video, 27 10-year-old children from local schools use dance to convey the intricate processes by which a gene is converted, via messenger RNA, into a protein such as haemoglobin, and to show the effects that the sickle-cell mutation has on the behaviour of the red blood cell. The children wear specially printed colour-coded T-shirts and baseball caps to identify themselves as the individual DNA bases, amino acids, etc. The use of a high-angle camera enables a unique bird's-eye view of the cellular events underlying this painful disorder to be visualised. The video includes interviews with individuals who have sickle-cell anaemia and their families to explain the health issues related to this disorder, and is presented by athlete and Olympic gold medallist Linford Christie. Copies were distributed to all health centres and secondary schools in Haringey and to all the children involved in the project.

Evidence

Meta-analysis has shown dance and movement therapy to be effective in the treatment of psychiatric patients and anxiety.[5] Most other evidence is of an experiential nature.

Music therapy

Definition

Music therapy is the prescribed use of music by a qualified person to effect positive changes in the psychological, physical, cognitive or social functioning of individuals with health or educational problems.

History

The idea of music as a healing influence that could affect health and behaviour is at least as old as the writings of Aristotle and Plato. Five hundred years before Christ, the followers of Pythagoras developed a science of musical psychotherapy. A daily programme of songs and pieces for the lyre made them feel bright and energetic on rising, and another set of pieces relieved them of the cares of the day and prepared them for agreeable dreams when they retired to sleep. Plato believed that musical training was a more potent instrument than any other because 'rhythm and harmony find their way into the inward places of the soul, imparting grace, and making the soul of him who is rightly educated graceful'. The Bible recounts that young David was summoned to play the harp for a tormented King Saul: 'Whenever the spirit from God came upon Saul, David would take his harp and play. Then relief would come to Saul; he would feel better, and the evil spirit would leave him' (I Samuel 16:23).

Anyone who has played in an orchestra or sung in a choir will know that participating in music with others enhances group solidarity as well as promoting individual well-being. The twentieth-century discipline began after the First and Second World Wars when community musicians of all types, both amateur and professional, went to military hospitals around the country to play for the thousands of combatants suffering both physical and emotional trauma from the wars. The patients' notable physical and emotional responses to music led doctors and nurses to request the hiring of musicians by the hospitals. It was soon evident that hospital musicians needed some prior training before entering the hospital and so the demand grew for a college curriculum. The first music therapy degree programme in the world was founded at Michigan State University, USA, in 1944.

Theory

Studies with electroencephalography suggest that music creates a level of coherence between the electrical activity of different areas of the brain.

Practice

According to the American Music Therapy Association website,[6] music therapists:

- assess emotional well-being, physical health, social functioning, communication abilities and cognitive skills through musical responses
- design music sessions for individuals and groups based on client needs, using music improvisation, receptive music listening, song writing, lyric discussion, music and imagery, music performance and learning through music
- participate in interdisciplinary treatment planning, ongoing evaluation and follow-up.

The following groups are said to benefit from music therapy:

- children with developmental and learning disabilities
- the elderly with mental health needs, Alzheimer's disease and other age-related conditions
- people with substance abuse problems
- people with physical disabilities and/or acute and chronic pain
- mothers in labour.

Evidence

In a controlled study of 40 infants matched for gestational age, sex and birth weight, half had lullabies sung to them and were massaged once or twice a week until they were discharged.[7] The other 20 served as controls. The hospital stay was shortened by an average of 11 days for female infants and 1.5 days for male infants in the music and massage group compared with the control group. Infants of both sexes gained weight, although the amount was not statistically significant.

Music therapy also has a special place in the treatment of children who cannot easily communicate verbally; this includes autistic children as well as those with learning disabilities or brain damage. It is likely that music can provide an alternative channel of communication that prevents some children from retreating into, or remaining in, a state of total isolation.[8]

A few years ago, a researcher reported a study that showed that listening to Mozart's *Sonata for Two Pianos* (K448) significantly enhanced the ability of a subject to perform tests of spatial perception.[9] The report was widely publicised, and a number of investigators have since attempted to reproduce the findings with mixed results. According to a *JAMA* article,[10] a much larger study study found that it was not Mozart but movement that enhances performance ability. Whether the stimulus is auditory or visual, the key is movement, because movement gets attention and, with attention, performance improves. *JAMA* reported that 175 subjects were randomly selected and placed into one of seven groups each containing 25 persons. Those in six of the groups performed a spatial ability test before and after 8.5 min of exposure to one of the following: the Mozart sonata; audible rhythmic patterns with a steady pitch; random pitches with steady time intervals; environmental sounds, such as falling rain and singing birds; continually changing geometric patterns, such as those that appear on a computer screen-saver; and colour slides of abstract paintings. The control group sat for 8.5 min without exposure to any auditory or visual stimuli. The first five groups tested performed the spatial ability task equally well and significantly better than the controls and those viewing the abstract paintings. The Mozart listeners fared no better than the others.

A Swedish study investigated the possible influence of attendance at cultural events, reading books or periodicals, making music or singing in a choir as determinants for survival.[11] This was a simple random sample of 15 198 individuals aged 16–74 years. Of these, 85% (12 982) were interviewed by trained non-medical interviewers about cultural activities. They were followed up with respect to survival for approximately 8 years. It was concluded that attendance at cultural events may have a positive influence on survival.

Autobiographical recall in patients with dementia improves significantly when music is played. Foster and Valentine examined the recall of personal facts in 23 older adults with mild-to-moderate dementia.[12] Participants were tested in each of four auditory background conditions presented randomly, 1 week apart: quiet, cafeteria noise, familiar music (first movement of Vivaldi's *The Four Seasons*), and novel music (Fitkin's *Hook*). Questions were drawn from three life eras: remote (up to age 20; for example, where were you born?), medium-remote (approximately ages 20–50; for example, have you ever been married?) and recent past and present (for example, where do you live now?). Performance was significantly better with sound (mean percentage recall 67%) compared with quiet (61%), and with music (68%) compared with cafeteria noise (66%). There was no difference between familiar and novel music; recall for both was about 68%. Recall was also positively related to age of memory; it was better for remote past (80%) compared with medium-remote (68%) and recent past and present (48%). A typical question that participants were able to answer with the aid of background music but not without it was: 'Can you remember the name of the school your children attended?' – something from the middle period of their lives which they probably had not had occasion to think about much since then. It was concluded that music should be played when physicians are interviewing or attempting to get information from patients with dementia and should also be tried in combination with other treatments for dementia management.

Music therapy is a popular complementary treatment in hospitals in the USA, where randomised trials have supported its use for reducing pain and anxiety in the acute setting.[13,14]

Other mind–body interventions

Hypnotherapy

Hypnotherapy is an intervention based on the use of hypnosis (literally, 'nervous sleep'), a form of cognitive information processing in which a suspension of peripheral awareness and critical analysis cognition can lead to apparently involuntary changes in perception, memory, mood and physiology.[15] In simpler terms hypnosis may be considered as the induction of a deeply relaxed state, with increased suggestibility and suspension of critical faculties.[16]

The French physician Mesmer (1734–1815) was the first person to propose a mechanism for hypnosis that did not have a demonic basis to its theory. He suggested that hypnosis was due to magnetism radiating from himself. There have been many other hypotheses as to how hypnosis may work but none has been accepted as the definitive answer.

Hypnotherapy is often associated with the induction of a trance-like state during which behavioural modification may be suggested (e.g. stop smoking during pregnancy[17] or reduce eating). In fact it is now more widely used as an adjunct to psychological treatments.[18,19]

Hypnosis may be indicated if the patient has a high ability to become hypnotised and has a positive attitude towards hypnosis for the treatment of a condition in which alteration of perception, memory and mood can reduce the intensity of a symptom. Thus it may be used in suitable patients for the reduction of chronic pain, reduction in the memory of past pain and enhancing mood.

Apart from pain and headaches, hypnosis has been used for several other conditions,[20] including asthma, removal of warts and irritable bowel syndrome.[21]

Safety

It has been pointed out that hypnosis or deep relaxation has the capacity to exacerbate psychological problems by retraumatising those with post-traumatic disorders or by inducing false memories in psychologically vulnerable individuals.[16] Concerns have also been raised that it can bring on a latent psychosis, although the evidence is inconclusive. Hypnosis should be undertaken only by appropriately trained, experienced and regulated practitioners. It should be avoided in established or borderline psychosis and personality disorders, and hypnotherapists should be competent at recognising and referring patients in these states.

Training

The British Society of Medical and Dental Hypnosis runs basic, intermediate and advanced courses for doctors and dentists, and holds regular scientific meetings. There is no standard training in hypnosis for practitioners without a conventional healthcare background.

Meditation

Meditation is the intentional self-regulation of attention, a systematic focus on particular aspects of inner or outer experience and has developed in association with religious and spiritual contexts (e.g. Buddhist and Hindu rituals), the aim being to seek a full state of mind embodied in the concept of 'enlightenment'. Meditation can be broadly divided into two groups of practices:

- concentration or restrictive practices that emphasise the stabilising of attention when directed to a specific object or focus; typically, meditators concentrate on their breath or a sound (mantra) that they repeat to themselves
- mindfulness practices (e.g. Zen) that involve attention to all emotions, perceptions and sensations rather than focusing on one

particular aspect of life; this is said to cultivate a sense of open-mindedness in life.

In fact, it may be difficult to separate these two groups, as the first may be required before the second can be achieved. For example, in mindfulness practices individuals are taught to concentrate initially on a simple event, such as breathing, and then allow the mind to wander.

Transcendental meditation (TM)

Transcendental meditation was introduced to the west from the vedic traditions of India by maharishi Mahest Yogi and was popularised by the Beatles in the 1960s. In transcendental meditation the individual sits with eyes closed for 20 min each day, focusing on a word or syllable. Whenever distraction occurs the attention is directed back to the word. A refreshing state of restful alertness can be achieved with practice. Transcendental meditation has been used in the reduction of stress and various anxiety states. It has also been used, together with orthodox treatments, in the treatment of carotid artery disease.[22]

A group mindfulness meditation training programme is claimed to reduce symptoms of anxiety and panic, and help maintain these reductions in patients with generalised anxiety disorder, panic disorder or panic disorder with agoraphobia.[23] Meditation has also been used to enhance mood,[24] to treat hypertension[25] and for pain control.[26]

Relaxation

One example of a relaxation technique is sequential muscle relaxation, progressive relaxation or Jacobson relaxation. The subject sits comfortably in a dark, quiet room. He or she then tenses a group of muscles, such as those in the right arm, holds the contraction for 15 s, and then releases it while breathing out. After a short rest, this sequence is repeated with another set of muscles. Gradually, different sets of muscles are combined.

Another technique, the Mitchell method, involves adopting body positions that are opposite to those associated with anxiety (fingers spread rather than hands clenched, for example). In autogenic training subjects concentrate on experiencing physical sensations, such as warmth and heaviness, in different parts of their bodies in a learnt sequence. Other methods encourage deepening and slowing the breath, and a conscious attempt to let go of tension during exhalation.

Relaxation has been found to be beneficial in the treatment of chronic pain.[27] Some general practitioner practices in the UK offer relaxation classes to improve well-being in patients with mild anxiety or depression or who suffer from chronic physical complaints for which further treatment options are limited.[28]

Spiritual healing and prayer

Healers and their clients assume a cause-and-effect relationship between the application of a healer's intention to heal and any subsequent improvement in symptoms.[29] Healers believe that the power of healing is a therapy in its own right; non-believers are sceptical and reject this suggestion.

The difficulties of conducting research into the effectiveness of healing are significant – how, for example, does one know when a patient is better?[30] Some healers would say that some of the most significant changes following healing may not be measurable. The healing approach is to act with love and compassion and support patients during their suffering. Measuring such input is a problem, especially when it is complementary to other more orthodox treatments. A recent systematic review identified a total of 59 randomised controlled trials (RCTs) comparing healing with a control intervention on human participants. In 37 of these trials healing was used for existing diseases; the remaining 22 trials were excluded from the review, mainly because no identifiable symptoms were present.[31] The author stated that no firm conclusions could be drawn about the efficacy or otherwise of healing from the diverse group of RCTs reported in the literature. He suggested two possibilities for future healing research: pragmatic trials of healing for undifferentiated conditions on patients based in general practice and larger RCTs of distant healing on large numbers of patients with well-defined measurable illness. A double-blind randomised trial of distant healing for skin warts[32] found no evidence that healing practices had any beneficial effects.

The calming effect or coping strategy of prayer can be beneficial and, especially amongst those with religious faith, provide the necessary support at times of extreme stress and tension. There are four types of prayer, all of which may contribute to an overall effect:

- meditative prayer, which involves focusing on a single word, phrase or sound
- ritualistic prayer, which involves repeating passages of prose that form part of a religious service
- petitionary prayer, which involves making a request, e.g. for better health

- conversational prayer, which involves chatting or informing one's deity.

Blood pressure measurement offers a method of identifying an effective outcome due to prayer particularly in older people.[33]

Intercessory or third-party prayer has been practised since Professor John Tyndall caused much debate in 1872 when he proposed comparing mortality rates in London hospitals between patients who were prayed for and those who were not.[34] Every so often a trial adds to the controversy. For example, a double-blind RCT with a population of 393 cardiac patients split into an active (prayed-for) group and a control group showed that intercessory prayer appeared to be effective in reducing respiratory and cardiac symptoms.[35] More recently, results from an RCT have suggested that intercessory prayer might be an effective adjunct to standard medical procedures in coronary care.[36]

A randomised controlled study concluded that chronically ill patients who want to be treated by distant healing and know that they are treated improve in quality of life.[37]

Therapeutic touch

Therapeutic touch is an intentionally directed process of energy modulation during which the practitioner uses the hands as a focus to facilitate healing. It is largely passive in its application and requires no conscious participation by the patient.

Therapeutic touch is claimed to have three main effects:[38]

- a rapid relaxation response
- improved pain relief
- an acceleration of the body's own healing process.

Yoga

Yoga involves postures, breathing exercises and meditation aimed at improving mental and physical functioning. Some practitioners understand yoga in terms of traditional Indian medicine, with the postures improving the flow of prana energy around the body. Others see yoga in more conventional terms of muscle stretching and mental relaxation, with an ability to improve vitality.[39]

Commonly practised yoga methods are pranayama (controlled deep breathing), asanas (physical postures) and dhyana (meditation), which are mixed in varying proportions with differing philosophic ideas.

More information

Colour therapy

International Association of Colour Therapy (IAC)
46 Cottenham Road
Histon
Cambridge
CB4 9ES
Tel: 01223 563403
E-mail: mailto.iac@cix.co.uk

Colour Therapy Association (CTA)
PO Box 121
Chessington
KT9 2WQ
Tel/Fax: 020 8391 2380

Crystal therapy

Further information may be found at the following web site: http://www.gems4friends.com/~lorraine/therapy.html

Music therapy

MusicSpace Trust is a charity devoted to the provision of music therapy and the training of music therapy students

The MusicSpace Trust
The Southville Centre
Beauley Road
Bristol
BS3 1QG
Tel: 0117 963 8000
Fax: 0117 966 9889
www.hants.gov.uk/hampshire-musicspace/Trust.html

The American Music Therapy Association
8455 Colesville Rd,
Silver Spring
MD 20910
USA
Tel: 301 589 3300
www.musictherapy.org

References

1. de Craen A J M, Roos P J, Leonard de Vries A, Kleijnen J. Effect of colour of drugs. Systematic review of perceived effect of drugs and of their effectiveness. *BMJ* 1996; 313: 1624–1626.
2. www.gems4friends.com/~lorraine/therapy.html
3. American Dance Therapy Association website. http://www.adta.org
4. Berrol C. The neurophysical basis of the mind–body connection in dance/movement therapy. *Am J Dance Ther* 1992; 14: 19–29.
5. Cruz R, Sabers D. Dance therapy is more effective than previously reported. *Ann Psychother* 1998; 25: 101–104.
6. American Music Therapy Association website. http://www.namt.com
7. Standley J M. The effect of music and multimodal stimulation on responses of premature infants in neonatal intensive care. *Pediatr Nurs* 1998; 24: 532–538.
8. Bunt L. *Music Therapy: An Art Beyond Words*. London: Routledge, 1999.
9. Rauscher F H, Shaw G L, Ky K N. Listening to Mozart enhances spatial–temporal reasoning: towards a neurophysiological basis. *Neurosci Lett* 1995; 185: 44–47.
10. Marwick C. Music therapists chime in with data on medical results. *JAMA* 2000; 283: 731–733.
11. Bygren L O, Konlaan B B, Johansson S-E. Attendance at cultural events, reading books or periodicals, and making music or singing in a choir as determinants for survival: Swedish interview survey of living conditions. *Neurology* 2000; 55: 1935–1936.
12. Foster N A, Valentine E R. The effect of auditory stimulation on autobiographical recall in dementia. *Exp Aging Res* 2001; 27: 215–223.
13. Winter M J, Paskin S, Baker T. Music reduces stress and anxiety of patients in the surgical holding area. *J Post Anesth Nurs* 1994; 9: 340–343.
14. Koch M E, Kain Z N, Ayoub C, Rosenbaum S H. The sedative and analgesic sparing effect of music. *Anesthesiology* 1998; 89: 300–306.
15. Wickramasekera I. Hypnotherapy. In: Jonas W, Levin J S (eds) *Essentials of Complementary and Alternative Medicine*. Baltimore: Lippincott/Williams & Wilkins, 1999: 426.
16. Vickers A, Zollman C. ABC of complementary medicine. Hypnosis and relaxation therapies. *BMJ* 1999; 319: 1346–1349.
17. Vaibo A, Eide T. Smoking cessation in pregnancy: the effect of hypnosis in a randomised study. *Addict Behav* 1996; 21: 29–35.
18. Rhue J, Lynn S, Kirsch I (eds) *Handbook of Clinical Hypnosis*. Washington, DC: American Psychological Association, 1993.
19. Kirsch I, Montgomery G, Sapirstein G. Hypnosis as an adjunct to cognitive-behavioral psychotherapy: a meta-analysis. *J Consult Clin Psychol* 1995; 63: 214–220.
20. Wadden T A, Anderton C H. The clinical use of hypnosis. *Psychol Bull* 1982; 91: 215–243.
21. Harvey R F, Hinton R A, Gunary R M, Barry R E. Individual and group hypnotherapy in treatment of refractory irritable bowel syndrome. *Lancet* 1989; i: 424–425.

22. Zamarra J W, Schneider R H, Besseghini I *et al.* Usefulness of the transcendental meditation program in the treatment of patients with coronary artery disease. *Am J Cardiol* 1966; 77: 867–870.

23. Kabat-Zinn J, Massion A O, Kristeller J *et al.* Effectiveness of a meditation-based stress reduction program in the treatment of anxiety disorders. *Am J Psychiatry* 1992; 149: 936–943.

24. Smith W B, Compton W C, West W B. Meditation as an adjunct to a happiness enhancement program. *J Clin Psychol* 1995; 51: 269–273.

25. Eisenberg D M, Delbanco T L, Berkey C S *et al.* Cognitive behavioral techniques for hypertension: are they effective? *Ann Intern Med* 1993; 118: 964–972.

26. Kabat-Zinn J, Lipworth L, Burney R. The clinical use of mindfulness meditation for self-regulation of chronic pain. *J Behav Med* 1985; 8: 163–190.

27. Carroll D, Seers K. Relaxation for the relief of chronic pain: a systematic review. *J Adv Nurs* 1998; 27: 476–487.

28. Smith W P, Compton W C, West W B. Meditation as an adjunct to a happiness enhancement program. *J Clin Psychol* 1995; 51: 269–273.

29. Charman R A. Placing healers, healees and healing into a wider research context. *J Altern Complement Med* 2000; 6: 177–180.

30. Brown C K. Methodological problems of clinical research into spiritual healing: the healer's perspective. *J Altern Complement Med* 2000; 6: 171–176.

31. Abbot N C. Healing as a therapy for human disease: a systematic review. *J Altern Complement Med* 2000; 6: 159–169.

32. Harkness E F, Abbot N C, Ernst E. A randomised trial of distant healing for skin warts. *Am J Med* 2000; 108: 448–452.

33. Koenig H G, George L K, Hays J C *et al.* The relationship between religious activities and blood pressure in older adults. *Int J Psychiatry Med* 1998; 28: 189–213.

34. O'Mathuna D P. Prayer research: what are we measuring? *J Christian Nurs* 1999; 16: 17–21.

35. Byrd R C. Positive therapeutic effect of intercessory prayer in coronary care unit population. *South Med J* 1988; 81: 826–829.

36. Harris W S, Gowda M, Kolb J W *et al.* A randomised controlled trial of the effects of remote, intercessory prayer on outcomes in patients admitted to the coronary care unit. *Arch Intern Med* 1999; 159: 2273–2278.

37. Wiesendanger H, Werthmuller L, Reuter K, Walsch H. Chronically ill patients treated by spiritual healing improve in quality of life: results of a randomised waiting-list controlled study. *J Altern Complement Med* 2001; 7: 45–51.

38. Krieger D. *Accepting your Own Power to Heal. The Personal Practice of Therapeutic Touch.* Sante Fe, NM: Bear, 1993.

39. Wood C. Mood change and perceptions of vitality: a comparison of the effects of relaxation, visualization and yoga. *J R Soc Med* 1993; 86: 254–258.

Index